Baseball

STEPS TO SUCCESS

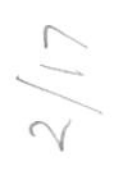

Kenny Thomas
DJ King

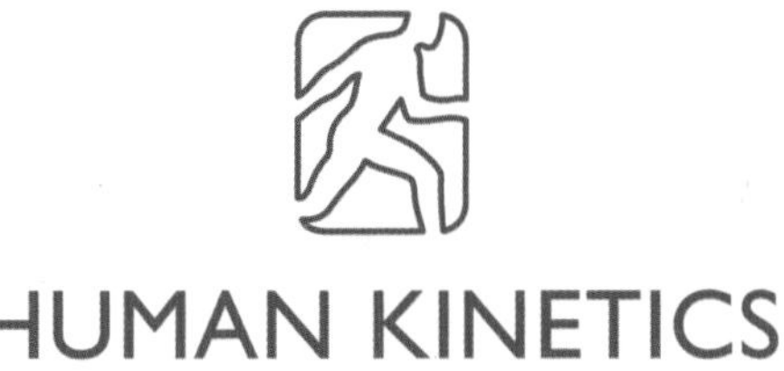

Library of Congress Cataloging-in-Publication Data

Names: Thomas, Kenny, 1955- author. | King, DJ, 1984- author.
Title: Baseball: steps to success / Kenny Thomas, DJ King.
Description: Champaign, IL: Human Kinetics, 2017.
Identifiers: LCCN 2016015819 (print) | LCCN 2016025296 (ebook) | ISBN9781492504573 (print) |
ISBN 9781492541158 (ebook)
Subjects: LCSH: Baseball--Coaching. | Baseball--Training. |
Baseball--Physiological aspects.
Classification: LCC GV875.5.T56 2016 (print) | LCC GV875.5 (ebook) | DDC
796.357--dc23
LC record available at https://lccn.loc.gov/2016015819

ISBN: 978-1-4925-0457-3 (print)

The web addresses cited in this text were current as of September 2016, unless otherwise noted.

Acquisitions Editor: Justin Klug
Developmental Editor: Kevin Matz
Managing Editor: Ann C. Gindes
Copyeditor: Bob Replinger
Senior Graphic Designer: Keri Evans
Cover Designer: Keith Blomberg
Photograph (cover): iStock.com/Stefano Tiraboschi
Photographer (interior): Neil Bernstein; Photographs © Human Kinetics
Visual Production Assistant: Joyce Brumfield
Photo Production Manager: Jason Allen
Senior Art Manager: Kelly Hendren
Illustrations: © Human Kinetics
Printer: Walsworth

We thank the City of Aiken, South Carolina, and the University of South Carolina Aiken for assistance in providing the locations for the photo shoot for this book.

Printed in the United States of America 10 9 8 7 6 5 4 3 2 1

The paper in this book was manufactured using responsible forestry methods

Human Kinetics
Website: www.HumanKinetics.com

United States: Human Kinetics
P.O. Box 5076
Champaign, IL 61825-5076
800-747-4457
e-mail: info@hkusa.com

Canada: Human Kinetics
475 Devonshire Road Unit 100
Windsor, ON N8Y 2L5
800-465-7301 (in Canada only)
e-mail: info@hkcanada.com

Europe: Human Kinetics
107 Bradford Road
Stanningley
Leeds LS28 6AT, United Kingdom
+44 (0) 113 255 5665
e-mail: hk@hkeurope.com

Australia: Human Kinetics
57A Price Avenue
Lower Mitcham, South Australia 5062
08 8372 0999
e-mail: info@hkaustralia.com

New Zealand: Human Kinetics
P.O. Box 80
Mitcham Shopping Centre, South Australia 5062
0800 222 062
e-mail: info@hknewzealand.com

E6435

Baseball

STEPS TO SUCCESS

Contents

Climbing the Steps to Baseball Success

Baseball is a sport that requires players to engage continuously in developing fundamental skills and knowledge of the game. Baseball players of all levels and ages are constantly practicing the fundamental skills of throwing, catching, fielding, and hitting. The ability to execute these fundamentals on a consistent basis helps separate players into different levels. Physical attributes such as body size, speed, and strength may help determine a proper fit to a specific position, but a baseball player can compensate for a lack of size, speed, or strength by developing the craft of the position chosen.

Each position on a baseball field has specific physical fundamentals and skills that players must continuously work on, but to develop the craft of a position, players must also develop their baseball IQ, or knowledge of the game. As a player advances to higher levels of the sport, the mental aspect of the game becomes more important. A player's baseball IQ is reflected in his ability to make on-field decisions. The combination of physical ability and baseball IQ is the general formula for determining the level of each player.

To define what success is within this sport, note that baseball is a game built on failure. For instance, if a batter fails to get a hit 7 times out of 10 attempts, he has statistically been successful. This unique aspect of the sport drives the use of statistical measurements to define success at the professional, collegiate, and high school levels. Unfortunately, for individual player development (especially for the younger ages playing the game), statistics do not necessarily define success. For many young players, development and success in this sport are directly affected by the ability to handle failure. Those who use failure as a learning tool have the ability to set goals that will help define their individual success. For most, success in baseball is directly correlated with consistency, regardless of the level of the player. Consistency can be developed over time by combining the player's physical ability, baseball IQ, work ethic, and ability to use failure as a tool for success.

The 10 steps detailed in *Baseball: Steps to Success* break down the fundamentals of individual play and give you drills and techniques that you can use to enhance your fundamental skill set. You will be shown proper techniques, common mistakes, and individual drill sets for throwing and receiving, fielding, pitching, catching, hitting, and baserunning. These fundamentals will be your foundation for developing into a complete player.

In this book, you will learn key components of baseball's fundamental skills as well as how to practice them. Every effort has been made to help you understand why performing skills a specific way is valuable. As you work through each of the skill elements, follow this sequence to maximize your learning:

1. Study the skill covered in each step, why it is important, and how to perform it.
2. Observe the photos of demonstrators modeling how to perform the techniques successfully.
3. Read and practice each drill and track your progress in each of the success checks at the end of the skill element chapters.
4. Have a qualified observer, such as your teacher, coach, or a trained peer, evaluate your skills after completing each set of drills and compare their assessment of your skill to your own.
5. Once you have achieved the indicated level of success in each skill element, you can move on to the next step.

While you may be anxious to move through the steps quickly, be sure to revisit skill elements to keep your game strong. You can always increase the challenge of each drill (or reduce it if you are struggling). Keep in mind that specific positions will require more training in individual skills.

Building on your foundation, the later chapters focus on the specifics of each position and the connection of the individual game to the team concept. These chapters take a closer look at infield play, outfield play, situational defense, and situational offense, combining physical demands with the proper mental approach. As you move through each step, you will find ways to develop your physical and mental game, so you'll gain the confidence and consistency needed for reaching your goals.

Acknowledgments

We would like to thank the following people and organizations for their help in making *Baseball: Steps to Success* possible:

- Phil Disher, Assistant Baseball Coach, University of South Carolina–Aiken
- Hope Beedle, Social Media Director for baseball, University of South Carolina–Aiken
- David Brinkley, Aiken Baseball Academy, Aiken, South Carolina
- Judy Thomas, wife of Coach Kenny Thomas
- Haleigh Taylor, Aiken, South Carolina
- Citizens Park and the City of Aiken, South Carolina

The Sport of Baseball

Baseball is an individual sport played within a team concept. Many of the steps to developing success in baseball rely heavily on individual development of specific skills. Unlike any other sport, in which certain individual weaknesses can be hidden within the nature of the team game being played, individual skill weaknesses in baseball can be highlighted during the course of a baseball game. The goal of *Baseball: Steps to Success* is to provide you with not only a fundamental knowledge of the sport but also a blueprint for individual development.

The following discussion is directed toward the beginner and amateur-level player, although we recognize that coaches, teachers, and parents may be reading this book. This discussion will be a helpful resource to them as well.

Known as America's pastime, baseball has spread internationally, grown in popularity, and become a cultural melting pot. Regardless of where the game is being played or what level or age group is playing, the game is based on a few basic principles. To move forward in developing a blueprint for development, we must first recognize that some readers may not be familiar with these basic principles. The following is an overview of how the game of baseball is played, including basic knowledge of how the game is structured. The discussion includes brief definitions of common terminology, an overview of basic rules, and a layout of the baseball field itself. We address equipment needs and proper fittings for different levels of players. We conclude with a brief discussion on the fundamentals of preparation.

PLAYING THE GAME: THE OBJECTIVE AND FIELD DIMENSIONS

The game is played by two teams competing to score the most points, or runs. At the end of each game, the team with the most runs wins. The home team is the team that plays defense first. The visiting team is on offense first. The objective for the offensive player is to start at home plate and attempt to reach each base safely, in order, and finish at home plate to score a run. If the player touches home plate before the third out of the inning is made, a run is scored.

Each field layout consists of a pitcher's mound surrounded by home plate and three bases, as seen in figure 1. Depending on the level of play, the distance between bases, as well as the distance from home plate to the pitcher's mound, varies. From the high school level to the professional level, the base distance is 90 feet (27.4 m) and the pitcher's distance is 60 feet 6 inches (18.4 m). These distances are shorter for younger ages.

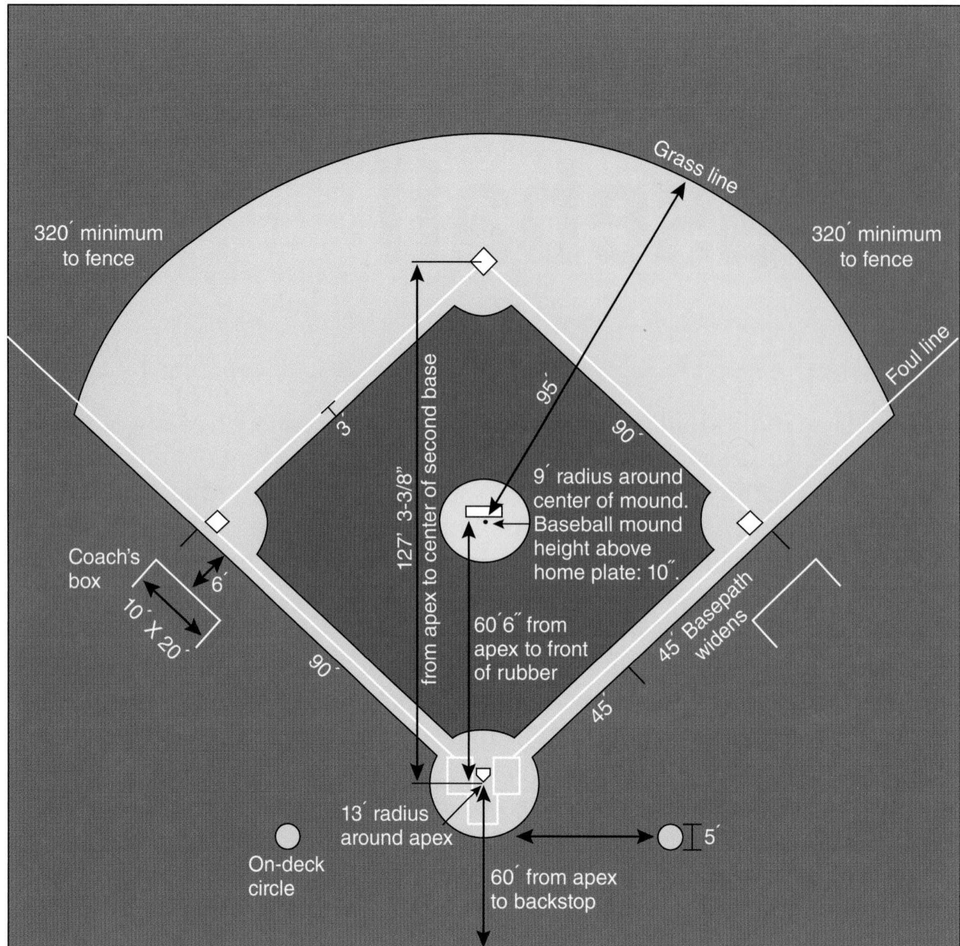

Figure 1 The field.

The outfield is enclosed by a fence or wall that stretches from the right-field foul line to the left-field foul line. A batted ball that travels over this wall in the air is a home run. There is not a specific, defined distance from home plate to the outfield wall. Each field is different. For younger ages, the field dimensions are usually smaller. At the higher levels of play, the outfield dimensions and the shape, height, and layout of the outfield wall are unique to each field or ballpark.

The defensive positions can be seen in figure 2. The foul lines stretch from home plate, through first base and third base, all the way to the right-field and left-field wall. These lines enclose the playing field and separate fair territory from foul territory. A batted ball played inside these lines is considered fair. If a batted ball lands outside the lines, it is considered foul. A ground ball that starts in fair territory must past the first-base or third-base bag inside the line to be fair.

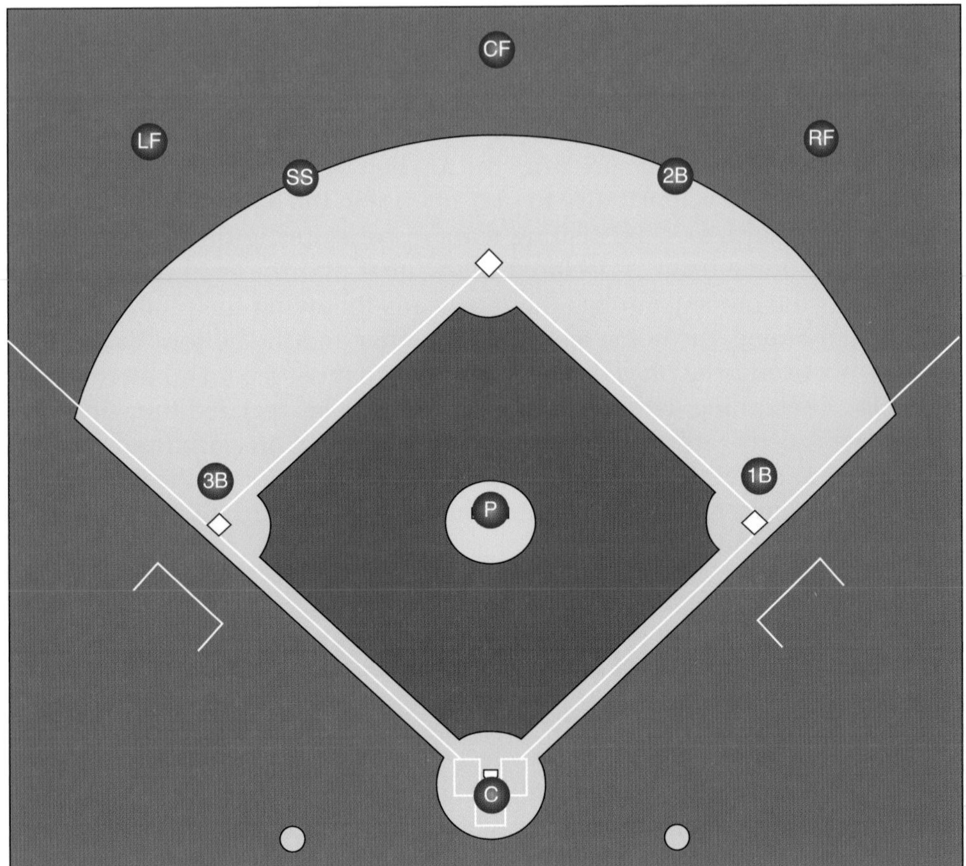

Figure 2 Foul lines and field positions.

INNINGS

In each game, a certain number of innings must be played. A professional game consists of nine innings. For all other levels, the number of innings varies depending on the rules set by the governing body of the league. An inning is played when each team has had the opportunity to play offense and defense. A half-inning is played with one team on offense and one team on defense. The top half of an inning has the home team on defense and the visiting team on offense. The bottom half of an inning is the home team's opportunity to play offense and the visiting team's chance to play defense.

During each half-inning, the offense is given the chance to score as many runs as possible before the defense records three outs. To score a run, the offense must have a player successfully touch each base, in order, finishing at home plate. After the player has rounded the bases and crossed home plate, a run is scored. To record an out, the defense must successfully stop an offensive player from reaching the next base. An out is recorded when an umpire rules that the batter or base runner did not reach the next base safely. The batter or base runner is then considered retired. When three outs have been recorded, that half-inning is over and the offensive side has been retired.

DECLARING A WINNER

The final inning of a game may be played out in full or in part, or just the top half may be played, depending on which team has the most runs entering the final inning. If the visiting team has the most runs after the top half of the final inning is played, the home team is given the opportunity to play offense in the bottom of the final inning. If the home team surpasses the visiting team in runs during the bottom half of the final inning, the home team is declared the winner and the final outs do not need to be played. If the home team has the most runs following the final out of the top half of the final inning, the home team is the winner and the bottom half of the final inning does not need to be played. The visiting team must record all three outs in the bottom of the final inning, while retaining the lead, to be declared the winner.

If the game is tied at the conclusion of the final inning, an extra inning or innings may be played to determine a winner. Each extra inning follows the structure of the final regulation inning played. Depending on the rules set forth by each league, some games may have to end in a tie.

SCORING THE GAME

Outs may be recorded in a multitude of ways. The most common are a strikeout, a fly out, a force-out, and a tag out, but there are far too many rules defining how outs are made for us to cover them all. A strikeout occurs when a batter accumulates three strikes during an at-bat. A fly out occurs when a fielder catches a hit in flight without it touching the ground first. A tag out occurs when a base runner is out because he is touched by the fielder who is holding a live ball either in hand or glove while the runner is advancing. A force-out is when a base runner is forced to leave his base—and thus to try to advance to the next base—because the batter became a runner. Although many outs are universal throughout the sport, each governing body specifically defines the characteristics of how certain outs are ruled by an umpire.

Errors are made by a player on defense. The official scorekeeper judges whether a defender has made an error. An error is generally defined as a fielder's physical misplay of a routine ball that allows a batter or base runner to advance to the next base or bases.

Detailed pitching statistics and offensive statistics can be kept, depending on the capabilities of the official scorekeeper and the wants of the coach. We will not dive into the complexity of this aspect of the game, but we will highlight some statistical measurements throughout our discussion about specific aspects of the development process.

EQUIPMENT NEEDS AND PROPER FITTINGS

Baseball equipment is a common topic among players, coaches, and parents at all levels of the game. The following section breaks down the basic needs of each player. Most equipment needs and fittings are determined by the age, size, position, and preference of each player.

BATS

- Bat sizes vary depending on the age of the player. At the high school and collegiate levels, the weight of the bat in ounces must be within three of the length of the bat in inches. For instance, a 33-inch (84 cm) bat must weigh no less than 30 ounces (850 g).
- For younger ages, bat size and barrel size are determined by the governing body of the league.

GLOVES

- Glove shapes, sizes, and dimensions vary depending on the age and position of the player. Styles include the following:
    - Catcher's mitt
    - First baseman's mitt
    - Infield glove
    - Outfield glove
- The size and style of the player's glove are determined by his specific needs.

CLEATS

- Players can choose from a wide variety of cleats, depending on age, feel, and functionality.
- At the higher levels of the game, metal spikes may be allowed. For lower levels, only rubber cleats may be allowed.
- Players at higher levels may also choose to wear molded cleats, depending on the playing surface.
- Functionality of the cleat becomes important at the higher levels. A player with speed may choose a lighter weight cleat, whereas a bigger player may choose one with more support.

OTHER POSSIBLE EQUIPMENT

- Catching equipment
- Batting helmets
- Batting gloves
- Baseball pants
- Socks or stirrups
- Bat bag or equipment bag
- Protective cup or jock strap

FUNDAMENTALS OF PLAYER PREPARATION

As we move into step 1, we want to highlight the importance of preparation. As a player moves to higher levels of this sport, the daily preparation process becomes a more important factor in the development process. For younger players, basic pregame and prepractice stretching routines are commonly seen. For the more advanced players, stretching, conditioning, strength training, and nutrition become vital to the steps to success.

The professional baseball player of today is a more physical, more conditioned, and stronger athlete than the typical baseball player of past generations. This change is credited largely to the growing popularity of healthy living. The health craze is spreading throughout amateur levels of sport as well. The focus of off-field training is to prepare mind and body so that the player has the best opportunity to perform consistently at the highest level of his ability.

That being said, success and results do not happen overnight, nor do they happen by reading this book. Success and results will come over time as you take these steps and combine them with the inner will to prepare, the physical ability to perform proper repetitions, and the mental toughness to use failure as a developmental tool.

Key to Diagrams

P	Pitcher
C	Catcher
1B	First baseman
2B	Second baseman
3B	Third baseman
SS	Shortstop
LF	Left fielder
CF	Center fielder
RF	Right fielder
R	Runner
B	Batter
——→	Path of runner or fielder
- - - - - -→	Path of ball
∿∿∿	Imaginary line for leads

Throwing and Catching

The game of baseball can be broken down into three specific areas of focus—offense, defense, and pitching. In step 1, we take a close look at throwing and catching the baseball, which are the fundamentals of playing defense and pitching. As simple as these skills may seem, if they are done incorrectly, the player will develop bad habits and, over time, will develop poor technique. In some cases, injury may occur. Because of the growing numbers of Tommy John and labrum surgeries among baseball players at all levels, arm injuries seem to have become as much a part of the game as Cracker Jack and hot dogs. Our goal in step 1 is to demonstrate proper throwing technique for the beginner and amateur player to slow this rate of injury in the game and give you a solid foundation for developing success.

Before we begin to play catch, we need to address the overhead motion of throwing a baseball. This motion, although it may seem routine, is not a natural movement for the arm. To prevent injury, the arm must be properly trained and cared for throughout the development process. In this discussion, we focus on finding the natural arm slot for each player and training the body to repeat the throwing motion within the same arm slot.

Because throwing a baseball is not a natural movement for the body, you should be aware that over the course of a career, each person's throwing shoulder will be affected internally. Today, many specialists focus on the conditioning and training of the thrower's arm. In addition, many online resources that focus on this topic are available to the player, coach, and parent. The idea is that those who are involved in a player's development should be aware of how the shoulder and elbow function in the throwing arm and what actions and reactions to look for to prevent injury.

Injury prevention, or prehabilitation, is a fast-growing and popular new method for training the professional and collegiate level athlete, especially in the area of arm care. Many of the methods used to prehabilitate the arm are done off the field. As we touched on in the introduction, some of these steps are proper nutrition and sleeping habits. Other off-the-field methods involve weight training and conditioning. Regarding weight training and conditioning, many theories and programs have been designed for player or position specificities. As you advance to higher levels of this sport, we highly recommend studying and implementing a program that caters to your needs.

Now that we have generally addressed the preparatory off-field actions for arm care, let's look at how the prehabilitation process works on the field. With any complete program for arm care or arm development, a throwing program is usually the focal point. Throwing programs, along with weight training and conditioning programs, are generally player and position specific. Position-specific throwing programs are used because each position requires different arm actions. For example, an outfielder typically has a longer throwing motion than a catcher does. Therefore, each player has to train his arm to meet not only his individual demands but also the demands of the position he will be playing. For pitchers, throwing programs vary depending on numerous factors such as arm angle, arm strength, and usage. We discuss this pitching more in step 3.

Every arm is different. For advanced players, arm angle, arm action, arm strength, and arm health vary widely, but at the beginning and amateur levels of this sport, the variety is usually narrower. As with learning to count, add, or spell, at this stage of development, players acquire the fundamental actions of throwing that will remain with them throughout their careers. After a player reaches a certain stage of physical development, usually in the later years of high school or the early years of college, the fundamental mechanics of the throwing motion typically cannot be changed without risk of injury. For that reason, we need to break down the basic techniques of throwing for beginner and amateur players to find a natural arm slot and create a proper foundation for the first step to success.

THE BASEBALL: GETTING A GRIP

A standard baseball is roughly 9 inches (23 cm) around and 5 ounces (142 g) in weight. The 108 double stitches make up the signature horseshoe pattern around the ball. These seams are used for specific grips; each grip has a different purpose when throwing. To begin, we look at the two standard fastball grips.

The four-seam grip (see figure 1.1) is the most common way to throw a baseball, and it is the suggested grip for all position players to use because it is allows the thrower the most control of where the ball will go. The control factor is the reason that the four-seam grip is the most common fastball grip for pitchers, especially in the amateur levels. When the ball is released, four seams will be rotating with backspin. These four seams guide the ball straight.

The two-seam grip (see figure 1.2) is a common fastball grip for pitchers because with only two seams rotating, the ball is likely to drift from side to side, or what is called run. The two-seam grip is therefore a preference pitch for pitchers but not a recommended grip for position players.

Figure 1.1 **GRIPPING A FOUR-SEAM FASTBALL**

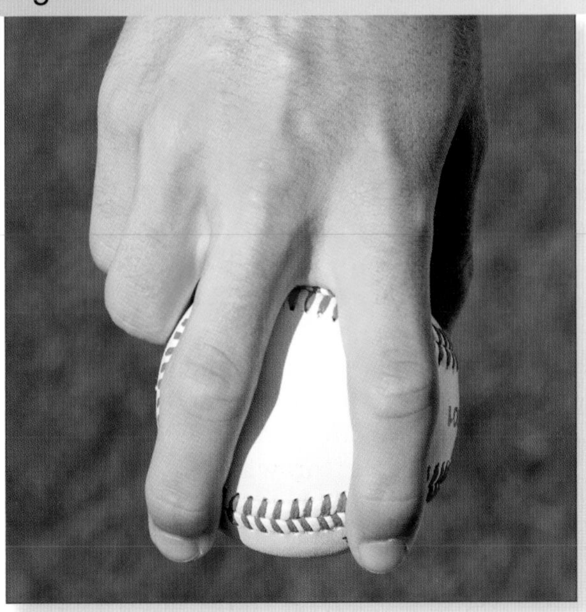

1. Place the index and middle fingers over the horseshoe, or half-circle, seams.
2. The thumb should be under the ball.

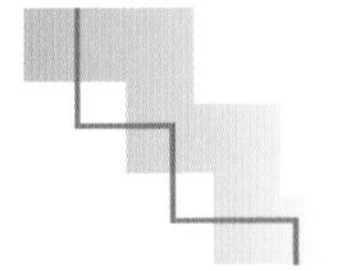

MISSTEP

You may not be comfortable with the thumb completely under the ball.

CORRECTION

The thumb can be placed diagonally under the ball, giving you a more comfortable feel for better accuracy.

Figure 1.2 **GRIPPING A TWO-SEAM FASTBALL**

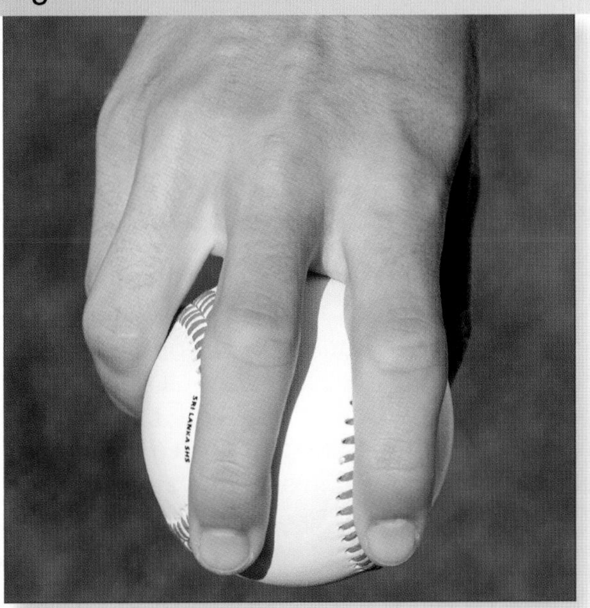

1. Place the index and middle fingers on the two seams away from the horseshoe.
2. The thumb should be directly underneath the baseball and cross the seams where they are closest together.

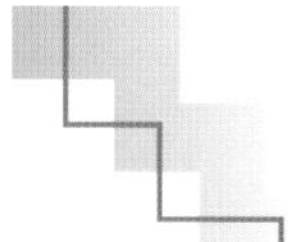

MISSTEP

You may use the two-seam grip when throwing as a position player.

CORRECTION

You need to concentrate on finding and feeling the four-seam grip as you transfer the ball out of the glove.

Grip Drill **Flip and Grip**

With your throwing hand, flip a baseball into the air and catch it in your glove. When you reach into the glove, try to find the four-seam grip on the ball, without looking, as you pull the ball out. Repeat the flip, this time grabbing the two-seam grip.

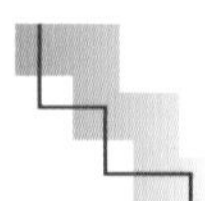

TO INCREASE DIFFICULTY

- Do this drill without a glove. Catch the ball in the throwing hand and spin quickly to the grip you prefer.

Success Check

- When doing this drill with the four-seam grip, you want to make sure that the flight of the ball stays perfectly in line and that you cannot see any of the seams when the ball is rotating.
- When doing this drill with a two-seam grip, you want to see that the ball has parallel lines during its rotation. If some movement occurs in the flight of the ball when using the two-seam grip, that is OK.

Score Your Success

Flip the ball five times, catch it with your glove, and grip two or four seams. Each successful attempt without looking earns 1 point.

Your score ____ of 5

Flip the ball five times and catch it in your throwing hand. Spin the ball to the two- or four-seam grip without looking or using two hands. Each successful attempt earns 1 point.

Your score ____ of 5

Total ____ of 10

THROWING MECHANICS AND ARM ACCURACY

Now that we have a grip on the ball, let's discuss the mechanics of the throwing motion (see figure 1.3 *a* through *e*). As we stated before, overhead throwing is an unnatural action for the arm. For beginners, however, it is an unnatural motion for the whole body because throwing a baseball requires the entire body to move in a single fluid motion. The method of getting the feet in coordination with the hips, the shoulders, and the arm, simultaneously, may seem impossible for someone who has never done it before, and the early attempts can be quite amusing to watch.

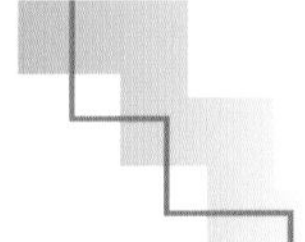

MISSTEP

You struggle to hit the target consistently.

CORRECTION

Are you looking at your target when you throw? Your body rotation with the hips may be off time with the arm, or you may need to lengthen or shorten your stride length.

Beginners need to focus on staying in line with the target. Misguided momentum and direction often result in an unsuccessful throw. For most, misdirection is caused by looking away from the target. Typically, the beginner looks down at his feet or at the ground, mainly because of the uncertainty of how the rhythm should feel. After the back foot is set and the power angle is achieved, the eyes should be on the target. Repeat the actions and add a step or two as you go. If you are confident with the results and the motion feels fluid, you may also want to add a shuffle with the feet. This shuffle will speed up the arm action and train your body to stay in unison at a much faster pace. Can you shuffle and stay in direction with the target while you throw? Does your arm angle stay the same as you throw, even though the pace is faster? Remember to keep the elbow up and to finish properly. Many different body movements make up this throwing motion; therefore, inconsistency could result from numerous causes that require different corrections. To help you find your corrections, let's look at a few drills that may help you find the corrections that benefit you the most.

To get started, we will break down the throwing motion into seven basic and universal steps that can be used throughout all levels of the game. These drills are designed to teach feel of the ball in the hand, proper mechanics, and natural arm slot. These seven steps simplify the throwing motion by eliminating movement throughout the body. After we train the arm motion, we will slowly add movement and direction throughout each step, finishing at a successful start to your throwing program.

One final note is always to remember to look at your target when you throw. The goal of playing catch is to hit your partner in the chest. Obviously, we want him to catch the ball, but the chest is the general area that we want to aim for when we throw because it is the easiest place for players to catch the ball. If you cannot see your target, you will rarely hit your target. Now grab a ball and let's begin!

Figure 1.3 **THROWING MOTION**

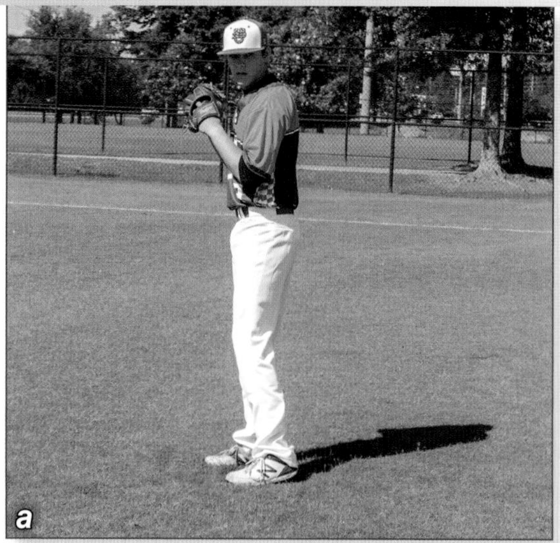

a

Setup

1. Turn your body so that the hip and shoulder opposite the throwing-arm side point to the target.
2. The feet should be slightly wider than shoulder-width.
3. The knees should be bent in an athletic position.

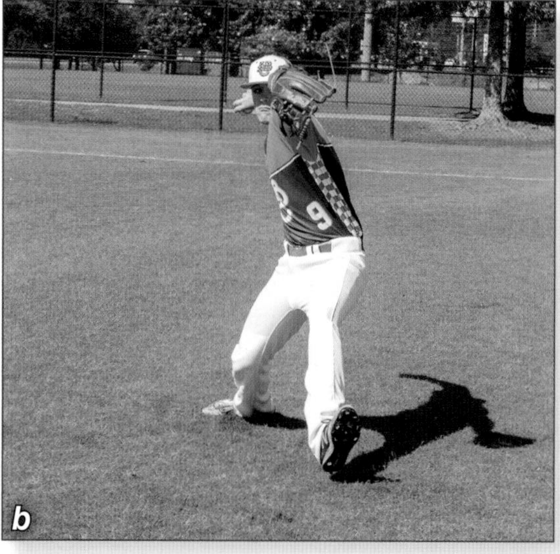

b

Stride

1. The front foot steps and points to the target.
2. Keep the weight on the back foot.
3. The front elbow should point at the target while the shoulders tilt back slightly.
4. Eyes should be on the target.

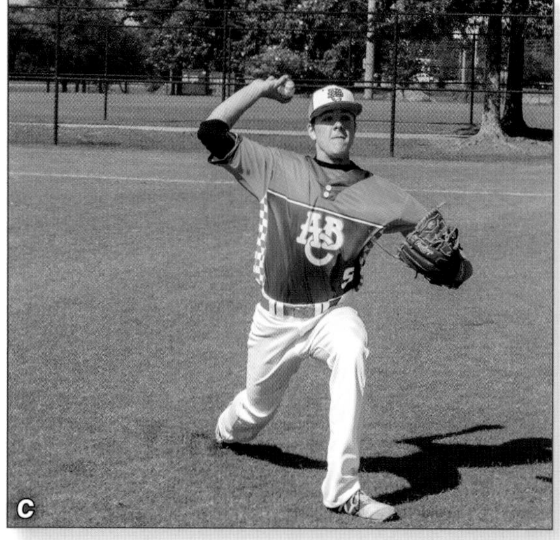

c

Rotate to Power Position

1. Rotate the hips to point the chest at the target.
2. The shoulders will rotate with the throwing motion of the arm.
3. Drive your weight from the back foot forward.
4. The arm should be in the natural arm slot at the power position.

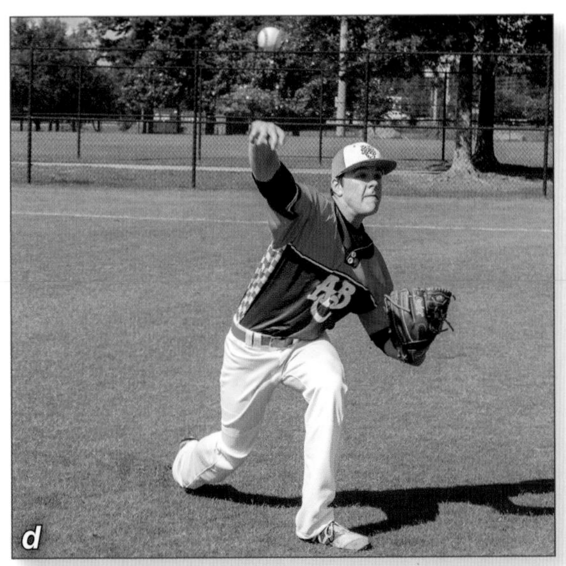

Release

1. Release the ball at the target.
2. The glove-side arm should be controlled beside your body.
3. The back foot will rise.
4. Maintain balance on the front foot.

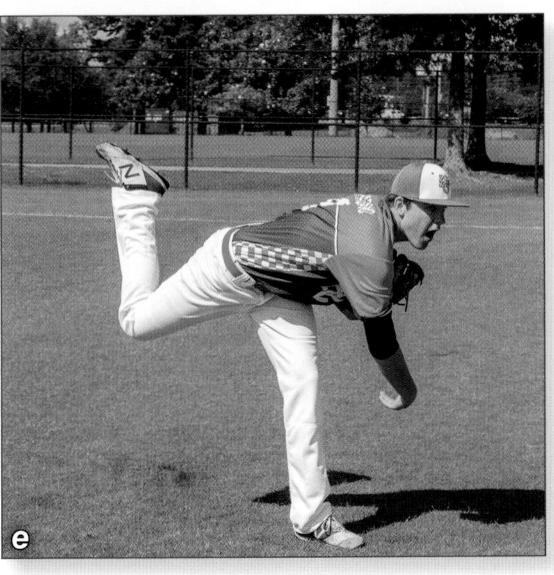

Follow-Through

1. The throwing arm will finish the motion across the body.
2. The glove-side arm should finish centered, or tucked next to the chest.
3. The back foot will land.
4. The body should be in a proper athletic position, facing the target at the finish.

Throwing Drill 1 **Wrist Flips**

As we noted before, we begin our drills by simplifying the throwing motion and starting with minimal body movements. Wrist flips can be done standing or on both knees, while facing your partner. The distance between you and your partner will be relatively close, 10 to 25 feet (3 to 8 m), depending on your level. The glove needs to be under the throwing elbow, with the glove arm at shoulder height as shown (see figure 1.4*a*). With the throwing elbow at rest on the glove, the ball should be in the throwing hand with a four-seam grip. Using only the movements of the wrist and forearm, flip the ball to your partner's chest (see figure 1.4*b*). As you flip the ball, you will feel the release point and be able to see the four-seam spin.

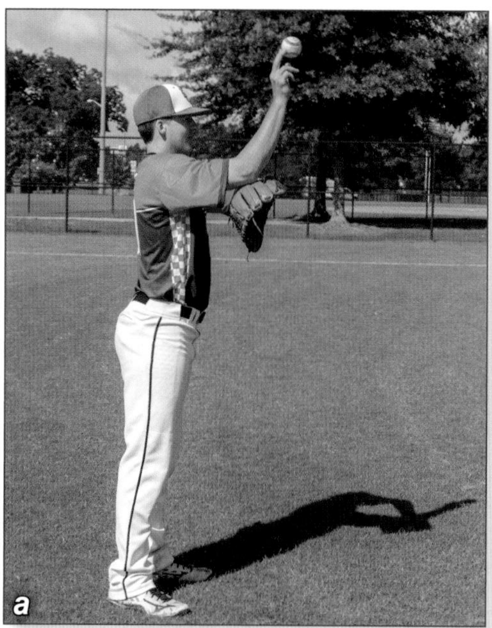

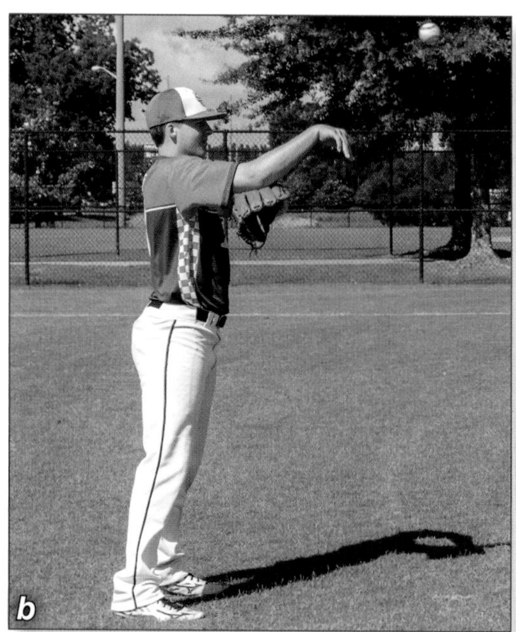

Figure 1.4 Wrist flips.

Success Check

- The ball has good spin and proper four-seam rotation.
- The ball hits the target at the partner's chest.

Score Your Success

You earn 1 point each time you hit the target with proper four-seam rotation.

Your score ____ of 10

Throwing Drill 2 **Double-L**

The double-L is a drill that emphasizes the elbow-up phrase commonly used with beginners. By keeping the elbow even or above the shoulder when throwing (see figure 1.5), less stress will occur on the elbow throughout the delivery. Another common trait of beginners is a weak glove side. As the ball is released, the glove arm falls by the leg, and the head and shoulders are typically at an angle. This action may cause added pressure on the throwing arm as well. The double-L trains the glove-side arm, head, and rest of the upper body in the proper direction and finish to minimize stress on the throwing arm while increasing feel and control.

For Throwing Drill 2, the distance between you and your partner should increase to 30 to 45 feet (9 to 14 m). You do the double-L while standing with your feet slightly past shoulder-width apart, your knees slightly bent, and both feet pointed in the direction you are facing, otherwise known as the athletic position. As seen in figure 1.5, the shoulders are level. The throwing arm is in an L-shape above the shoulder, and the glove-side arm is in an inverted L-shape below the shoulder, creating the double-L. Your back should be straight, and you should slightly pinch your shoulder blades together, activating the muscles in the thoracic spine. At this point, the ball should be in the throwing hand with a four-seam grip.

This position starts with the arm at the highest point in the throwing motion, allowing the functional movements of the rest of the upper body. When the ball is thrown to the target from this position, the upper body should bend at the waist, forcing the chest toward the ground. The glove should simultaneously be brought to the center of the chest. As the ball is released and the throwing arm follows through, this chest-down, glove-to-center position should be maintained. This position is the proper finish that you should attempt to achieve every time you throw the baseball.

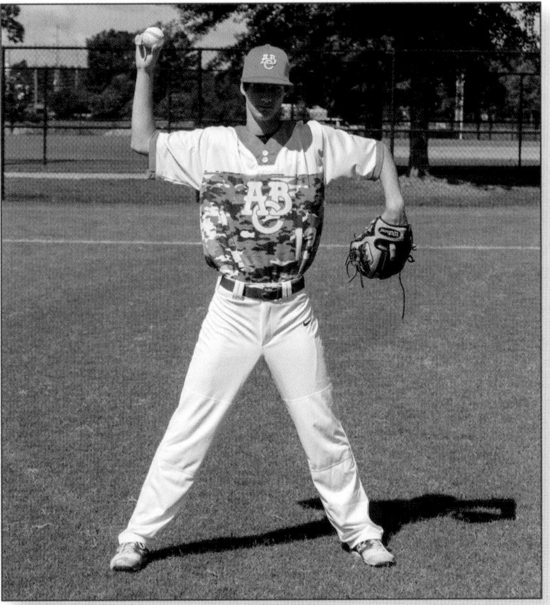

Figure 1.5 Double-L drill.

Success Check

- The ball has good spin and proper four-seam rotation.
- The ball hits the target at the partner's chest.
- The proper finish is achieved.

Score Your Success

You earn 1 point for every target hit with proper four-seam rotation.

Your score ____ of 10

Throwing Drill 3 **Center and Separate**

Throwing Drill 3 will keep you facing the target while remaining in the athletic position. You should remain at the same distance or slightly farther from your partner than you were in Throwing Drill 2, staying roughly 45 feet (14 m) from your target. The starting point for drill 3 requires the throwing hand to be inside the glove, holding the ball with a four-seam grip, while resting in the center of the torso (see figure 1.6*a*). From this position, your hands separate and move directly to the double-L position from Throwing Drill 2 (see figure 1.6*b*). As you pinch your shoulder blades together, you should continue in one fluid motion through the double-L position, release the ball to the target, and finish in the proper position with the chest down and the glove back in the center of the torso.

The center and separate drill allows us to begin to train the entire arm action from ball in glove to the finish of the arm swing. By using only the upper body, the beginner can more easily feel the natural rhythm of the upper body as the throwing arm travels, as well as get the throwing arm into a healthy arm slot with the elbow above the shoulder.

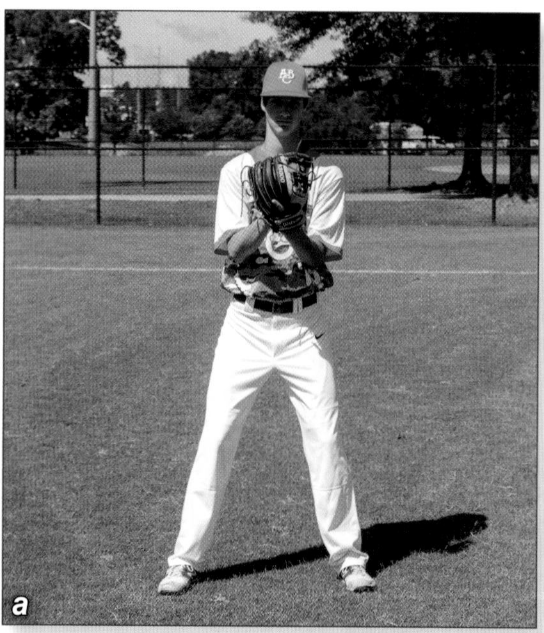

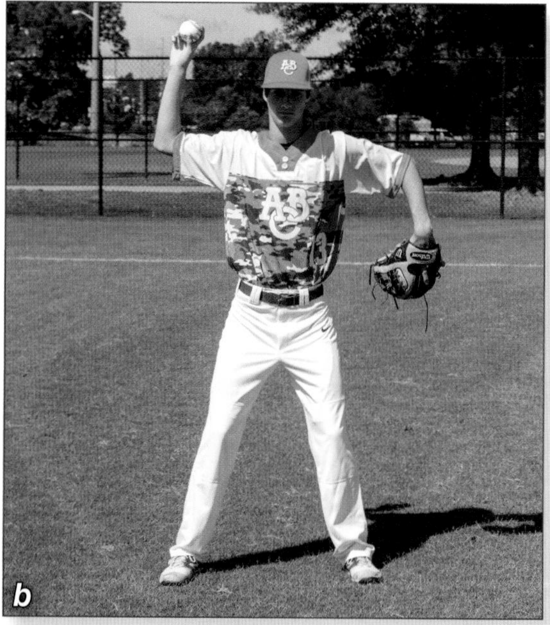

Figure 1.6 Center and separate drill.

Success Check

- The ball has good spin and proper four-seam rotation.
- The ball hits the target at the partner's chest.
- The proper finish is achieved.

Score Your Success

You earn 1 point for every target hit with proper four-seam rotation.

Your score ____ of 10

Throwing Drill 4 **Center, Rotate, and Separate**

In this drill, you remain at the same distance and in the same starting position as you were in Throwing Drill 3. For this drill, we add an upper-body rotation into the delivery. As the hands separate from the center of the body, you rotate your upper body so that your glove-side shoulder and elbow are pointing at your target at the double-L position (see figure 1.7). As in Throwing Drill 3, you should continue in a constant, fluid motion through the release of the ball and into the finish position.

By adding the rotation with the upper body in this drill, we are again training the natural rhythm of the upper body in relation to the arm swing. Although the focus should remain on repeating the throwing motion in the same arm slot and finishing in the proper position, you may begin to notice that your glove-side knee can begin to turn with the rotation of the upper body. This is a positive sign that you are beginning to feel the natural movement of the body through the entire delivery. You may also notice that your arm swing from separation will lengthen, making a circular rotation as your approach the double-L position. This action is another positive sign that your entire upper body is functioning as one.

At this point, proper or improper functional movements will determine the result of the throw. For instance, if the throw was on target and the entire step felt like one fluid motion, then the mechanics of the delivery were likely executed properly. If the throw was not on target, then the motion itself probably did not feel fluid. Therefore, depending on the flight of the ball, you should be able to identify the mechanical flaw in the motion that caused the resulting throw. What did you feel within the delivery that you can adjust for your next repetition? This concept is important, especially for advanced pitchers, but we will address it now; if you can feel it, you can fix it. Throwing Drill 4 is your gateway to feeling your natural arm action and finding adjustments that you can make to correct yourself and avoid creating bad habits.

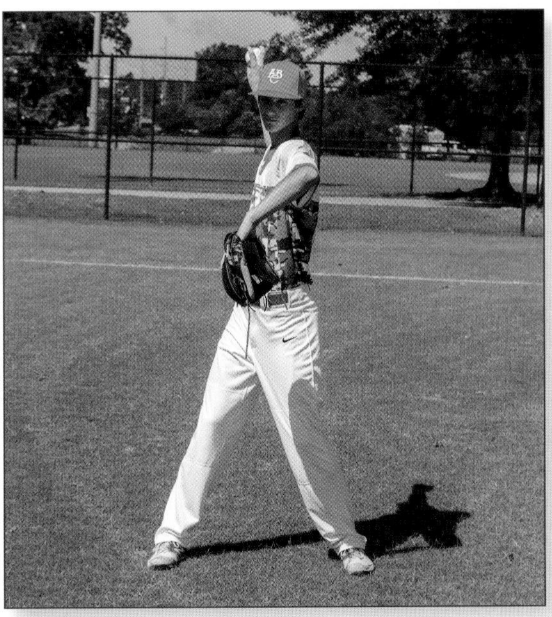

Figure 1.7 Center, rotate, and separate drill.

(continued)

Throwing Drill 4 *(continued)*

Success Check

- The ball has good spin and proper four-seam rotation.
- The ball hits the target at the partner's chest.
- The proper finish is achieved.

Score Your Success

You earn 1 point for every target hit with proper four-seam rotation.

Your score ____ of 10

Throwing Drill 5 **Power Angle**

For the power angle step, you now turn your body sideways so that your glove-side shoulder, hip, and foot are directed at the target (see figure 1.8*a*). From this drill forward, you should be at a comfortable distance of 30 to 45 feet (9 to 14 m), depending on level. For the higher levels, 60 to 90 feet (18 to 27 m) is a reasonable distance for the remaining drills. Your feet should be slightly less than twice shoulder-width apart, and your weight should be centered. This time, we will start with the hands in a W, or power angle position, with the shoulder blades pinched. You rock, or lean back, so that approximately 60 to 70 percent of your weight shifts to the inside of your back foot (see figure 1.8*b*). At this point, the shoulders should remain level. This shift allows the throwing arm and lower half to get in synchronization so that when the weight shifts forward, the throwing arm will transfer forward as well. After the weight begins to shift forward, the hips and the feet rotate to face the target, creating the double-L position with the upper body and moving into the proper finish (see figure 1.8*c*). For the first few repetitions, let the back foot remain in place during the finish. Doing this will allow you to feel the torso stretch as you reach to the target. For the latter repetitions, let the back foot rotate through into the original, proper follow-through and finish position. By doing this, you will feel the proper rotation of the lower half and be able to repeat the finish. Again, watch the flight of the ball and make the proper adjustments that you feel to correct the delivery.

When the weight shift occurs in the full throwing motion, the arm will make an action that is unique to each player. These arm actions are highly debated topics in the world of baseball, especially with pitchers. To learn your natural arm slot and the basic mechanics of throwing a baseball, we suggest that you keep several key points in mind. One, do what feels natural and is easiest on your arm. Two, keep your elbow up and repeat your delivery. Finally, keep it fluid. As we have seen many players do, mimicking arm actions that are not natural or trying to make the ball move by changing the arm slot will quickly lead to arm troubles and bad habits. So for this drill, we start from the power angle so that you can feel the correct, natural position for your arm to get to in the delivery process.

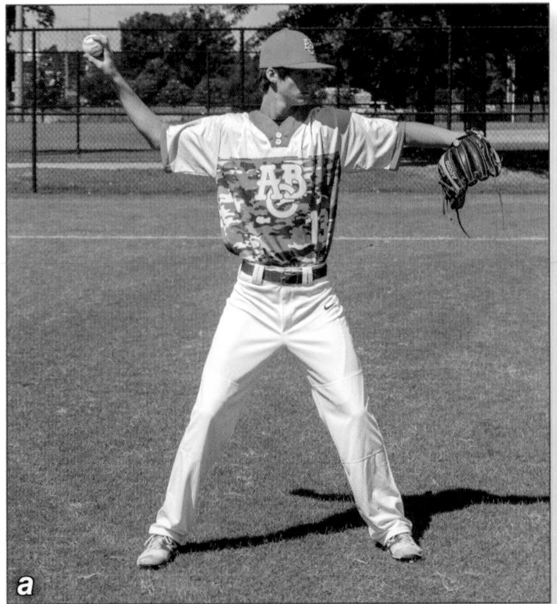

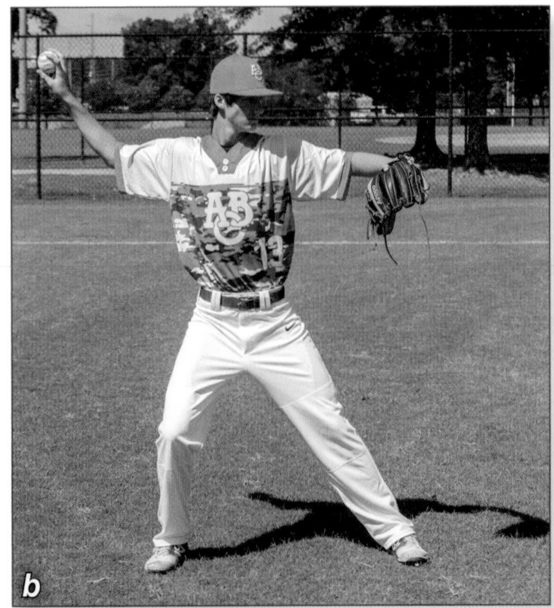

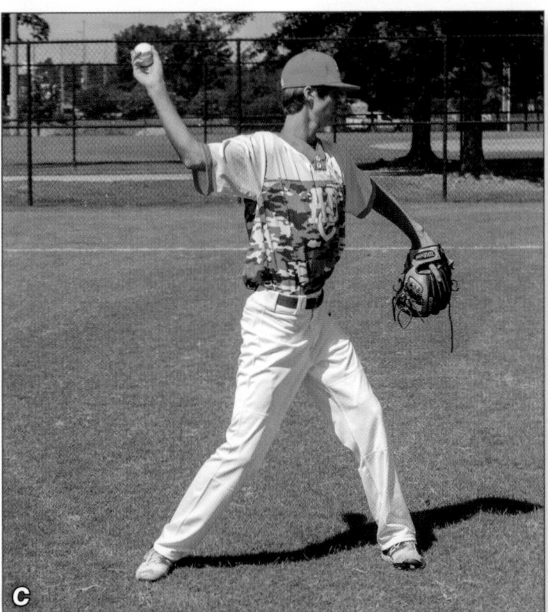

Figure 1.8 Power angle drill.

Success Check

- The ball has good spin and proper four-seam rotation.
- The ball hits the target at the partner's chest.
- The proper finish is achieved.

Score Your Success

You earn 1 point for every target hit with proper four-seam rotation while the back foot remains in place.

Your score ____ of 10

You earn 1 point for every target hit with proper four-seam rotation while the back foot finishes through the delivery.

Your score ____ of 10

Throwing Drill 6 **Stride**

In this drill, you again start in the sideways position, but your feet should be at a comfortable distance about shoulder-width apart (see figure 1.9*a*). With the hands centered and your weight slightly on the back foot, the lower half of your body will be fully incorporated into the delivery (see figure 1.9*b*). This action is called the stride. As the hands separate, you step to the target with your front foot. Your throwing arm will make its natural path, and when the front foot lands, your body should be in the power angle position (see figure 1.9*c*). A fluid motion should continue through the release and into the proper finish.

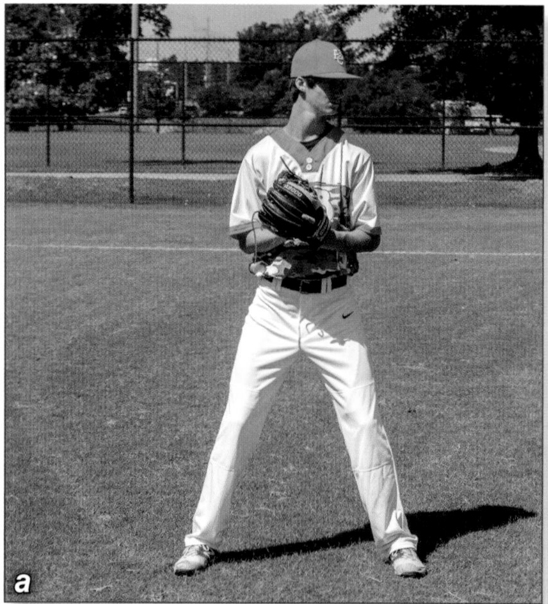

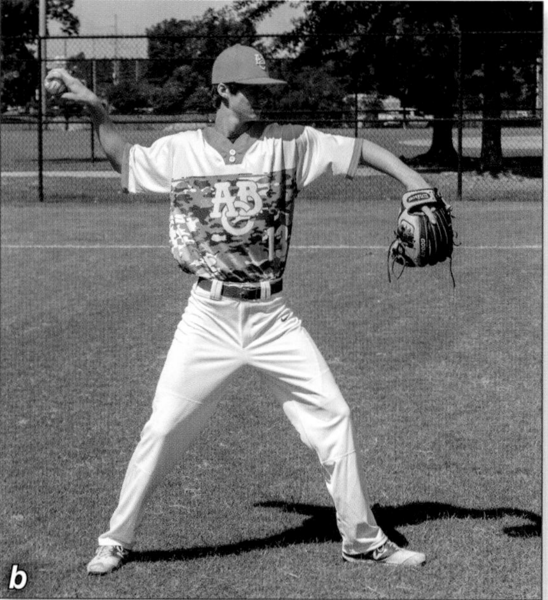

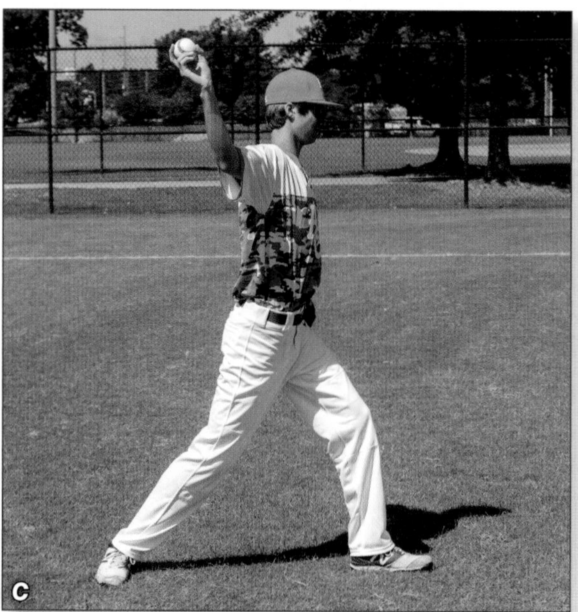

Figure 1.9 Stride drill.

The incorporation of the stride gives many beginners the most trouble, simply because they are moving the feet for the first time in the delivery. A common issue is stride length. Stride length varies by the person, the position, and the type of throw being made. For playing catch, the length should be the same as the power angle length or slightly wider. The other issue is timing of the rotation from power angle to double-L. A common mistake is rotating the hips too soon before the front foot lands, which causes misdirection and arm drag. If you feel either of these issues affecting the results of your throw, you can fix the issue with a small timing adjustment.

Success Check

- The ball has good spin and proper four-seam rotation.
- The ball hits the target at the partner's chest.
- The proper finish is achieved.

Score Your Success

You earn 1 point for every target hit with proper four-seam rotation.

Your score ____ of 10

Throwing Drill 7 **Step and Throw**

The final drill is to involve your feet fully with the delivery of the ball. For this drill, you face your target, then center your hands and grip the ball (see figure 1.10*a*). Take a step toward your target with your back, throwing-arm-side foot (see figure 1.10*b*). Your body will rotate to point the glove side at the target and shift the weight onto the back foot (see figure 1.10*c*). From this position, you stride and finish the throw in one fluid motion.

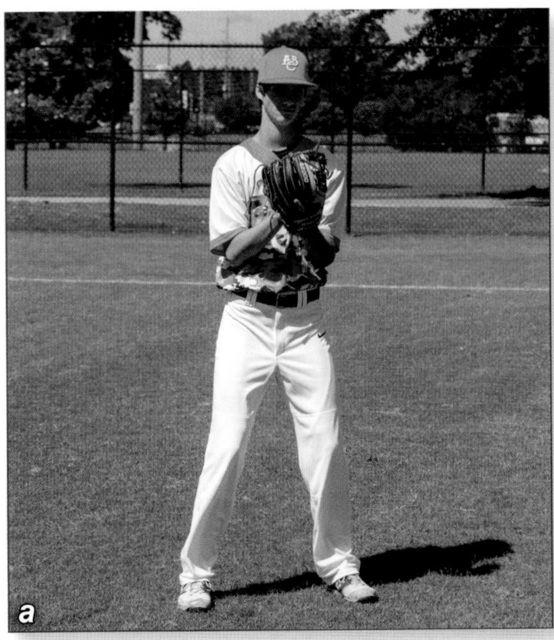

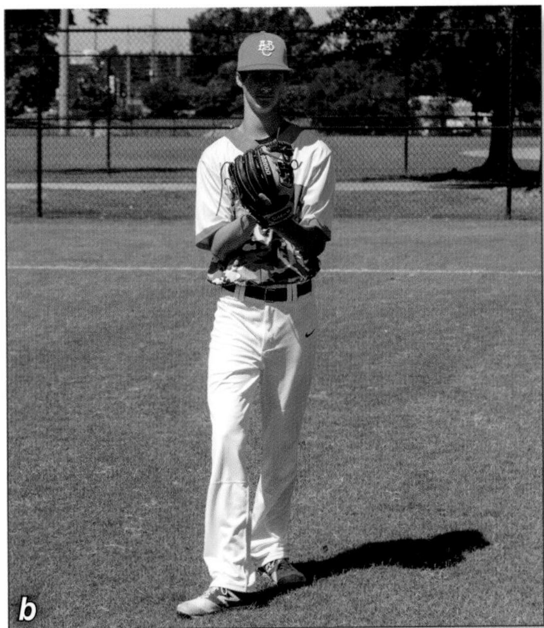

Figure 1.10 Step and throw drill.

(continued)

Throwing Drill 7 *(continued)*

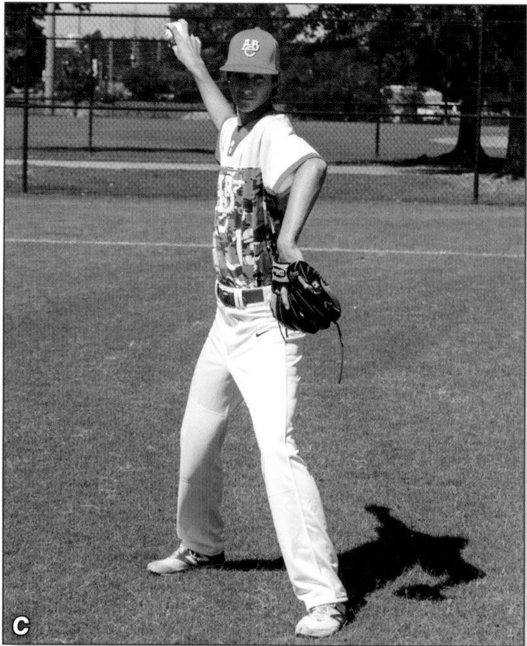

Figure 1.10 Step and throw drill.

Success Check

- The ball has good spin and proper four-seam rotation.
- The ball hits the target at the partner's chest.
- The proper finish is achieved.

Score Your Success

You earn 1 point for every target hit with proper four-seam rotation.

Your score ____ of 10

CROW HOP

We need to cover one final throwing technique before we move on to the bulk of the throwing program—the crow hop (see figure 1.11). The crow hop is a technique used to incorporate the maximum amount of energy and direction into a throw. The crow hop is started facing the target. The number of steps taken before the hop may vary, but the steps must be forceful.

Figure 1.11 **CROW HOP**

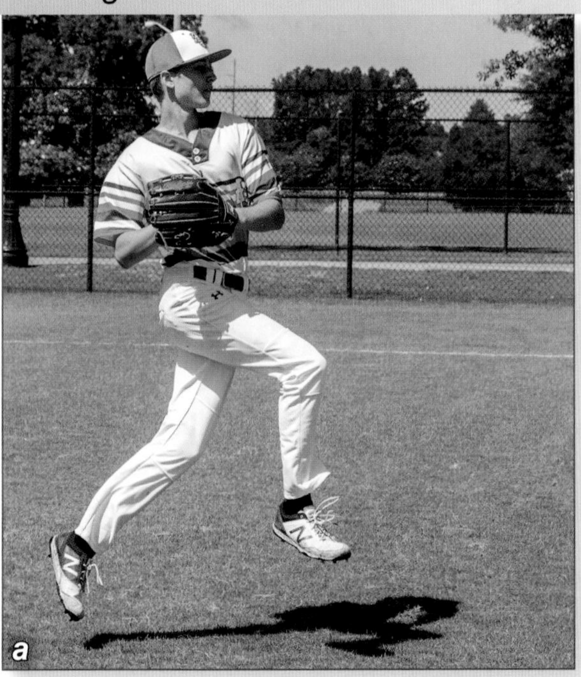

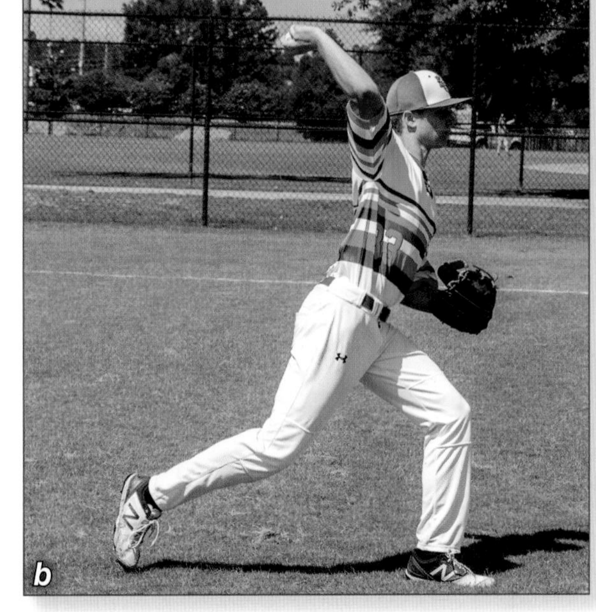

1. The hop is created in stride with a raise of the back leg (throwing-arm side) and a simultaneous, forceful push with the opposite leg. This should create a slight lift, or hop, landing on the back leg (figure 1.11*a*).
2. As the hop occurs, the hands should break as the body rotates into the proper throwing position.
3. As the back foot lands, the throwing motion should take over with the full momentum of the body (figure 1.11*b*).

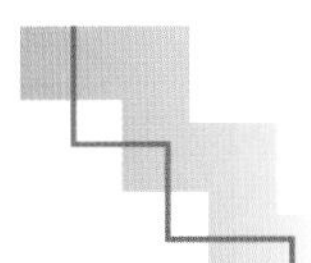

MISSTEP

The initial step in the crow hop is too high in the air.

CORRECTION

The distance of the initial crow hop step needs to be farther outward rather than upward.

Throwing Drill 8 **Practicing the Crow Hop**

Practice your technique because the crow hop will be useful for the long toss program as well as for outfield play. The best way to go about practicing your crow-hop technique is to have someone hit or roll ground balls to you in the outfield, perform the technique at game speed, and throw to a specific target.

Success Check

- The ball has good spin and proper four-seam rotation.
- The ball hits the target at the partner's chest.
- The proper technique is used, allowing maximum energy to be released through the ball.

Score Your Success

You earn 1 point for every target hit with proper four-seam rotation.

Your score ____ of 10

ARM STRENGTH AND THROWING PROGRAMS

Now that you have made it through the basic drills that begin our throwing program, you are ready to start increasing the distance between you and your partner. This distance increase will loosen, or warm up, your arm. The structure of the throwing program that follows the warm-up drills will fluctuate depending on many factors. In the broad spectrum of things, age and experience will be the biggest determining factors of the kind of structure to be implemented. As the experience level increases, other factors may be derived from position-specific requirements, individual arm strength and health, or a universal team program set by forth the coach.

Long toss is the term used to describe throwing at an extended distance. For high school and above, the distance element within most throwing programs typically stretches to a distance of 150 feet (45 m) in 30-foot (9 m) increments. Long toss is usually described as throwing at a distance beyond this mark. Throwing at these extended distances requires close to, if not all of, a player's maximum effort if the goal is to keep the flight path of the ball relatively low. To hit the target at these distances, the entire body must function not only at maximum effort but also with perfect fluidity throughout the throwing motion.

Debate continues over the functionality of long toss and its relationship to arm strength, arm conditioning, and arm health. The primary target for the long toss debate focuses on pitchers at higher levels of the sport. This topic will be discussed more in step 3. The theory behind long toss is that it builds arm endurance. Throwing at maximum effort and maximum distance requires the entire body, especially the arm motion, to function properly, thereby conditioning the arm to handle the body's maximum output. Some believe that this effort strengthens the arm as well. Either way, long toss is an important tool in the development process. It does not require daily attention; rather, it is to be used to fit the needs of each player.

Many throwing programs are out there to fit each player's individual needs, but whatever program is used, the health of the athlete's arm must not be put in danger. Unproven throwing programs or programs created by someone who isn't familiar with arm care or athletic training can do more harm than good.

RECEIVING THE BASEBALL

We next focus on fielding the baseball at various positions, but before we can move on to this discussion, we must backtrack to the beginning of our throwing program and focus on the proper techniques for catching the baseball. Receiving fundamentals are vitally important to the steps to success because they will remain with you throughout your career. So let's look at the fundamentals for catching the baseball and the techniques that you can use to improve your game.

For beginners, catching a baseball is not an easy task, largely because of the fear of getting hit by the ball. This fear derives from the lack of experience with tracking a ball in flight. Beginners must get used to the depth perception of a little round ball traveling toward them at a rapid pace. Easier said than done, we understand. So how do we overcome this fear and teach the eye to follow the ball to the glove? Let's take a look!

Principles of Catching

Although you see it done all the time, much more than meets the eye goes into the simple act of catching a baseball. Positioning, technique and using the proper-sized equipment (figure 1.12) are crucial to being able to catch a baseball properly.

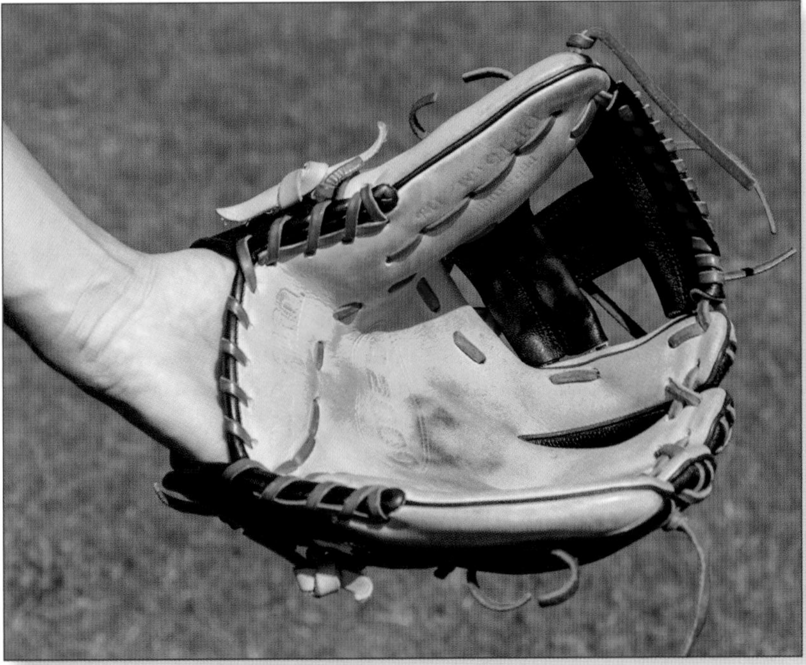

Figure 1.12 A glove that fits properly, with the hand being in the correct position within the glove.

Glove sizes for experienced players depend on functionality for the position of each player. For the beginner, glove size should depend on the size of the hand and the size of the player. Smaller players just beginning to learn the sport often attempt to use gloves that are too big for their hands. Bigger is not always better, especially when learning to catch a baseball. The glove must be functional for the player using it. If the glove is too big, moving it quickly to the ball may be hard, if not impossible.

Finding a glove that fits means finding a glove that can be easily controlled; in other words, the glove should be an extension of the hand. The smaller the glove is, the more functional it will be. An added benefit of a smaller glove is the training of eye-hand coordination. As anyone in baseball will tell you, eye-hand coordination is the backbone of success in all areas of this game.

Making the Catch

"Use two hands" is a directive heard in every ballpark and field around the globe. For professionals, it is often used as a punch line to highlight the lack of use of this basic skill when a player drops the ball. For beginners, "Use two hands" stresses the importance of controlling the baseball in the glove. We often witness beginners attempt to catch a ball thrown to the side of the body using the single glove hand. When playing catch, using two hands should begin before the ball has been thrown.

Beginners who attempt to catch the ball to the side of the body often close their eyes or turn their head in the opposite direction. As with throwing a baseball to a target, catching a baseball is nearly impossible when you cannot see it. Using the thumb-to-thumb technique, you need to trust your natural reactions because if your eyes are tracking the ball, the glove hand will naturally move with the eyes to the ball in flight. A ball traveling at you becomes dangerous when you turn your eyes or head from it. You can rarely catch what you cannot see, but you can definitely be struck by it. So eliminate the fear of being struck and trust your eyes; they will guide your hands to where they need to be.

Just giving your partner a good target at the chest does not mean that he will always hit it. Honestly, the target is often missed even at higher levels of the game. As the distance between you and your partner increases during a throwing program, the likelihood that the ball will be thrown to your chest will inevitably decrease. Knowing this, you must learn to incorporate your feet into the process of receiving the baseball. The purpose of moving your feet is to accomplish a common goal with any ball in motion, which is to keep the ball in front of you. A ball in front of you is easier to see and therefore easier to catch. For a ball thrown to your side, move your feet so that you center the ball with your body (see figure 1.13).

Figure 1.13 **MAKING THE CATCH**

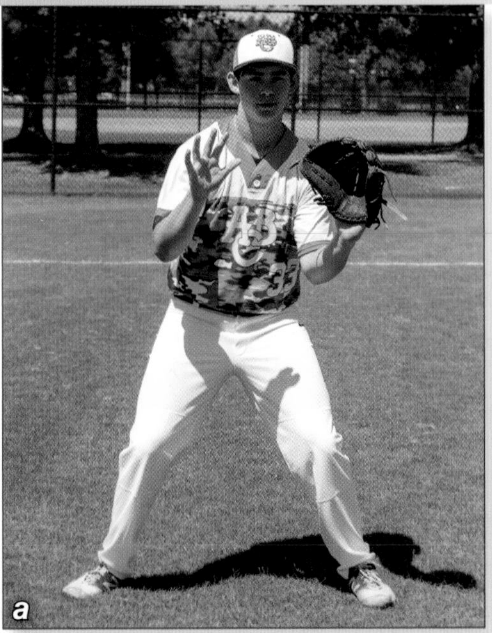

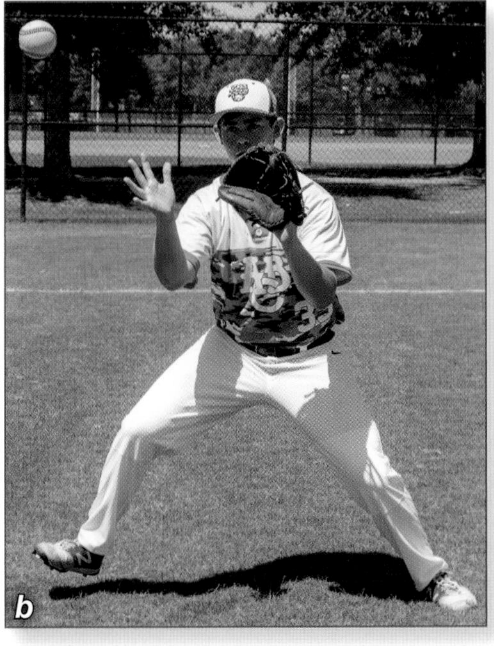

1. As we discussed earlier, the goal of throwing the baseball should be to hit your partner in the chest. As the receiver, you want to show your partner the target (glove) in the center of the chest because this is the easiest place to catch the baseball.
2. Give the target by placing the glove and the throwing hand side by side in a position called thumb to thumb. From this position, you can catch a ball thrown at the target in the glove (see figure 1.13*a*).
3. Be in an athletic position as you give your target.
4. Move your feet to center your body with the ball (see figure 1.13*b*).
5. The throwing hand should follow the ball into the glove and secure the catch.

(continued)

Figure 1.13 *(continued)*

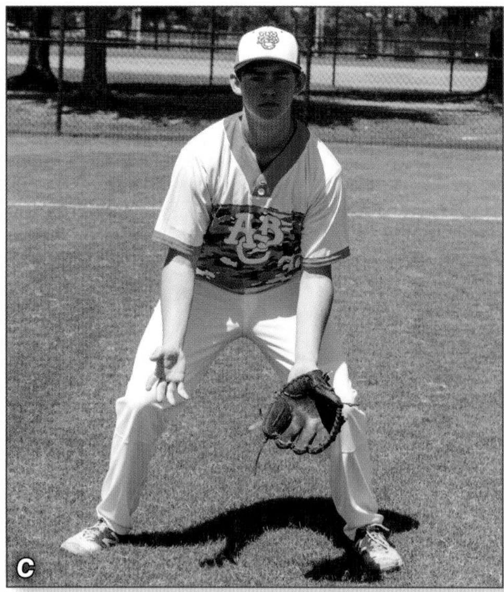

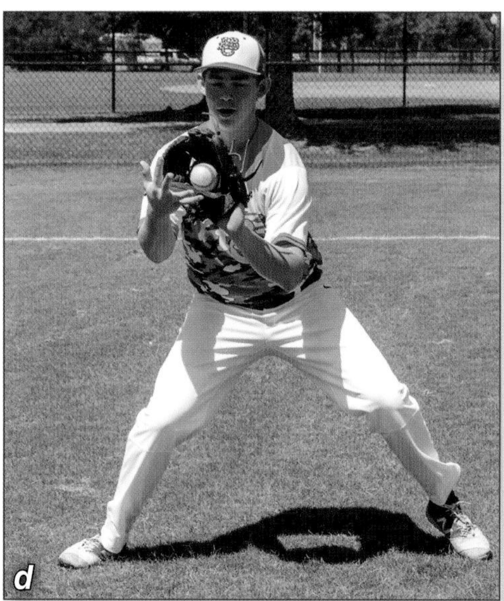

6. For a ball that is thrown below the waist, invert the thumb-to-thumb position so that the glove is turned over, making the reception easier (see figure 1.13*c*).
7. Watch the ball from the release point.
8. Watch the spin of the ball.
9. Watch the ball into the glove (see figure 1.13*d*).
10. As discussed in "Getting a Grip," you now locate the four-seam grip, leading to what is called the transfer of the ball from glove to hand.

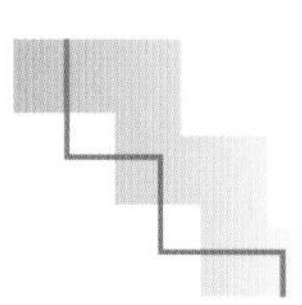

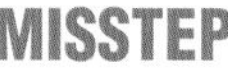

MISSTEP

The ball hits your glove and falls out.

CORRECTION

Be sure to secure the ball. Squeeze the catch while securing the ball with your throwing hand.

MISSTEP

You completely miss the ball with your glove.

CORRECTION

Watch the ball all the way as it comes toward you.

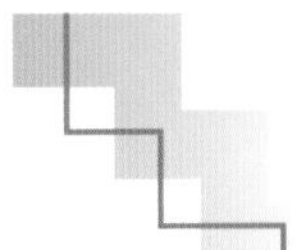

MISSTEP

You miss the ball while turning your body to the side.

CORRECTION

Move quickly to get in front of the ball to make the catch.

Catching Drill 1 **Transfers**

The transfer drill tests your ability to catch the baseball and quickly get into the throwing position with the proper four-seam grip. To do this, have your partner throw the ball to you. You must move your feet to position yourself in front of the ball (see figure 1.14). As you make the catch, you should be rotating your body into the throwing position. You should take the ball from the glove, grip it, and place it in position to throw as your body reaches the throwing position. After you are in the proper throwing position, reset and start over.

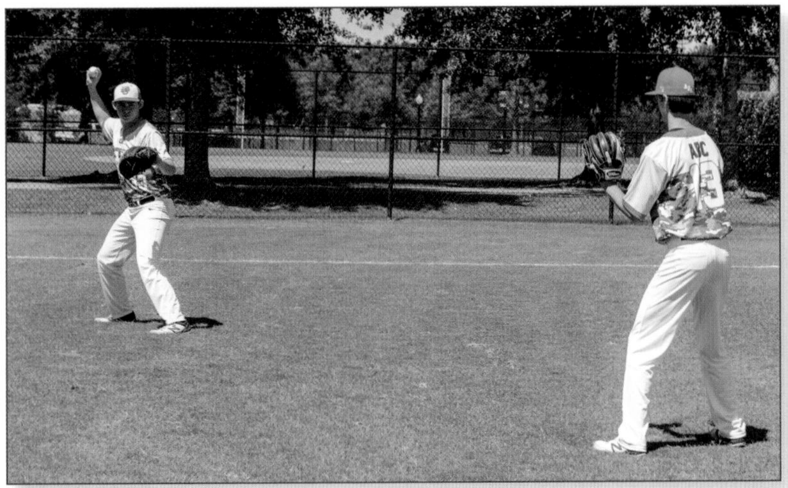

Figure 1.14 Transfers drill.

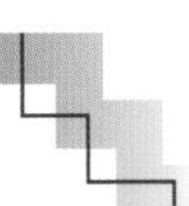

TO INCREASE DIFFICULTY

- Have your partner throw the ball to different locations away from your body, forcing you to move your feet and adjust your glove.

Success Check

- You caught the ball in front of your body.
- You transferred the ball from glove to hand quickly while getting into throwing position.
- You have a four-seam grip.

Score Your Success

You earn 1 point for every successful transfer that you end in the throwing position with the four-seam grip.

Your score ____ of 10

Catching Drill 2 **Rapid Fire**

The rapid-fire drill is a continuation of the transfer drill, except that there is no reset. After you make the catch and transfer the ball (see figure 1.15*a*), you throw the ball in rhythm with the body (see figure 1.15*b*). Notice that you will slowly close the distance with your partner. After 10 throws each, stop and reset your position.

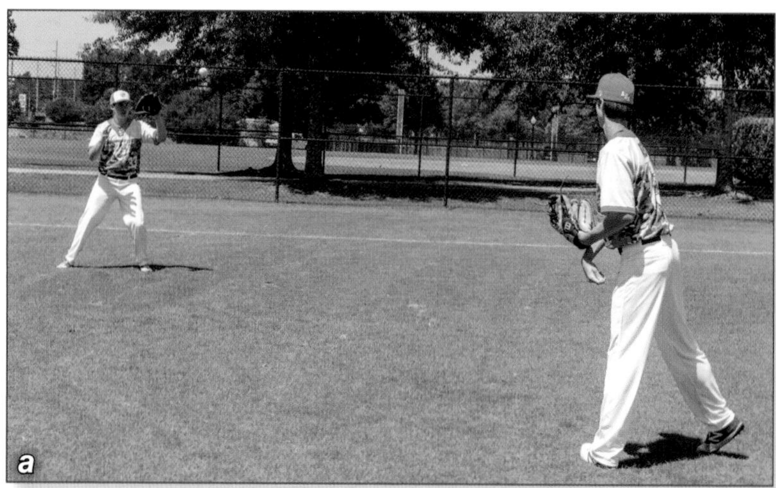

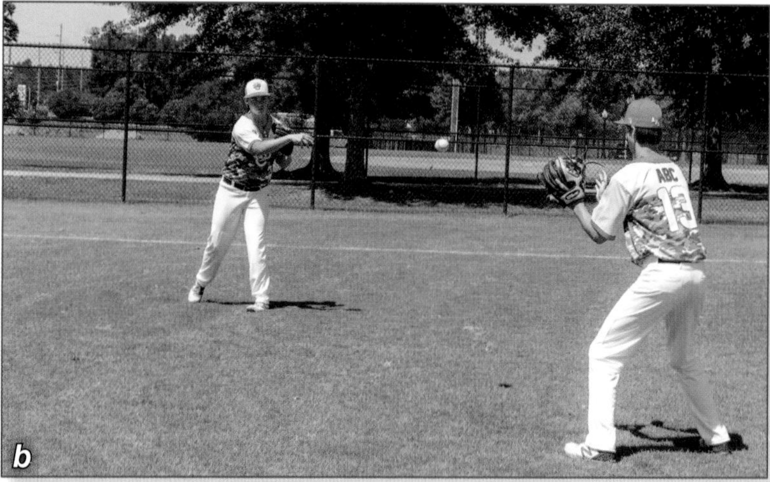

Figure 1.15 Rapid-fire drill.

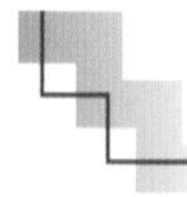

TO INCREASE DIFFICULTY

- Increase the speed at which you are moving.

Success Check

- You center every catch with your body.
- Your footwork and transitions are in time.
- Your throws are hitting the target.

Score Your Success

You earn 1 point for every successful transfer and throw that is on target.

Your score ____ of 10

Catching Drill 3 **Relays**

The relay drill requires three or more people. Stand between your two partners facing the one with the ball (see figure 1.16*a*). As the first partner throws the ball, you need to catch and transfer while rotating your glove side and getting into throwing position in the direction of your second partner (see figure 1.16*b*). After you throw the ball to your second partner, you must reset your feet to receive a quick rapid fire, relaying the ball back to the first partner.

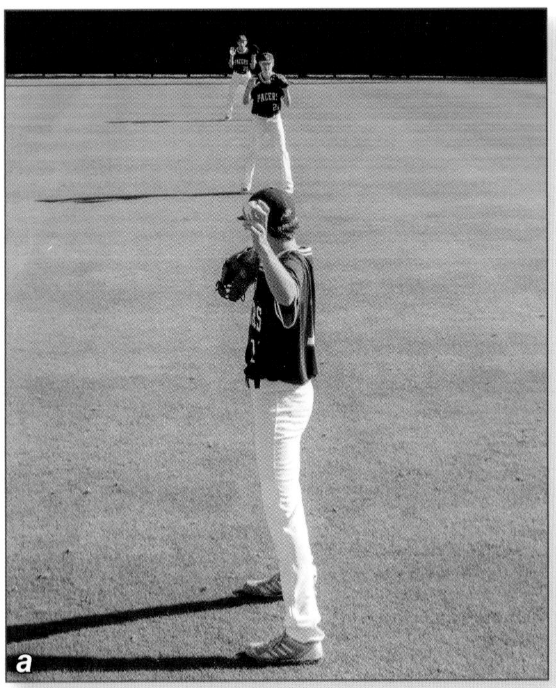

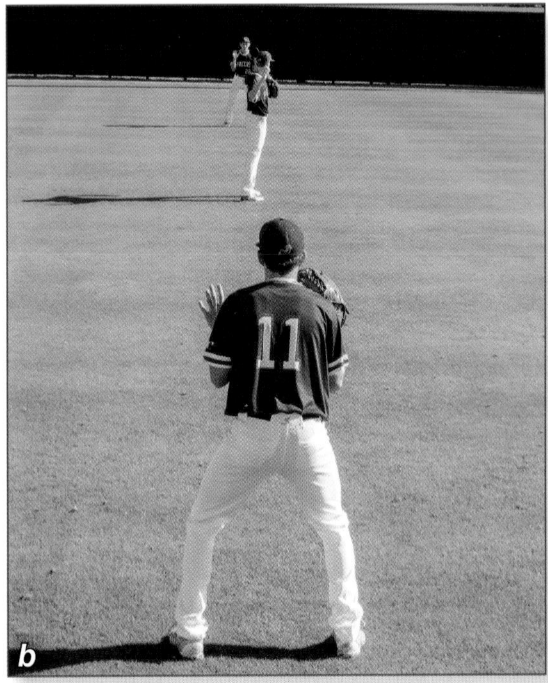

Figure 1.16 Relay drill.

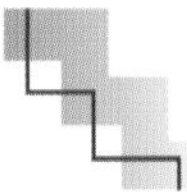

TO INCREASE DIFFICULTY

- Increase the relay speed of each partner.

Success Check

- Your footwork allows you to get into the proper position for the next throw.
- Your transitions are quick.
- You throw each ball with a four-seam grip, hitting the partner in the chest.

Score Your Success

You earn 1 point for every successful relay made without a drop or a bad throw.

Your score ____ of 10

SUCCESS SUMMARY

In step 1, we have discussed the fundamentals of throwing and catching, which are the foundation for pitching and defense. We have discussed the importance of proper preparation in regard to arm care along with the importance of proper mechanics and routine throwing programs as they pertain to arm development. We also addressed the proper techniques for catching the baseball, which leads to the next step.

Grip Drill

1. Flip and Grip	_____ out of 10

Throwing Drills

1. Wrist flips	_____ out of 10
2. Double-L	_____ out of 10
3. Center and separate	_____ out of 10
4. Center, rotate, and separate	_____ out of 10
5. Power angle	_____ out of 20
6. Stride	_____ out of 10
7. Step and throw	_____ out of 10
8. Practicing the crow hop	_____ out of 10

Catching Drills

1. Transfers	_____ out of 10
2. Rapid fire	_____ out of 10
3. Relays	_____ out of 10
Total	_____ **out of 130**

If you scored 90 or more points, congratulations! You have mastered the basic mechanics of throwing and catching. If you scored fewer than 90 points, you may want to continue practicing your technique to ensure proper arm slot and continued arm health. You should continue to practice your fundamental glove work technique as well. By practicing these drills, you will develop the technique needed to take the next step to success.

STEP 2

Fielding

Now that you are warmed up and have learned to move your feet to receive the ball, we are ready to discuss the fundamentals of fielding the baseball. In this discussion, we break down proper techniques for fielding ground balls and fly balls. We show you drills that will help you learn the proper body movements to field the baseball. As we move forward, we show position-specific drill sets for more advanced players. We also dive into fielding preparation techniques for being a successful defensive player.

As with our throwing and catching step to success, fielding the baseball is a broad area that encompasses the entire defensive side of the game. Therefore, our goal is to give you the physical and mental building blocks you need before we move into the details of playing each position. These building blocks are the solid foundation on which you can build further success.

"Ninety percent of the game is half mental," according to Yogi Berra. You should notice that the foundation we are going to build in this discussion is not entirely focused on the physical movements of fielding the baseball. We want to take advantage of the simplicity of our physical drills and incorporate a mental approach that coincides with the physical development taking place. As noted in the introduction to this book, physical ability must combine with baseball IQ to increase your level of play. The fielding discussion is our first chance to implement a mental approach to a physical drill. By doing so, we create both positive habits and a mentality that will allow you to expand your knowledge, feel, and awareness of the game.

Learning how to field the baseball properly is an obvious yet vital beginner step to playing the game. To develop baseball IQ, beginners must learn the fundamentals of position-specific fielding as well. Typically, at this point beginners find a position that fits their physical abilities. As coaches, we can usually identify the physical ability of players easily, especially at younger ages. Those with lesser physical skills commonly play an outfield position at an early age simply because it is easier for them to defend themselves when a ball is hit at them. From the outfield, they can also see the game in front of them to learn how to play defense. So for the Little League parents in the audience, do not feel discouraged if your son is not the shortstop. Instead, encourage him to learn the position and the fundamentals and flow of the game, because he is developing his baseball IQ for the future.

The time to learn position-specific fielding fundamentals will come soon, but before a ball is hit for you to field, we must work backward and break down the basic techniques you will use as a defender. As with all the fundamental topics we discuss, preparation for each skill must be addressed. The preparation for the fielding discussion began with our previous talk on throwing and catching. By this time, you have found a glove that you are comfortable with. You have learned to move your feet to keep the ball in front of you. You have also learned to find a grip on the ball while transitioning from catch to throw. Lastly, you know to look at your target and hit him in the chest. Now you are ready to climb the next step to success. Let's look at the next step in preparing to field the baseball.

MENTAL AND PHYSICAL PREPARATION

Due to the time between pitches, baseball is a relatively slow-paced game when compared with other sports. Defenders should use the time between pitches to clear the mind and to mentally prepare for the next pitch. In a professional game, the defensive players may appear to be staring into space and wandering around aimlessly between pitches, but most are mentally preparing themselves for what may happen next. So, what are they thinking about, and why do they have to refocus?

Let's say you focus your eyes and attention on a ball that someone is holding still. Over time your focus will diminish and the initial focal point will blur. Eventually, you will have to adjust your eyes and refocus before the ball is thrown to you. Beginners must learn and develop this concept over time. This is the first step that we discuss as we begin our fielding drills.

PREPITCH FOCUS AND SETUP

If you were to ask a group of T-ball players to get in the defensive ready position, most would probably get into an athletic position with their hands on their knees. If you were to watch a T-ball game, some would remain in this position as long as the ball was not hit in their general direction. Although this position is a good start, we want to take it a few steps further. The following basic drill is used with beginners, typically in a practice or camp setting.

Ready Position

This drill is designed to help beginners understand the proper timing of when to give full attention and when to relax and refocus. You will use this process throughout your career, just as the professionals do.

Your body should be in the ready position at the moment the pitch is thrown. This position is simply an athletic position with the hands off the knees and in front of the body (figure 2.1). From this position, you should be able to move quickly in any direction.

Figure 2.1 **READY POSITION**

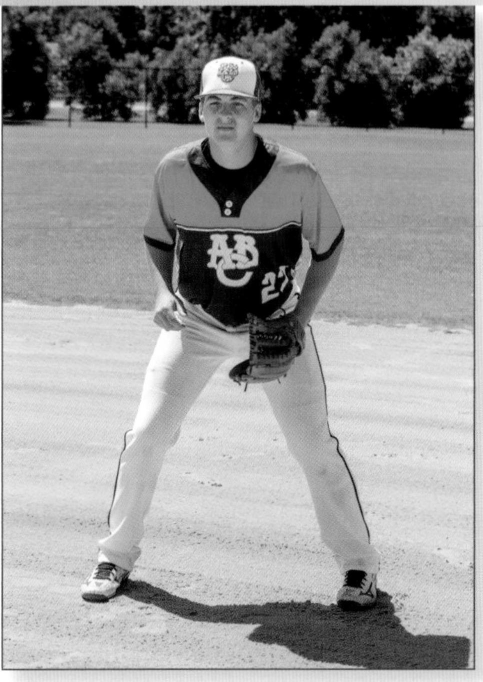

1. Legs are shoulder-width apart with knees bent.
2. Hands are in front of the body.
3. Eyes are looking forward.

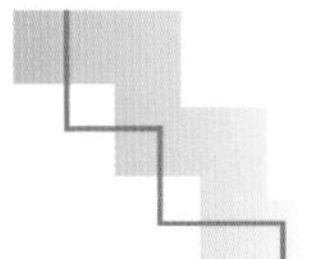

MISSTEP

You are in the ready position too long or not long enough.

CORRECTION

You can use the creep technique to ensure proper timing.

Creep Technique

One of the best ways to ensure that you are in an athletic and ready position on every pitch is to implement the creep technique (figure 2.2). The creep technique is a series of small steps that puts you in the most athletic position possible as the pitch is being delivered. You keep your feet moving so that you are able to react more quickly if the ball is put into play.

You should enter the ready position as the pitcher delivers the ball, allowing you enough time to see the flight of the ball and react immediately to contact. For this timing to take place properly, we need to look at a few steps before getting into position.

The focus circle is a way to show the player visually where he should be and when to focus his attention. Let's start at shortstop.

Figure 2.2 CREEP—FOCUS CIRCLE

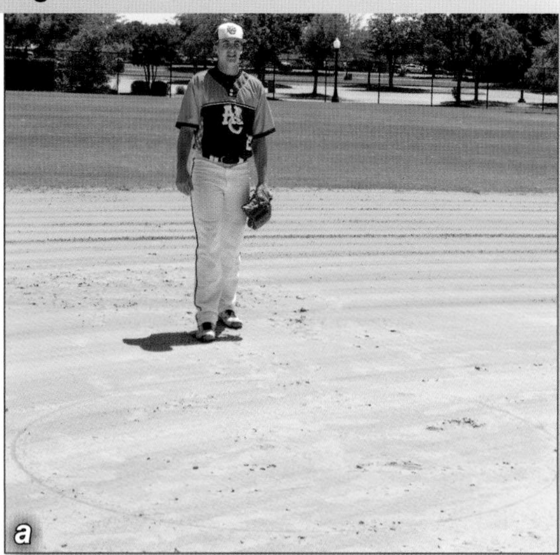

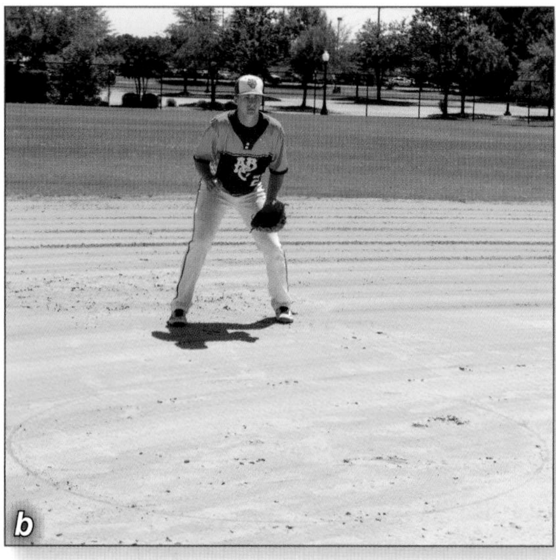

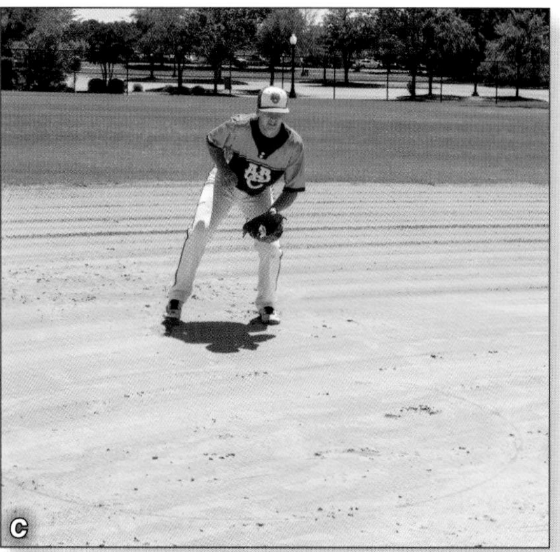

1. Draw a circle or half-circle on the ground approximately 3 to 4 feet (1 m) wide (figure 2.2*a*). This circle should be at the position on the field where you want the defender to be when the pitch is delivered. The player stands behind the circle (approximately 5 to 10 feet [1.5 to 3 m]) while getting prepared.
2. As the pitcher begins his delivery, the defender begins to creep, or slowly walk, toward the circle. The defender lowers toward an athletic position with the hands (or at least the glove) in front of the body (figures 2.2*b-c*). Creeping keeps the defender's feet moving; otherwise, his feet are still, which slows his reaction time. By creeping into the ready position, he will be able to react with his feet more quickly.

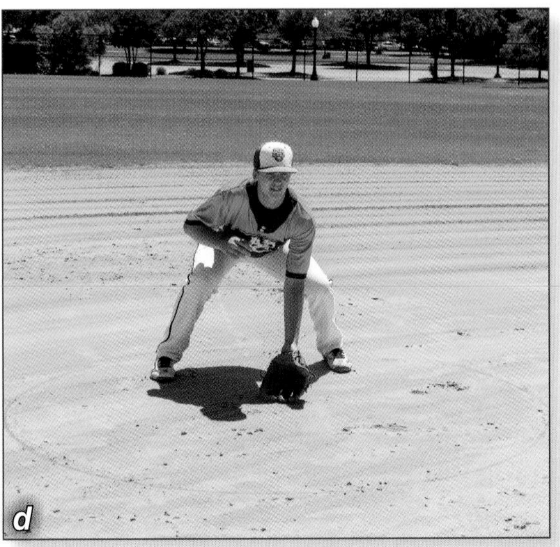

3. As the defender reaches the circle, the pitcher should be in the delivery, close to releasing the baseball. After the defender creeps inside the circle, he should be fully focused on the baseball while quickly setting the feet and body into the ready position as the pitcher releases the ball (figure 2.2*d*). At this point, the defender is in the best position to react.
4. Clear, refocus, and reset. If no action occurs on the pitch, the defender can then rest his focus and work back to the starting position behind the circle.

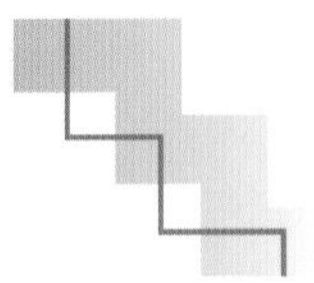

MISSTEP

The proper timing of the creep can be difficult to find, causing you to be out of position.

CORRECTION

To be sure that you are getting into the ready position just before the pitcher releases the ball, find the number of steps you are comfortable taking and repeat them every pitch. Repetition will iron out any flaws with your timing.

FIELDING GROUND BALLS

The process of prepitch preparation has you focused and in the proper ready position as a defender. Now, we can discuss the proper technique for fielding the baseball. Because we are still at shortstop, let's begin with grounders.

Learning to field ground balls is a step-by-step process for beginners. In this section we will choreograph the proper timing with the proper positioning as you approach the ball, field the ball, and continue through the throw. To begin this process, we must first have you feel the proper body positioning at the point of reception. The repeated, proper execution of this positioning is vitally important to your growth as a defender, primarily because it allows you to adjust your positioning as the ball travels while also keeping the ball in front in case of a bad hop. As you continue through the steps, you will add movement and speed to the process, creating fluidity with the entire motion.

Before we begin, we must address an important concept. Ground balls come in many different forms, and they are defined in accordance with how they relate to the position of the defender. In this section, we address the common forms of ground balls to create proper body control and positioning. As we continue into the pitching, infield, and outfield play steps, we will add to our drill sets to address position specificities. Let's look at the various styles of ground balls and the fielding positions that we are looking to achieve.

- Routine: a ground ball directly at the defender
- Forehand: a ground ball to the glove side of the defender
- Backhand: a ground ball to the throwing-hand side of the defender
  - Open backhand: a ball fielded on the backhand side without crossing the feet
  - Closed backhand: a ball fielded on the backhand side with the feet crossed
- Short hop: a ball that bounces slightly out of catching distance and is received just after the bounce
  - Forehand short hop: a short hop to the glove-hand side of the defender
  - Backhand short hop: a short hop to the throwing-hand side of the defender
- Chopper: a batted ball with high bounces or hops, the first of which is typically off the ground near home plate
- Infield slow roller: a weakly batted or bunted ball that forces the defender forward
- Outfield play ground balls: a ground ball hit to the outfield
- Pitcher ground balls: a ground ball hit near the pitcher

Routine Ground Balls

A routine ground ball (figure 2.3) can best be described as any ground ball that is hit directly to the defender, or that the defender is able to position himself directly in front of and thus field on the midline of his body. It is the most common type of ground ball. Developing the ability to field a routine ground ball is the foundation on which becoming a good defender is built.

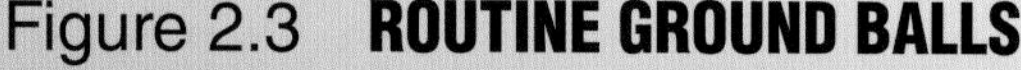

Figure 2.3 **ROUTINE GROUND BALLS**

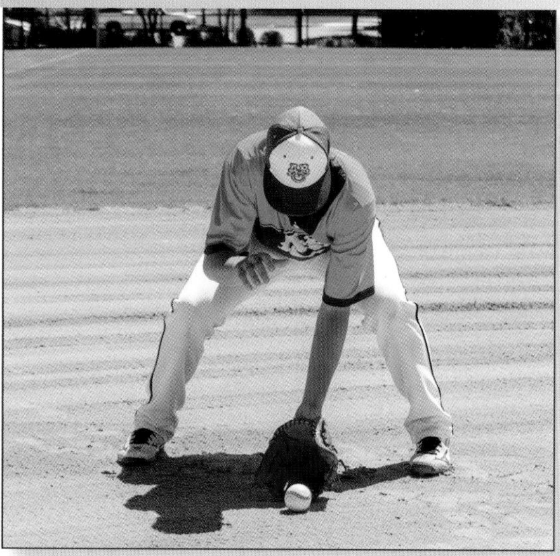

1. First, get into the triangle stance. The triangle is created with the feet and the glove hand as shown. Notice that the feet are squared to the ball, the body is lowered, the head is down with the eyes on the ball, and the glove is slightly off center toward the glove side of the body. Also, notice the flexion in the wrist and elbow of the glove-side arm.
2. The throwing hand at reception should be over the glove in the alligator position as shown.

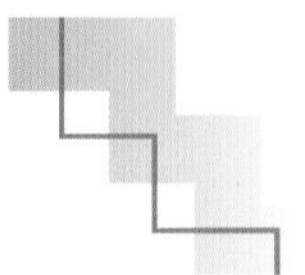

MISSTEP

You bend too much at the waist, putting yourself into an unbalanced position.

CORRECTION

Be sure that your center of gravity is low and that your chest is centered between your knees to ensure the best positioning.

Fielding Drill 1 **Triangle Position**

The coach or partner should be approximately 10 feet (3 m) away while rolling the ball. As the ball is delivered, the glove works through the baseball (see figure 2.4). The throwing hand secures the ball in the glove, preparing for transition. Relax and repeat.

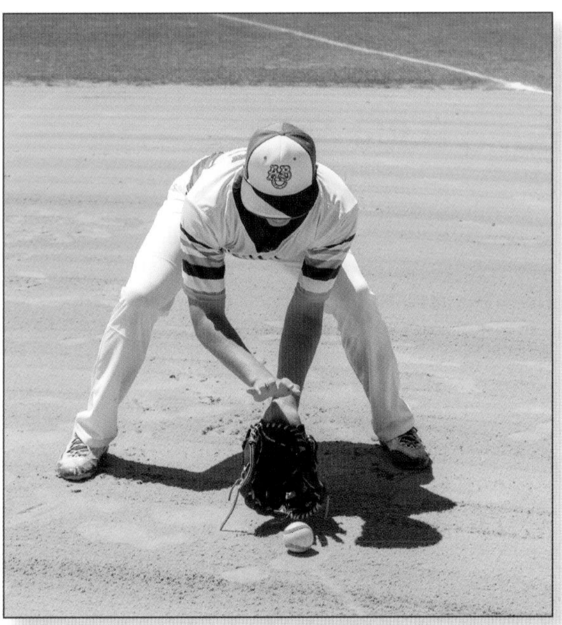

Figure 2.4 Triangle position drill.

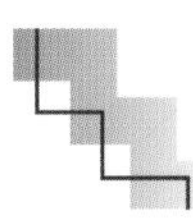

TO INCREASE DIFFICULTY

- The drill can be done without a glove, using the bare hand to ensure proper technique.

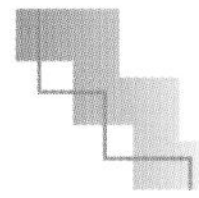

TO DECREASE DIFFICULTY

- The drill can be done on two knees so that the focus is on the use of the hands or glove.
- The coach can increase the distance and hit the ball.

(continued)

Fielding Drill 1 *(continued)*

Success Check

- The ball was fielded cleanly, without a drop.
- The triangle position remained throughout the catch.
- You made the catch in front of the body with the glove working through the ball—that is, while moving your glove hand forward toward the ball and getting into a throwing position. You watched the ball into the glove rather than turned your head away from the catch.
- The throwing hand secured the ball after the catch.

Score Your Success

You earn 1 point for every clean catch in the triangle position.

You earn 1/2 point if you make the catch out of position—that is, if the glove funnels under the body and between the feet or the head turns away from the catch.

Your score ____ of 10

Forehand Ground Balls

Once you have established the ability to field routine ground balls, the next type of ground ball to be introduced is the forehand ground ball (figure 2.5). A forehand ground ball is any ball to a player's glove side that they are unable to position their body in front of and thus have to field with an outstretched arm. It is the second most common type of ground ball and slightly more difficult to field than a routine ground ball.

Figure 2.5 **FOREHAND GROUND BALLS**

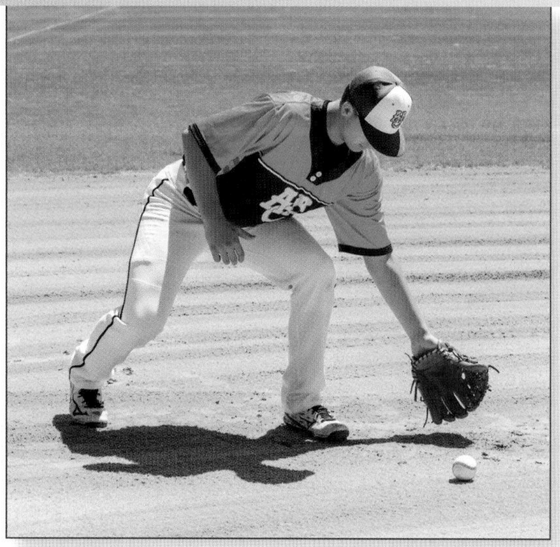

1. To begin, from the triangle fielding position, turn both feet in the direction of the forehand side.
2. From this position, lower your body so that your glove is on the ground outside the foot. Your legs should make the A-shape as shown.

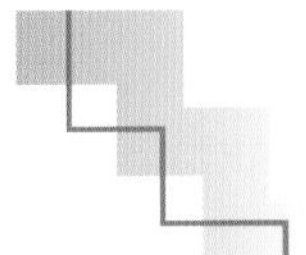

MISSTEP

Your position is too high, making it difficult to field the ball.

CORRECTION

Make sure that you have ample bend in the knees so that your body is much lower to the ground, giving you more reach and putting you in a better position to field.

Fielding Drill 2 **Forehand**

From 10 feet (3 m), your partner rolls a ball to your glove so that you can feel the proper positioning as you field the forehand grounder (see figure 2.6). The glove should work through the baseball as you field it. Relax and repeat.

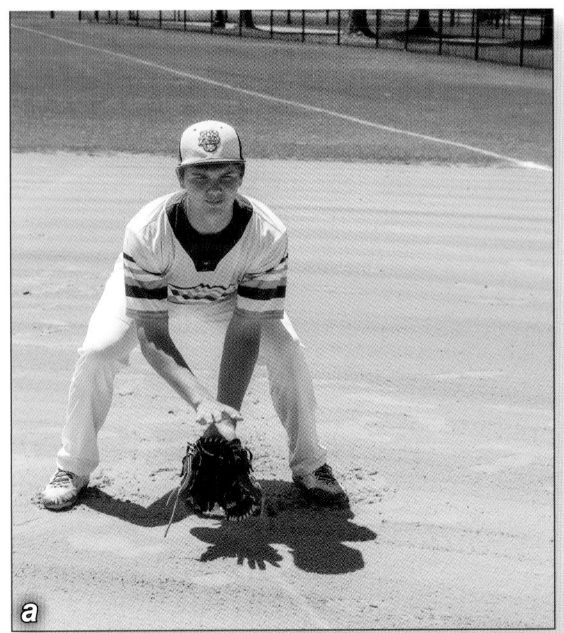

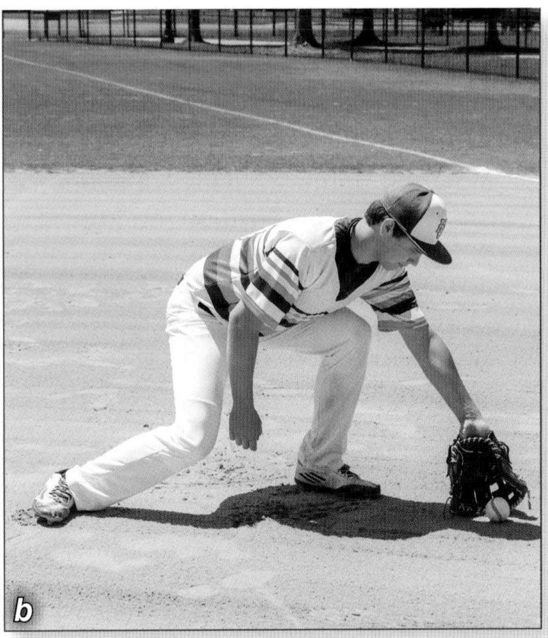

Figure 2.6 Forehand drill.

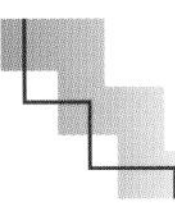

TO INCREASE DIFFICULTY

- The drill can be done without a glove, using the bare hand to ensure proper technique.

TO DECREASE DIFFICULTY

- The drill can be done on one knee so that the focus is on the use of the hands or glove.
- The coach can increase the distance and hit the ball.

(continued)

Fielding Drill 2 *(continued)*

Success Check

- The ball was fielded cleanly, without a drop.
- The forehand position remained throughout the catch.
- The glove worked through the ball—that is, you moved your glove hand toward the ball and worked through the ball to get into a throwing position.

Score Your Success

You earn 1 point for every clean catch in the forehand position.

You earn 1/2 point if you make the catch out of position.

You earn 1/2 point if the glove works backward while making a clean catch.

Your score ____ of 10

Backhand Ground Balls

The next type of ground ball is on the throwing side of the infielder, referred to as a backhand ground ball. Players can use two different techniques to field backhand ground balls—open backhand and closed backhand.

You can use two different positions for fielding backhand ground balls. The first position is with the glove turned over and grounded, in front of the back foot, as shown in figure 2.7. This is the open position because the legs are still open to the ball. You use this position for ground balls that are to the backhand side, yet you can still get your body in front and your feet in good position to throw.

The closed backhand position is for the ground ball that makes you field the ball at a larger distance toward the backhand side. The closed position gets its title because the body is closed off to the front (see figure 2.8).

Figure 2.7 **OPEN BACKHAND GROUND BALLS**

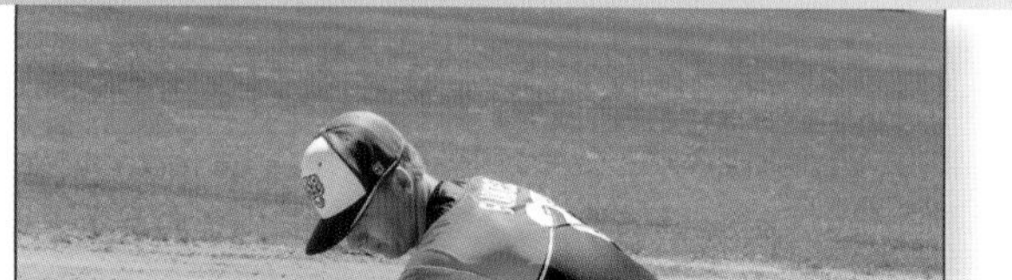

1. From the triangle position, turn the feet toward the arm side. Place the glove in front of the back foot as shown.
2. The legs should again make the A-shape.

Figure 2.8 CLOSED BACKHAND GROUND BALLS

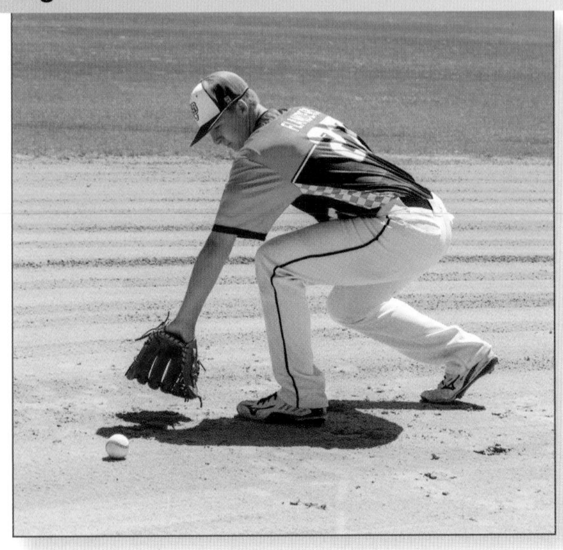

1. From the open backhand position, switch the positioning of your feet and turn your body so that your glove-side foot is now on the backhand side. (The setup is similar to that of the forehand position, although you will field a ball traveling from the opposite direction.) Notice the A-shape with the legs.
2. You should have the glove turned over and grounded outside the front foot.

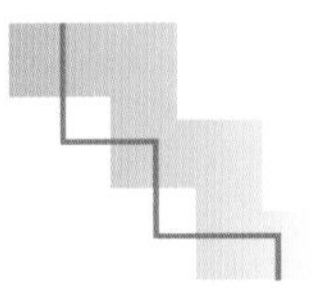

MISSTEP

Your glove and your head are far above the ground.

CORRECTION

Make sure that your glove is almost on the ground in the initial fielding position and that your legs have plenty of flex so that your eyes can be close to where you are fielding the ball.

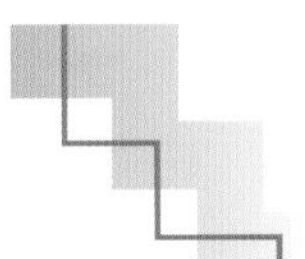

MISSTEP

The ball is fielded too much in the middle of your body and not out in front of the lead foot.

CORRECTION

Make sure that you are using proper timing to ensure that the ball is being fielded out in front of the lead foot.

Fielding Drill 3 **Open Backhand**

From 10 feet (3 m) away, have your partner roll the ball to your glove. Use an athletic positioning of the legs, with the weight slightly on the back leg yet still balanced. As the ball approaches, field the ball by working the glove through it (see figure 2.9). Relax and repeat.

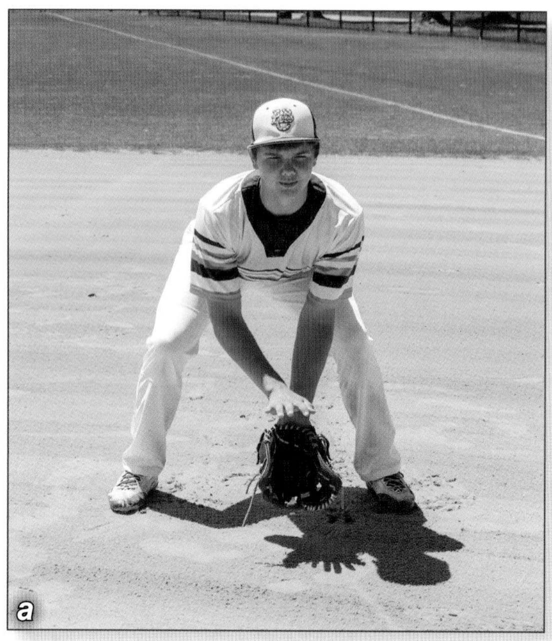

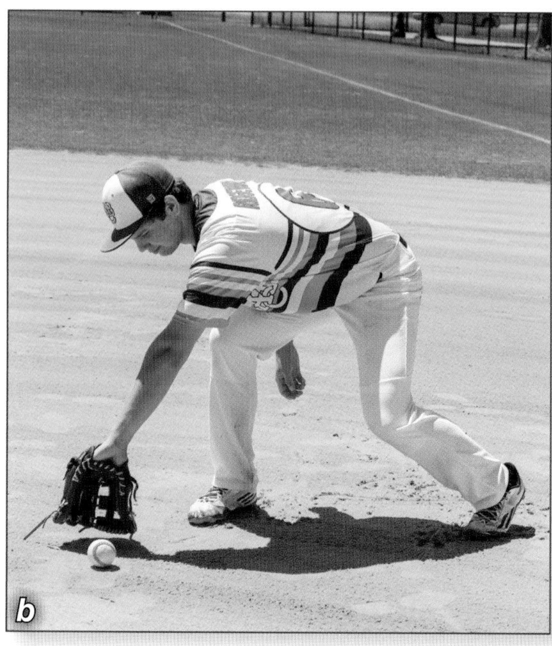

Figure 2.9 Open backhand drill.

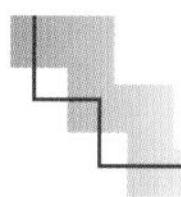

TO INCREASE DIFFICULTY

- Increase the distance and have the partner or coach hit ground balls.

TO DECREASE DIFFICULTY

- Start the fielder in the open backhand position and take the footwork and movement out of the drill.

Success Check

- The ball was fielded cleanly, without a drop.
- The open backhand position remained throughout the catch.
- The glove worked through the ball.

Score Your Success

You earn 1 point for every clean catch in the open backhand position.

You earn 1/2 point if you make the catch out of position.

You earn 1/2 point if the glove works backward while making a clean catch.

Your score ____ of 10

Fielding Drill 4 **Closed Backhand**

From 10 feet (3 m) away, have your partner roll a ball to the glove. Field the ball by working the glove forward and through the baseball (see figure 2.10). Relax and repeat.

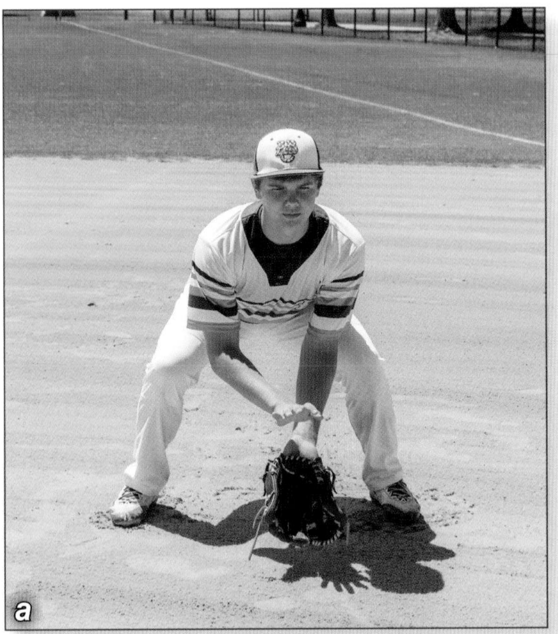

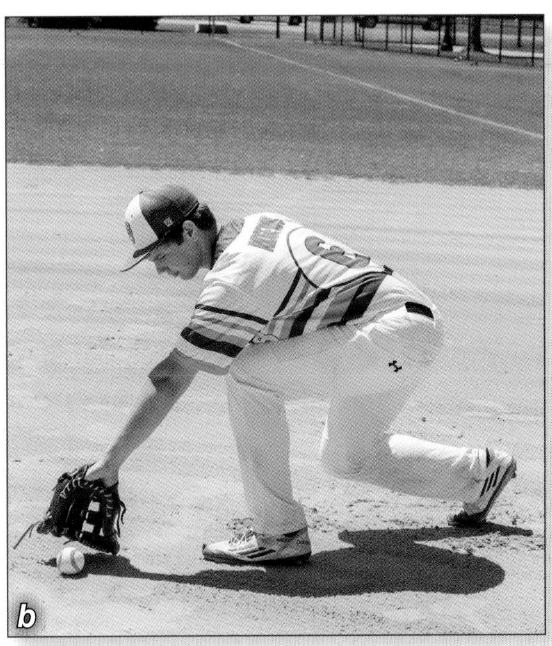

Figure 2.10 Closed backhand drill.

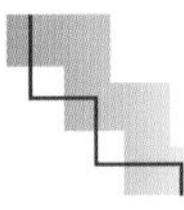

TO INCREASE DIFFICULTY

- Increase the distance of the drill and have the partner or coach hit ground balls.

TO DECREASE DIFFICULTY

- Start the fielder in the closed backhand position and take the footwork out of the drill.

Success Check

- The ball was fielded cleanly, without a drop.
- The closed backhand position remained throughout the catch.
- The glove worked through the ball.

Score Your Success

You earn 1 point for every clean catch in the closed backhand position.

You earn 1/2 point if you make the catch out of position.

You earn 1/2 point if the glove works backward while making a clean catch.

Your score ____ of 10

Short Hops

Most ground balls do not roll smoothly along the ground; rather, they bounce. In some instances, the defender may be caught between hops or have a line drive land just out of reach. As a defender, you must field these short hops as well. Figure 2.11*a* illustrates the forehand technique and figure 2.11*b* illustrates the backhand technique.

Figure 2.11 SHORT HOPS

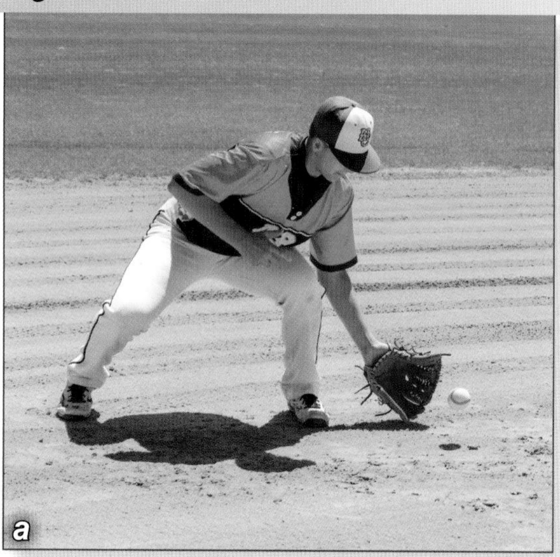

a

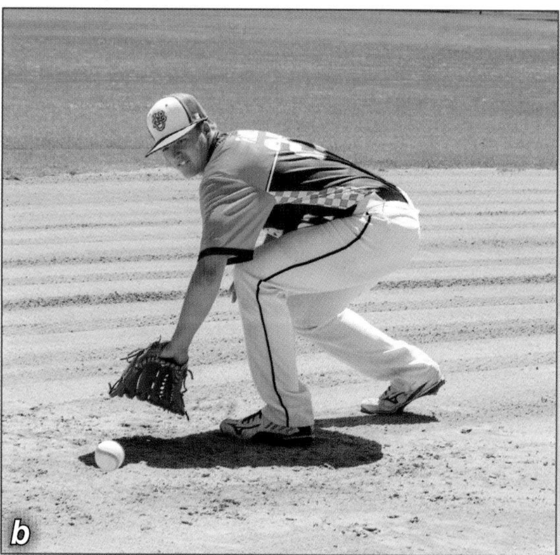

b

1. For any short hop, the defender must start with the same technique, footwork, and positioning as discussed and practiced earlier.
2. After he determines that the ball is going to be a short hop, the defender must change his glove work so that he is working back through the ball on the same angle that the ball is approaching him. This approach is the best way to avoid letting the ball get too deep into the defender's body, which makes it far more difficult to field.

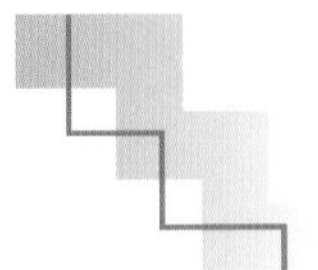

MISSTEP

You field the ball with the same softening glove work that you would on a routine ground ball—that is, on the same angle through the hops, instead of adjusting to the quick hop of the ball as it approaches.

CORRECTION

Be sure that you use positive glove actions—that is, moving your glove quickly and to the ball—back through the ball on the same angle that the ball is approaching you.

Fielding Drill 5 **Short Hops**

To practice short hops, you again go through the stationary fielding drill set positions, but this time, instead of rolling ground balls, your partner throws the ball, creating a short hop. (You may want to increase the distance slightly between you and your partner for this drill.)

1. Triangle position: short hop directly at a defender (see figure 2.12*a*)
2. Forehand position: short hop to the forehand side (see figure 2.12*b*)
3. Open backhand position: short hop to the open backhand position (see figure 2.12*c*)
4. Closed backhand position: short hop to the closed backhand position (see figure 2.12*d*)

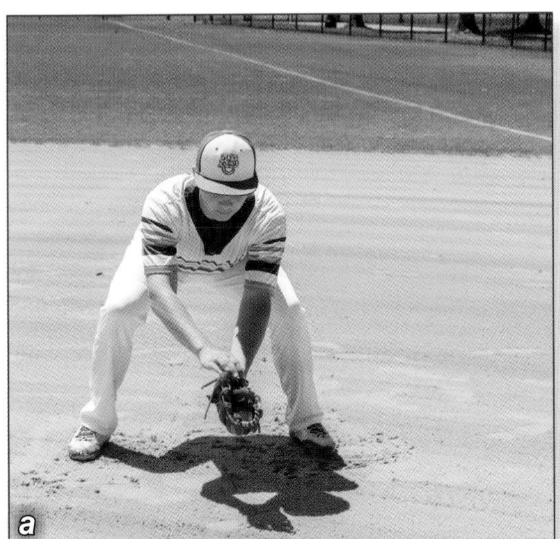

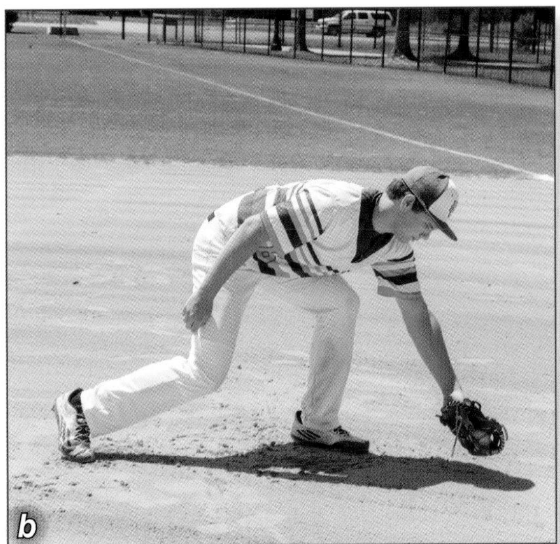

Figure 2.12 Short hops drill: *(a)* triangle position and *(b)* forehand position.

(continued)

Fielding Drill 5 *(continued)*

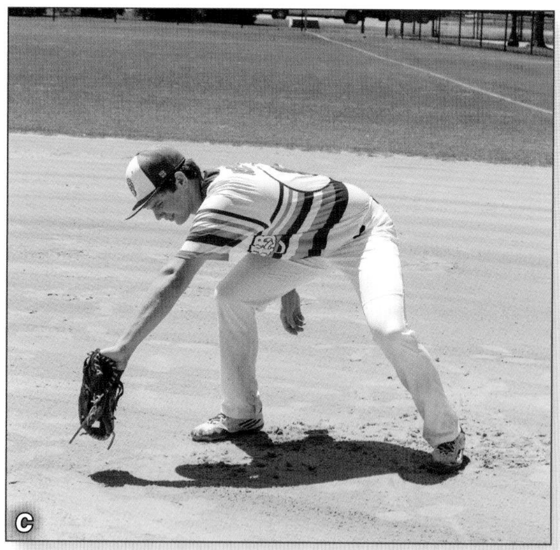

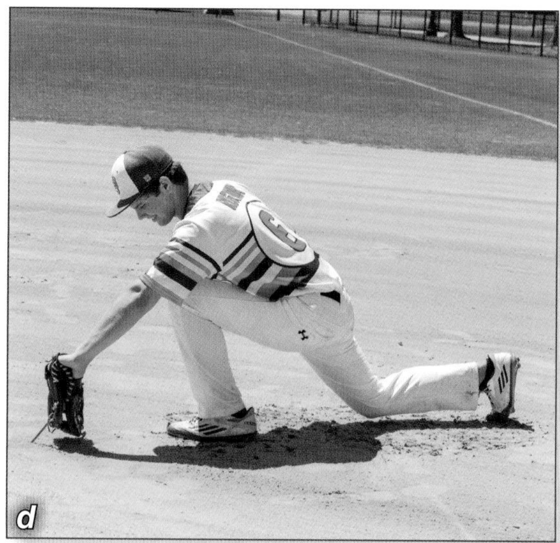

Figure 2.12 Short hops drill *(continued)*: *(c)* open backhand position and *(d)* closed backhand position.

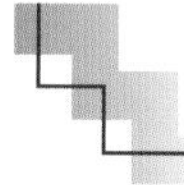

TO INCREASE DIFFICULTY

- Increase the distance of the drill and have the partner or coach hit ground balls.

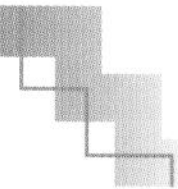

TO DECREASE DIFFICULTY

- Have the defenders decrease the distance between themselves and have them perform the drill on two knees so that the focus remains on the glove action.

Success Check

In each position, make sure that the legs are in the proper balanced position. Also, be sure that the glove is working through the ball. With short hops, working through the ball and using the proper glove positioning and wrist flexion is an individual skill that must be practiced repeatedly on a daily basis. You can separate yourself from the competition by consistently handling the short hop. Again, this is a skill, not a talent, and you must practice it.

Score Your Success

Use the same scoring methods used with fielding drills 1 through 4.

Triangle position—Your score ____ of 10

Forehand position—Your score ____ of 10

Open backhand position—Your score ____ of 10

Closed backhand position—Your score ____ of 10

Total ____ of 40

Choppers

A chopper is a ground ball that initially hits the ground close to home plate, which causes the initial hop to be much higher than it is on any other ground ball (see figure 2.13). A chopper usually takes only a few bounces before it is fielded, but it often results in a close play at first base because of its slower pace.

Figure 2.13 CHOPPERS

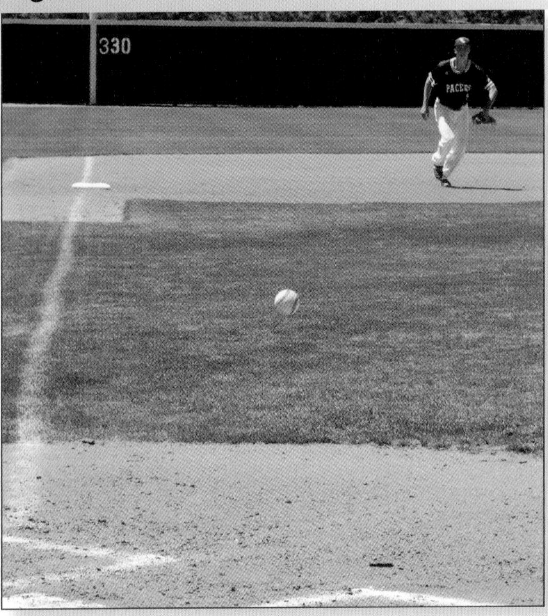

1. When he determines that the ground ball is a chopper, the defender needs to close ground aggressively between himself and the ball.
2. Ideally, all choppers are fielded above the waist, slightly on the defender's glove side.
3. The defender needs to be sure that he is using proper timing so that he is fielding choppers above the waist and not turning them into short hops, which are far harder to make a play on.

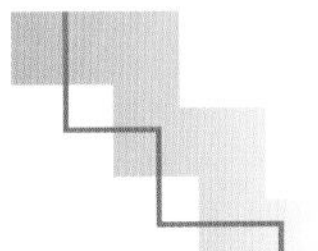

MISSTEP

You field the ball as a short hop.

CORRECTION

Make sure that you are being aggressive when initially closing ground between yourself and where you will field the ball. An aggressive approach allows you to pick the hop you want to receive.

Fielding Drill 6 **Choppers**

To practice fielding choppers, have the defenders start at their normal infield positions. A coach can then either hit or throw choppers to the defenders and have them field them in the proper manner. Because the chopper is a specific type of ground ball that requires recognition from the defender to make the proper play, adjusting the level of difficulty is not recommended. Instead, have players practice choppers as they would see them during the game, so that they are also practicing the cognition required to make these plays.

Success Check

- The defender is aggressive in closing the space between his initial position and where he will field the ball and is using the proper timing so that he can field the ball on the big hop rather than on a short hop.
- The ball was fielded cleanly, without a drop.
- The forehand position remained throughout the catch.
- The glove worked through the ball.

Score Your Success

You earn 1 point for every clean catch above the waist.

You earn 1/2 point if you make the catch below the waist.

Your score ____ of 10

Infield Slow Rollers

An infield slow roller is any ball that is put into play with far less pace than a normal ground ball and that requires the defender to field the ball much closer to the plate than normal (see figure 2.14). The slow roller is one of the most difficult ground balls to defend, and it requires precision to be defended successfully.

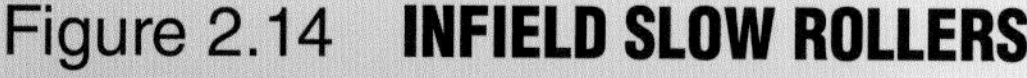

Figure 2.14 **INFIELD SLOW ROLLERS**

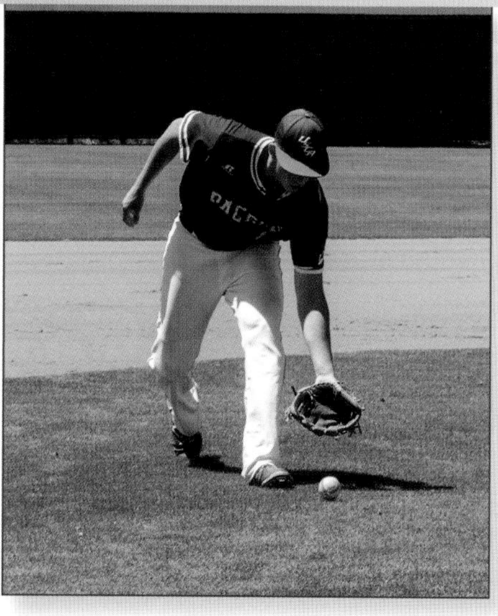

1. After the defender determines that the ball is going to be a slow roller, he needs to close the space aggressively between his initial positioning and the ball.
2. As the defender approaches the ball, he needs to be sure to slow his body to a speed that he can control.
3. At this point, the defender should be bent at the waist. He should field the ball on the glove-hand side.
4. If the defender is making a throw, he should make it from this bent-over position immediately after fielding the ball.

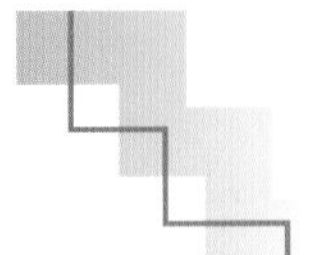

MISSTEP

You are not fielding the ball cleanly or are fielding it too close to your feet.

CORRECTION

Be sure that your bend at the waist is ample and that you are fielding the ball with both hands on the glove-hand side.

Fielding Drill 7 **Slow Rollers**

To practice fielding slow rollers, have two defenders start 20 feet (6 m) from one another. The first partner has the ball and rolls it to the second partner, who is in the ready fielding position. The second partner works through the slow roller, fielding it off the glove side of his body and bending at the waist. The partners then reset and repeat the drill.

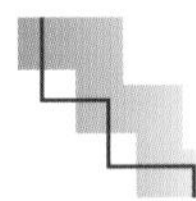

TO INCREASE DIFFICULTY

- Increase the distance of the drill and change the direction of the ground ball (i.e., make some of the slow rollers to the defender's right and some to his left so that not every slow roller is directly in front of him).

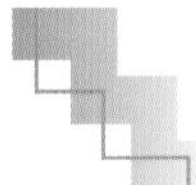

TO DECREASE DIFFICULTY

- Start the defender in the bent fielding position. Roll him slow rollers and have him practice fielding them with his throwing hand directly over the glove.

Success Check

- The ball was fielded cleanly, without a drop.
- The bent position remained throughout the catch.
- The throwing hand was directly over the glove.

Score Your Success

You earn 1 point for every clean catch in the bent position.

You earn 1/2 point if you make the catch out of position.

You earn 1/2 point if the throwing hand was not over the glove during the catch.

Your score ____ of 10

Outfield Ground Balls

Outfield ground balls are any balls that must be defended by an outfielder but have already made contact with the ground. The most important aspect to defending ground balls in the outfield is always to remain in control and not rush through the fielding process. Players can defend outfield ground balls in three ways—on a knee in the center of the body (see figure 2.15), with the infield triangle method (see figure 2.16), and in a do-or-die fashion by receiving the ball out in front of the body off the glove-side foot (see figure 2.17).

Figure 2.15 ONE-KNEE

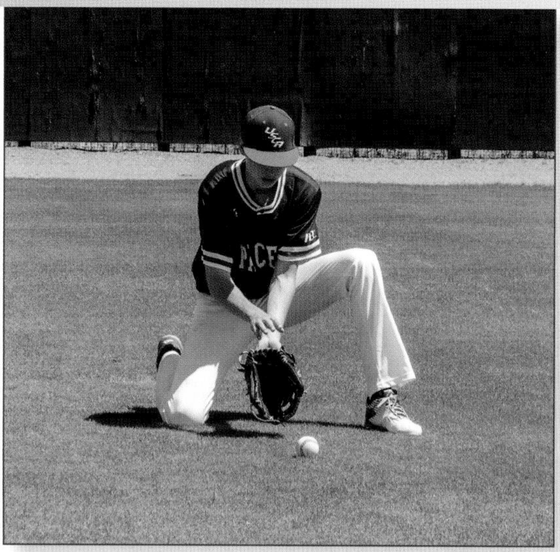

1. When the ball simply needs to be fielded and thrown back into an infielder, an outfield ground ball may be defended on a knee.
2. The outfielder must position himself in front of the ball so that he can receive it in the center of the body.
3. The glove-side leg should be bent, and the arm-side knee should be on the ground.
4. The ball is received out front with the throwing hand over the top of the glove.

Figure 2.16 INFIELD TRIANGLE

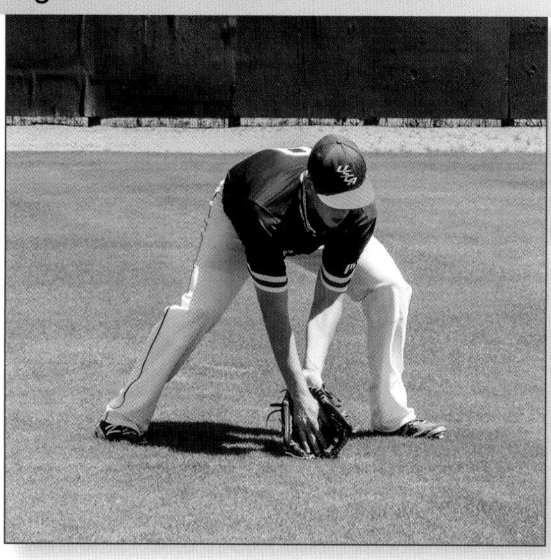

1. With an aggressive runner or when the ball needs to be fielded and thrown quickly into the infield, the infield triangle technique should be used.
2. The outfielder gets into the triangle stance. The triangle is created with the feet and the glove hand as shown. Notice that the feet are squared to the ball, the body is lowered, the head is down with the eyes on the ball, and the glove is slightly off center toward the glove side of the body. Also, notice the flexion in the wrist and elbow of the glove-side arm.
3. The throwing hand at reception should be over the glove in the alligator position as shown.

Figure 2.17 **DO OR DIE**

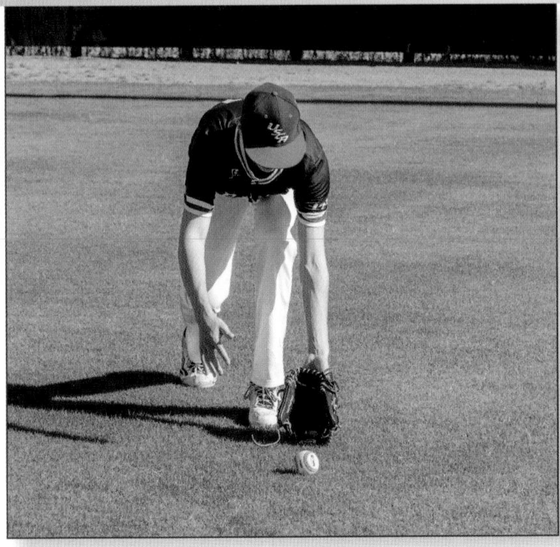

1. When the ball must be aggressively defended and thrown into the infield, the do-or-die technique should be used.
2. In the do-or-die technique, little time passes between receiving the ball and making the throw.
3. The outfielder should aggressively close the space between his initial position and the ball.
4. The outfielder should field the ball out in front of the glove-side foot with the throwing hand in a comfortable position near the waist.
5. From there, the outfielder goes into his crow hop and makes a throw.

Fielding Drill 8 **Outfield Ground Balls**

To practice each type of outfield ground ball, have two players partner up and roll each other ground balls in the outfield grass. They should rotate through the series of three ground balls described earlier so that they are able to practice fielding each type of outfield ground ball.

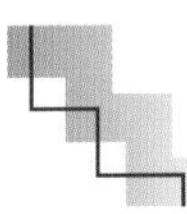

TO INCREASE DIFFICULTY

- Increase the distance between the person delivering the ground ball and the one receiving it, or have the partner hit ground balls rather than throw them.

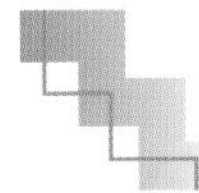

TO DECREASE DIFFICULTY

- Start the outfielder in the fielding position that is to be practiced and have him receive the ball without using any footwork, focusing solely on receiving the ball.

Success Check

- The ball was fielded cleanly, without a drop.
- The glove position remained throughout the catch.

Score Your Success

You earn 1 point for every clean catch in the proper position

You earn 1/2 point if you make the catch out of position.

Your score ____ of 10

Pitcher Ground Balls

After the pitcher has delivered the pitch to the plate, he essentially becomes another infielder and thus needs to know how to field a ground ball properly. Pitchers should treat ground balls just as any other infielder does and should use the techniques discussed earlier (see figure 2.18). The only difference between a pitcher and any other infielder is the way that he gets into his fielding stance. Because pitchers cannot use the creep technique, they must be sure to end their delivery in an athletic and ready position.

To practice pitcher ground balls, the pitcher starts on the mound and goes through his normal delivery, but without a ball. After he has completed the delivery, a coach or partner can roll him a ground ball and he can practice fielding it just as an infielder would. The technique, types of ground balls, and steps to success are exactly like those of the other infielders. The drills described earlier can be used for pitcher ground balls, except that the pitcher would go through his motion rather than use the creep.

Figure 2.18 **PITCHER GROUND BALLS**

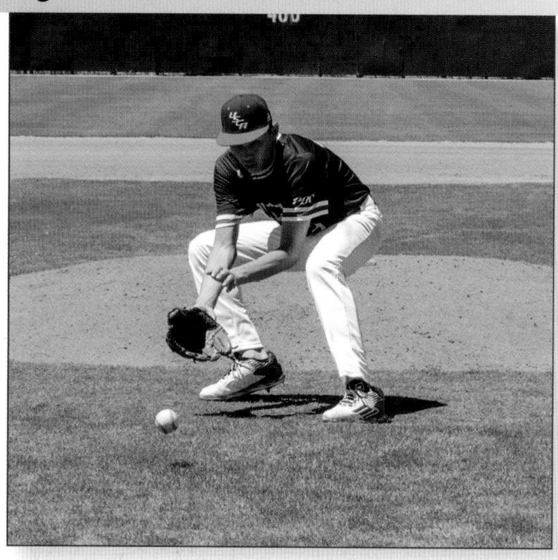

1. After delivering the pitch, the pitcher must be sure to get his body square to the plate, with both feet facing the hitter and the knees bent in a strong ready position.
2. The glove must be positioned out front and in the center of the body, in the same manner as the other infielders.
3. Pitchers need to start low and stay low while they are receiving ground balls because the mound can alter the hop and direction of the ground ball and make the ball more difficult to receive.

Ground Ball Footwork

One of the biggest keys to fielding ground balls successfully and consistently is having the proper footwork and rhythm when receiving the ball. Appropriate footwork and rhythm allow defenders to be in the right position to field the ball cleanly and gives them momentum to throw the ball to the desired location. If the proper footwork is not in place, a player's ability to field the ball cleanly or throw it accurately can be severely hindered. No ground ball should ever be fielded without some sort of rhythm and movement of the feet through the baseball.

As the player is approaching the ball and readying himself to receive it, the feet should be constantly moving in a controlled manner. The movement should be through the ball and in the direction of where the ball is to be thrown. The footwork should go like this: Right foot strikes the ground, the ball is received in the proper manner, left foot strikes the ground.

Fielding Drill 9 **Adding Footwork**

Now that the proper fielding positions are in place, let's add some movement to the drill sets. To do this, we revert to the prepitch focus and setup section as your partner expands the distance between you to 20 to 30 feet (6 to 9 m). You creep into the focus circle. After you are in the ready position, your partner rolls the ball. When the ball is rolling, you move your feet toward the direction of the path of the ball, field the ball with the proper technique according to the direction you are moving, transition the ball from glove to hand, and, finally, make a good throw to the target. The following are the sets that you will work through.

1. Routine ground balls: triangle position (see figure 2.19*a*)
2. Forehand ground balls (see figure 2.19*b*)
3. Open backhand ground balls (see figure 2.19*c*)
4. Closed backhand ground balls (see figure 2.19*d*)

In each of these drill sets, we need to discuss footwork and the art of working through the baseball. The stationary drill set is a great tool for the defender because it focuses on the proper body positioning at the point of reception. But to build consistency in fielding ground balls, the added movement of the feet is imperative. By keeping the format of the drill sets the same, adding footwork allows the defender to work on the most important factor in fielding consistency—timing.

Timing for the defender is a combination of footwork and proper positioning at the point of reception. As we have said before, rarely does a ball roll smoothly along the ground, so the defender is usually fielding a ground ball that is bouncing. To do this with consistent success, the defender must correlate the movement of his feet with the movement of the ball, placing himself in the proper position at the appropriate time to receive the ball.

1. For each of the four fielding positions, you start by creeping into the focus circle. As the ball is delivered, you move your feet toward the ball, reading the path and the hops that the ball is taking.
2. As you approach the ball, get your body into the proper fielding position. You should reach the fielding position slightly before the ball arrives.
3. After you field the ball, hold and check the positioning.
4. Relax and reset behind the focus circle.

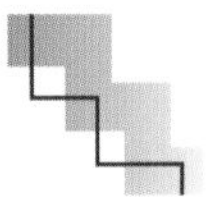

TO INCREASE OR DECREASE DIFFICULTY

- The intensity of the drill can be changed to make it either more or less difficult by changing the pace at which the ball is moving or the fielder is moving.

(continued)

Fielding Drill 9 *(continued)*

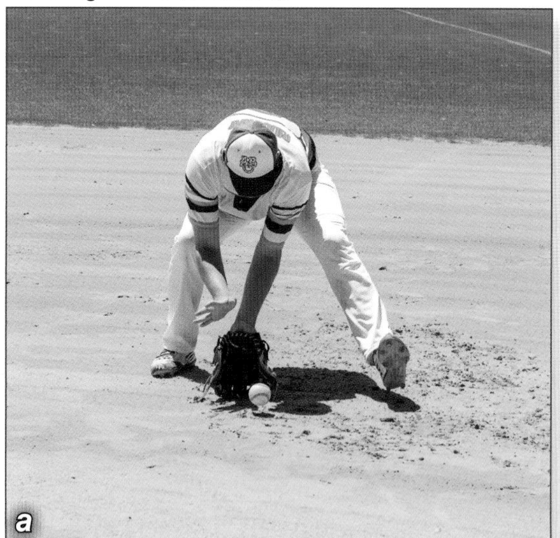
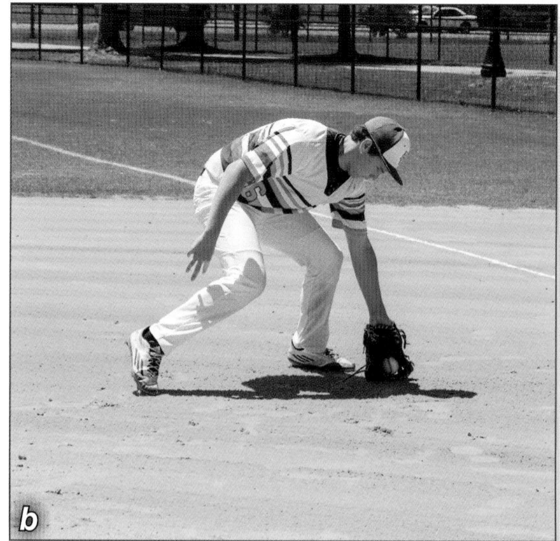
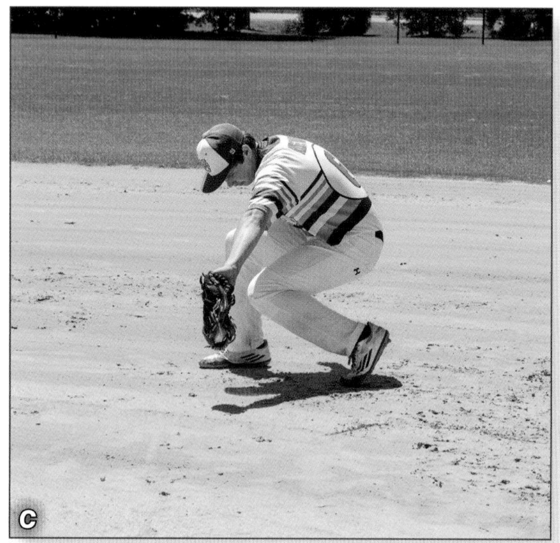
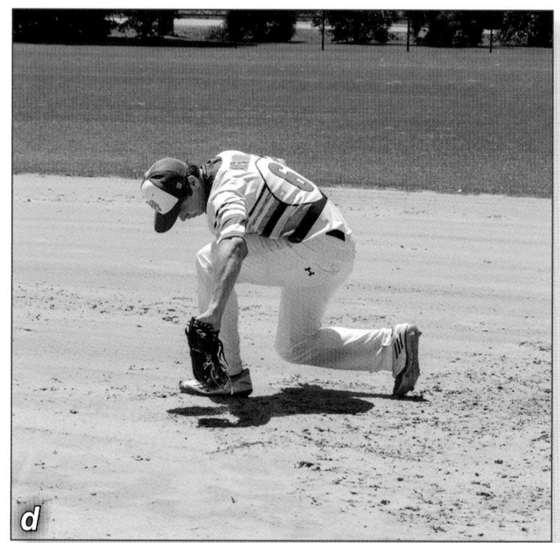

Figure 2.19 Adding footwork drill.

Success Check

- You fielded the ball in the proper position.
- You reached the proper fielding position slightly before making the catch.
- You worked through the ball with the glove.

Score Your Success

You earn 1 point for every ball fielded cleanly in the proper position.

You earn 1/2 point if you field the ball but the timing is off with getting into position.

Triangle position—Your score ____ of 10

Forehand position—Your score ____ of 10

Open backhand position—Your score ____ of 10

Closed backhand position—Your score ____ of 10

Total ____ of 40

Transitioning and Making a Good Throw

The ability to cleanly field a ground ball is only half of a defender's job. Equally as important is the ability to transition the ball from the gloved hand to the throwing hand, use proper foot work, and make a strong accurate throw to the appropriate base (figure 2.20).

Figure 2.20 **TRANSITIONING AND MAKING A GOOD THROW**

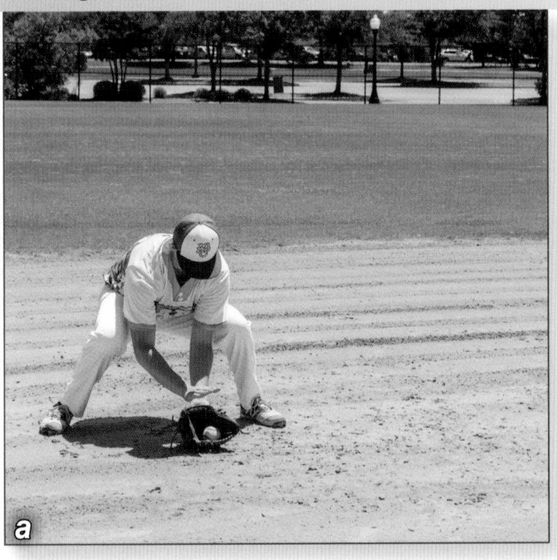

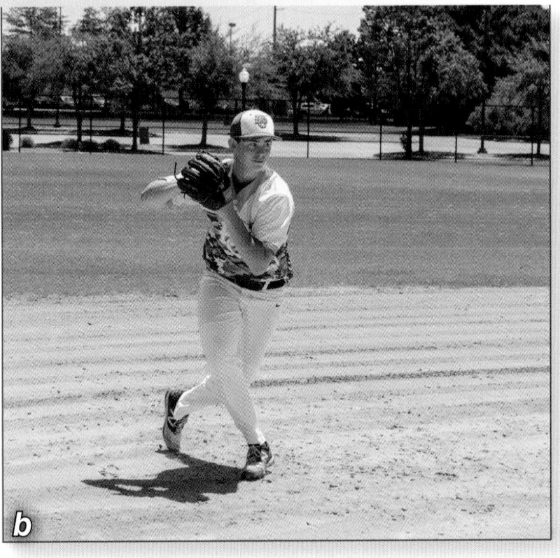

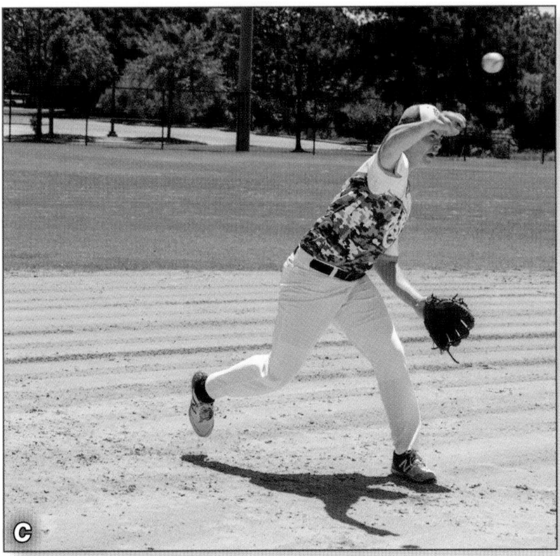

1. After you have fielded the ball properly (figure 2.20*a*), you have to make the exchange from glove to throwing hand and transition into making a good throw.
2. After you field the ball and complete the right, left footwork (figure 2.20*b*), you move the ball from the glove to the throwing hand. This exchange takes place in the center of the body.
3. During the exchange of the ball, the feet should continue to move and should be shuffling in the direction in which you will throw the ball. The shoulders should be pointing to the target. This shuffle step allows you to keep your momentum going to the target and allows you to make a strong throw (figure 2.20*c*).

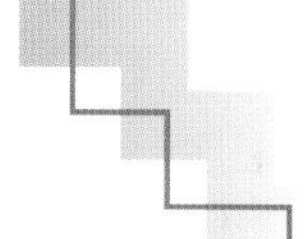

MISSTEP

You cannot make an accurate or strong throw to the desired target.

CORRECTION

Make sure that you are continuously shuffling your feet toward the desired target and that your shoulders are remaining pointed to where you intend to throw the ball.

Fielding Drill 10 **Transitioning and Making a Good Throw**

In all the drill sets, we have emphasized working through the ball with the glove. Now that we have added footwork into the process, the same concept is used with the feet as we begin to add speed and fluidity to the entire process. In this section, we work through all four fielding positions again. Let's look at how it works, again starting at shortstop.

1. As with the last section, you repeat the entire process of moving into the proper position and fielding the ball.
2. After you field the ball, hold and check the position for several moments.
3. From the fielding position with the ball in the glove, transition the ball into the throwing hand (four seams), while simultaneously shuffling your feet and turning your body toward first base.
4. Keep the feet moving and stay low, in an athletic position, as you make a good throw to your target.
5. Relax and repeat.

Success Check

When you begin your repetitions, you can break down the movements by pausing after the catch. This pause allows you to feel the proper positioning and footwork through the transition and throw. As you become more comfortable, you can speed up the process and create fluidity. For this to happen, the feet must continue to move through each of the fielding positions. This movement takes great timing and coordination. You must also work through the baseball with the feet, the body, and the glove. As you add continuous footwork through the process, be sure to stay down on the ball through the catch and throw. When your body rises up during the process, the timing and fluidity are upset, usually creating an error on the catch or throw. Remember to field the ball in front and trust your timing. After each repetition, relax and refocus the mind while you evaluate the previous result.

Score Your Success

You earn 1 point for every ball fielded cleanly in the proper position.

You earn 1/2 point if the ball is fielded but the timing is off with getting into position.

You earn 1 point for every quality throw to the first baseman.

Triangle position—Your score ____ of 20

Forehand position—Your score ____ of 20

Open backhand position—Your score ____ of 20

Closed backhand position—Your score ____ of 20

Total ____ of 80

FIELDING FLY BALLS

Now that we have broken down the steps of fielding the basic types of ground balls, you should feel comfortable moving your feet and getting your body into the proper fielding positions. You should also feel confident in working through the ball and making a good throw. As a defender, however, you will have to field other kinds of batted balls as well. We now turn our focus to catching fly balls.

Catching a fly ball is not simple, although compared with fielding a ground ball, the mechanics are far less complex. At the higher levels of play, fly balls are typically considered easy outs (you will see this topic again later in the discussions of offense). The fact is that less movement is required to catch a routine fly ball versus fielding a routine ground ball and making a good throw. Regardless of the differences, at the beginner levels learning to catch a fly ball can be an adventure. In this brief discussion, we look at the fundamentals of catching fly balls. We discuss beginner drills and establish a few guidelines that you will carry with you through other defensive-specific steps.

Let's look back at our discussion on catching the baseball. For beginners, we talked about keeping your eyes on the ball and tracking it into the glove. We also talked about the thumb-to-thumb position. You should use these two key elements when learning to catch fly balls. Along with noting these elements, we must also establish a few guidelines before we begin.

Just like learning to play catch, tracking a fly ball involves using depth perception and following the ball all the way into the glove. To do this, the player needs to understand the usual flight paths when the ball is hit in the air. First, let's look at the routine fly ball with backspin. This ball will have a simple path into the air and back down. The second is a fly ball with topspin. This ball will take a sharper downward angle after it has reached its highest point. We will discuss the topspin and sidespin fly balls later.

At the beginner levels, we like to establish a couple of guidelines before we begin the drill set. First, always try to keep the ball in front (see figure 2.21*a*). As young players learn to track fly balls, they often try to catch the ball overhead. This approach typically leads to their missing the ball as it lands behind them. After they can recognize flight paths, they will be able to position themselves accordingly.

The second guideline we establish builds on the thumb-to-thumb positioning. We like to see the ball caught with this technique but modified slightly so that the ball is caught just to the glove side of the head (see figure 2.21*b*). At the point of reception, the feet should be offset so that the glove-side foot is in front of the other. This adjustment is usually tough for beginners who like to keep their feet squared and still, but we will get there step by step.

To help the beginner learn, tennis balls or soft baseballs may be used for these drills. This modification gives the player the confidence to position himself correctly without fear of being hit by a regular baseball. For the player to learn the idea of keeping the ball in front, his first step after the ball is put into the air should be backward.

Figure 2.21 FLY BALL TECHNIQUE

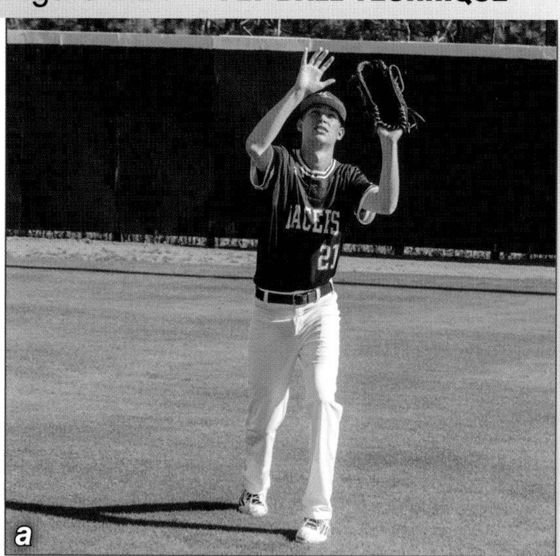

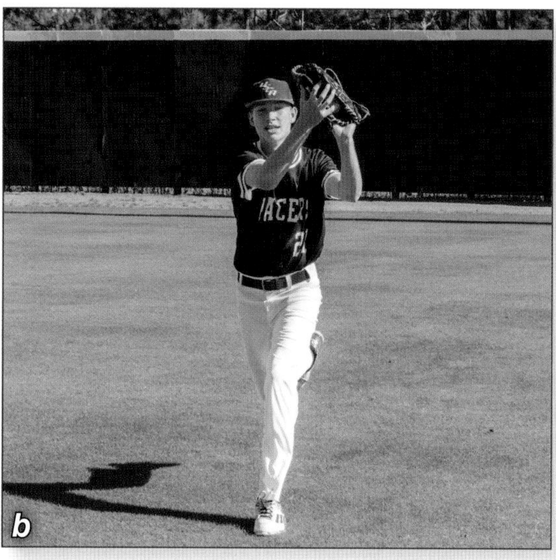

1. The initial step for every outfielder should be a drop step back to ensure that he is behind the ball.
2. As the fly ball begins to approach the outfielder, he should present the glove in an open manner at his shoulder.
3. The throwing hand should be open and adjacent to the glove and in the thumb-to-thumb positon.
4. As he is receiving the ball, the outfielder should remain behind the ball but should work back through the ball much like an infielder does to create some momentum and make a strong throw.

Fielding Drill 11 **Routine Fly Balls**

At a distance of 60 to 90 feet (18 to 27 m), the coach or partner delivers a fly ball. If you are using a tennis ball, a tennis racquet is an easy way to put the ball in flight. Otherwise, at this distance, you may want to throw the ball into the air. After the ball is put into the air, the player moves into position behind the ball. To do this, he must recognize the flight path. When the player is in position, he should catch the ball using the proper two-hand technique as shown. Although you will not creep as much into the ready position as you would for a ground ball, a slight step into the ready position is recommended. Relax and reset.

This drill can be repeated as often as needed for the player to learn the proper technique and beginning ball-tracking skills. When the player is confident enough to move on, we recommend using real baseballs and increasing the distance. At this point the balls may be delivered by machine or a coach's or partner's hitting. We will add more to this process in the step on outfield play.

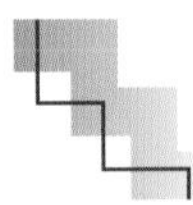

TO INCREASE DIFFICULTY

- Increase the distance from the coach or partner as well as the height of the fly ball.

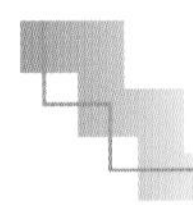

TO DECREASE DIFFICULTY

- Decrease the height of the fly ball and try to ensure that the ball is thrown or delivered directly to the outfielder.

Success Check

- You recognized the flight path and moved into position behind the baseball.
- You caught the ball in the proper position.

Score Your Success

You earn 1 point for every clean catch made behind the ball working forward.

You earn 1/2 point for every catch made while drifting backward.

Your score ____ of 10

SUCCESS SUMMARY

Learning the fundamentals of fielding may seem tedious, but the importance of developing proper technique could not be greater. By the end of this discussion, you should be capable of fielding ground balls and fly balls with the proper footwork and body positioning. You have learned the importance of clearing the mind and refocusing between pitches or repetitions. You have also learned what good timing feels like for the fundamental mechanics of your body when fielding the ball, allowing you to make the necessary adjustments when your timing is off. Let's review so that you can rate your development as a defender.

Fielding Drills

1. Triangle position	_____ out of 10
2. Forehand	_____ out of 10
3. Open backhand	_____ out of 10
4. Closed backhand	_____ out of 10
5. Short hops	_____ out of 40
6. Choppers	_____ out of 10
7. Slow rollers	_____ out of 10
8. Outfield ground balls	_____ out of 10
9. Adding footwork	_____ out of 40
10. Transitioning and making a good throw	_____ out of 80
11. Routine fly balls	_____ out of 10
Total	_____ **out of 240**

If you scored more than 205, congratulations! You have mastered the fielding drills and are ready to move on to the next step. If you scored fewer than 180 points, you may need to continue the repetitions while focusing on your positioning and timing.

Pitching

As you know by now, the game of baseball is separated into three areas of focus—offense, defense, and pitching. For the offensive-minded or defensive-minded audience, the format of *Baseball: Steps to Success* is designed to elaborate on specific fundamentals that are directly correlated with both of these areas. Step 1 and step 2 have set the foundation for the defensive area of focus and will be elaborated on later in our discussion. Step 5 and step 6 will set the foundation for the offensive area of focus and will be elaborated on as we move forward. We now shift gears and focus our attention on the third area of the game—pitching.

Pitching is arguably the most popular discussion concerning player development. To be honest, pitching in itself could have its own *Steps to Success* book, but to maintain our goal of setting a foundation for success in this sport, we need to keep our discussion focused on the fundamentals of this topic and on the specific factors that directly correlate with these fundamentals. Most pitching discussions concerning development consist of highly debated topics, most of which focus on arm care and arm health. This trending topic has currently become a fascination among parents and coaches of younger age groups; therefore, we will address this topic as well. But before we can formally address this matter, we must cover other areas first. Let's look at how our pitching discussion is broken down.

The art of pitching and developing as a pitcher encompasses many variables. First, we will discuss gripping the ball and throwing different pitches. Second, we will take a close look at the mechanics of pitching. Building on this foundation, we will then dive into the art of pitching in regard to the strike zone, getting outs, attacking hitters, and the mental approach to this part of the game. We will continue with fielding the pitcher position and look at the detailed areas that a pitcher needs to focus on as the ninth defender.

GETTING A GRIP: DIFFERENT PITCH GRIPS

Before we dive into the off-speed discussion, we must discuss a few important topics, especially for youth parents and coaches. The few points that we would like to address coincide with the popular topic of arm health and the current increase of Tommy John surgeries among pitchers of all ages. When we discuss steps to success, you need to understand that long-term success in this sport results from positive development over time. We often see youth parents and coaches strive for immediate success and accelerated development. With pitchers, especially youth pitchers, this can be a dangerous direction to take and a risky mind-set to have.

As we stated earlier, the overhead motion of throwing a baseball is not a natural movement for the body. Overhead throwing throughout a career will mean that scar tissue will be floating around the elbow and shoulder. The throwing arm needs to be trained over a long period to ensure growth and continued arm health. For youth pitchers, arm development and continued arm care have become a focus of national attention, with the implementation of pitch counts in many youth leagues. Many of us are concerned, however, that youth pitchers, although following pitch count regulations, are attempting to throw advanced pitches that are highly stressful on the throwing arm, even for adults. Our recommendation to youth parents and coaches is to monitor the growth process of each player. Even larger, older youth players may be incapable of handling the stress of trying to throw slider after slider.

As college coaches, we look at certain factors when recruiting a pitcher. As a parent, you must understand that your child is not going to play, professionally or collegiately, when he is not yet old enough to drive. As entertaining as youth baseball is, we ask that you understand that its purpose is to learn the game and its proper mechanics. Yes, it is a competitive sport, but jeopardizing a child's future because you want him to outperform other children is not a positive step to success. College and professional scouts look for several factors when evaluating a pitcher, but throwing a nasty slider when he is 12 years old is not one of them.

What these scouts do look at starts when pitchers are around age 16. Most of what they evaluate early concerns arm action. A consistent and fluid arm action with every pitch is important. Again, what is consistency derived from? As we begin to talk about throwing off speed, we need to stress the importance of the fastball and the repeatable action of the arm. The best pitch in baseball is probably a well-executed fastball. If a pitcher can command the fastball to both sides of the plate, he will set himself apart from many others. Remember, everything works off of the fastball.

So, why then do we need to throw other pitches? For hitters, timing is everything. Some experts define pitching as disrupting the hitter's timing. Off-speed pitches do just that. A consistent arm action with different pitches will create another factor that scouts evaluate—deception. We have already discussed the four-seam and two-seam fastball grips in step 1, so let's look at some other pitches you may want to add to your repertoire to develop some deception.

Off-Speed Pitches

The changeup is an important pitch at every level of the game, simply because it is thrown with the same arm action as the fastball. For youth, the changeup creates deception while protecting the arm; the young pitcher does not have to expose the arm to turning a baseball improperly while trying to throw a curve or slider. At higher levels, this advantage holds true as well. To be honest, the changeup is an extremely effective pitch that many pitchers in recent years have gotten away from. Now, with the arm care conversation in the public eye, the changeup is beginning to blossom again.

The changeup is one of many pitches that can disrupt a hitter's timing. Unlike many other off-speed pitches, the change is thrown with the same arm action as the fastball. The difference is the grip. The grip will slow the ball by 8 to 15 miles per hour (3.5 to 6.7 m/s), creating deception. By using the same arm action, the initial spin of the ball out of the hand will resemble a fastball, so the hitter has an extremely difficult adjustment to make. Figure 3.1 presents two variations of the changeup grip: the circle change *(a)* and the three-finger change *(b)*.

Figure 3.1 **CHANGEUP GRIPS**

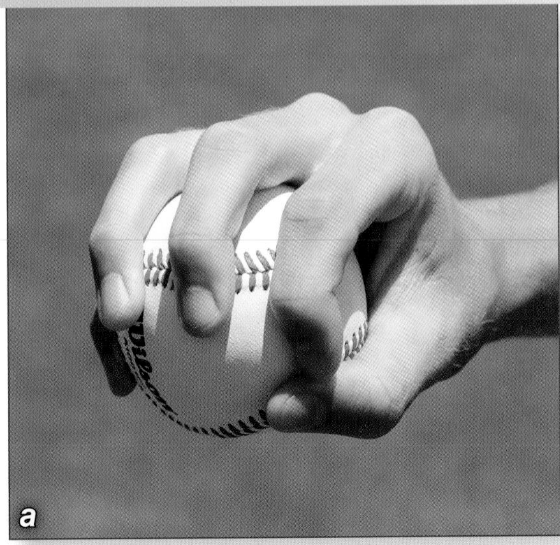

Circle Change Grip

1. The index finger and the thumb should make a circle, or the OK symbol, on the side of a four-seam grip.
2. The middle and ring fingers should cross the laces of the horseshoe.
3. The little finger should rest on the side of the ball.

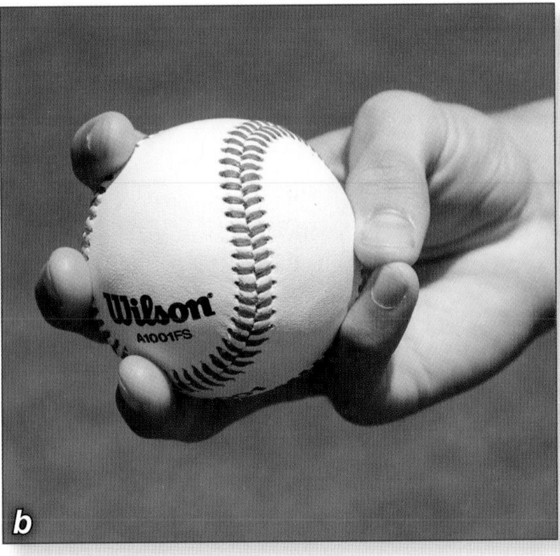

Three-Finger Change Grip

1. The index, middle, and ring fingers should cross the seams of the horseshoe.
2. The thumb and little finger should come together under the baseball.

The art of throwing the changeup is derived from mastering the release point and feel of the grip that works for you. Depending on the grip and your natural arm action, the flight path of a changeup should resemble that of your fastball. When the ball gets near the target, it should have a slight downward action. Some may have some run or cut as well. Most hitters describe this action as backing up, almost as if the pitcher pulls the ball back with a string as it approaches the target.

The concept that everything works off of the fastball is the backbone for throwing any off-speed pitch successfully, especially the changeup. We recommend that this be the standard pitch used when teaching youth pitchers the beginning stages of throwing off speed.

Cutter

The cutter, or cut fastball, is the first pitch after the changeup that we recommend teaching to a pitcher who is learning to throw off speed for the first time. The cutter is nice middle ground between the natural arm action of the fastball and the turning of the ball for more advanced breaking balls. Let's look at how the cutter is gripped in figure 3.2.

A successful cutter is thrown with the same arm speed as the fastball; therefore, with this grip and release, the velocity should not be very much lower than that of the fastball. The spin should be tight, and the cut action, a slight flat movement of the ball, should be small and late. With this grip, the hand turns slightly at the release point. As you get more comfortable throwing with the cutter grip, try to turn the hand a little more, releasing the ball with the fingers on the side as shown in figure 3.2. You can think of it as pulling a string downward. This action creates a slight sideways rotation on the baseball, causing the flight path to cut as it reaches the target. Remember, we are looking for tight spin and a little cut action with fastball velocity. You will have to figure out the feel at release to get the action you want on the baseball.

Figure 3.2 **CUTTER GRIP**

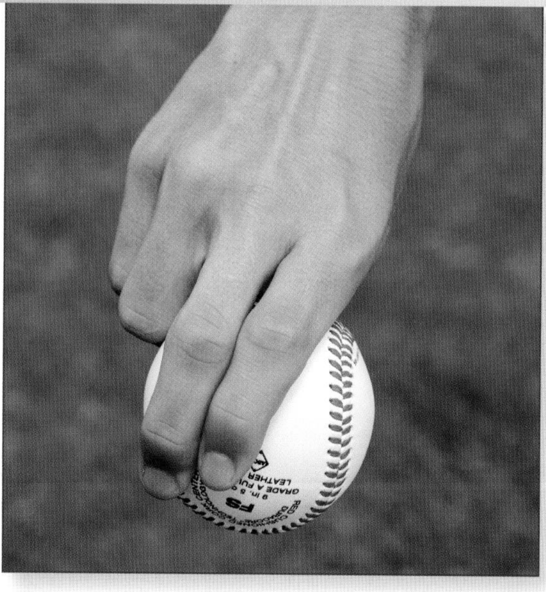

1. The index and middle fingers should be together, with the middle finger touching the inside seam of the horseshoe.
2. The thumb should be directly under or diagonally under the ball, touching the seam on the bottom of the horseshoe.

Slider

Building off what we just learned with the cutter, we turn now to the more advanced audience to talk about the slider (figure 3.3). To begin, we stress again that everything works off of the fastball. This concept has multiple meanings, one of which we will highlight in the next section. For now, the concept is used to refer to your pitching mechanics.

With pitchers of all ages, the mechanics often change during the delivery of a breaking ball. Several factors may cause this change in the mechanics. Some pitchers believe they must overcompensate with the body to get more break on the ball. Others may be uncomfortable and struggle with feeling the proper release, so they may slow down their delivery. Some may change arm slots by lowering the arm as they throw. Many other variations in the delivery can happen, but all variations that differ from the normal mechanics of throwing the fastball will cause added pressure on the arm and a lack of positive results with the pitches.

The only change that should happen from throwing a fastball to throwing a breaking ball should be with the grip, hand, and wrist. Getting back to the cutter, the only thing that we altered in the delivery was the grip and a slight turn of the hand at release. For a slider, the hand should turn a little more and a little sooner. The velocity should be slightly lower than that of the cutter, but you should have a slightly bigger break on the ball. A successful slider should have a late, side-to-side break. Some sliders may have a downward action as well, causing the ball to change planes, creating what we call depth.

Figure 3.3 **SLIDER GRIP**

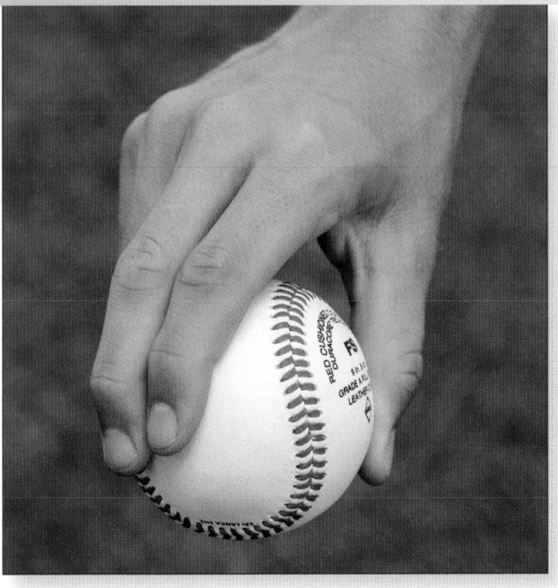

1. The index and middle fingers should be together, with the middle finger touching the inside seam of the horseshoe.
2. The thumb should be directly under or diagonally under the ball, touching the seam on the bottom of the horseshoe.
3. The ball should be placed more in the fingers rather than deep in the grip.

Curveball

As you advance, you should be capable of feeling the differences in releasing breaking balls. At this point, you should be able to adjust your release to create more or less break. With this foundation, the next pitch we discuss is the curveball (figure 3.4). The curveball spins forward, creating a downward bend in the trajectory. The release of the curveball has one adjustment from the slider. With the slider, the fingers rotate outside the baseball through the pitch, creating sidespin. For the curveball, that rotation incorporates a bend in the wrist, causing the fingers to rotate over the top of the baseball, creating topspin. Because of this heavy rotation at release and bend in the trajectory, the velocity of the curveball will typically drop 10 to 15 miles per hour (4.5 to 6.7 m/s) from that of the fastball.

Figure 3.4 **CURVEBALL GRIP**

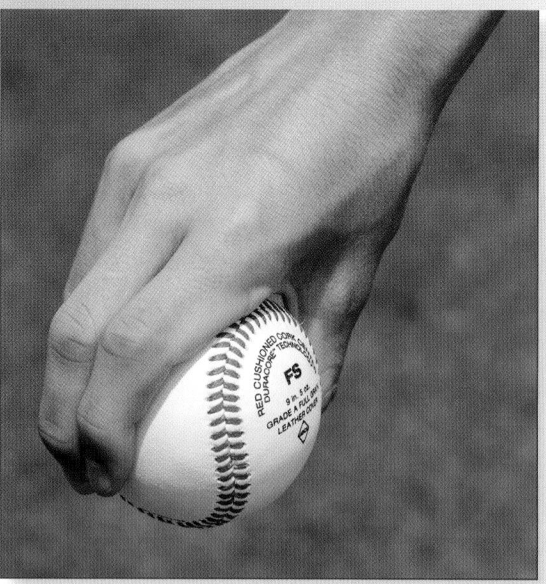

1. The index and middle fingers should be together, with the middle finger touching the inside seam of the horseshoe.
2. The thumb should be directly under or diagonally under the ball, touching the seam on the bottom of the horseshoe.
3. The ball should be placed deeper in the grip than it is with the slider.

MECHANICS

Baseball players come in all shapes and sizes. Pitchers are no exception to this rule. When you watch a baseball game, you will notice that all players, regardless of their body size and shape, use similar mechanics for hitting, fielding, and throwing. The mechanics of pitching a baseball, however, come in a wide variety. You may see a pitcher who delivers with a high leg kick and an arm swing that comes over his head as he throws a pitch. Another pitcher may have a small leg kick and an arm swing in a very low position to the side of his body. Certain factors cause pitchers to throw from these drastically different arm angles, but all pitchers have a feel of the baseball at the release point. As you are aware, the release point is near the end of the delivery process for throwing a baseball. To help you find your release point, we need to take a few steps back and start at the beginning. There are two legal pitching positions—the stretch, or set, position and the windup position. These two positions are covered here.

Stretch

At the higher levels of the game (high school and beyond), the most important pitch of every game is often delivered out of the stretch position. This fact is one reason why we teach beginner pitchers this position first. The other reason is that this position simplifies the delivery process and helps the arm get into a natural arm slot. Let's look at how the stretch position works. Follow the steps outlined in figure 3.5 and insert a pause after each one to ensure proper timing. After you become familiar with the process, add speed and rhythm to the delivery.

From the time when the leg is lifted, any timing variations with the body will affect the arm swing, potentially causing the arm to drag. Beginners need to learn and repeat the stretch position so that the motion and delivery become second nature. The rule of thumb for pitching mechanics is that if the pitcher can feel it, he can fix it. For beginners, the stretch is the easiest way to learn what the body must do to get into proper position. For the more advanced player, practicing the stretch will help simplify the delivery if an adjustment needs to be made.

Figure 3.5 **STRETCH POSITION**

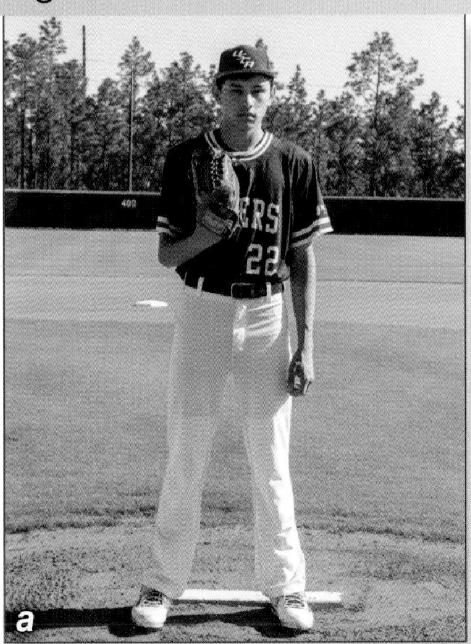

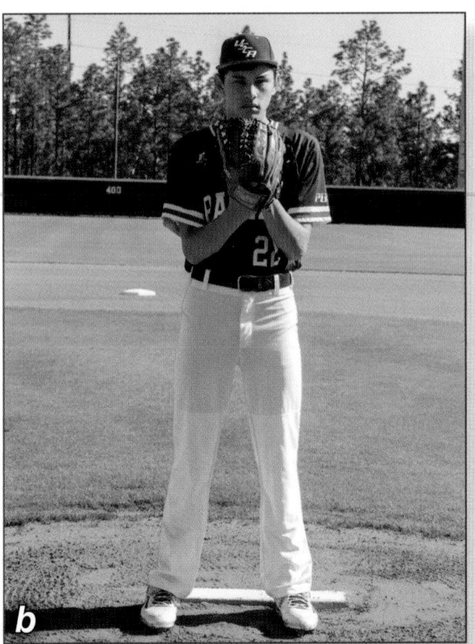

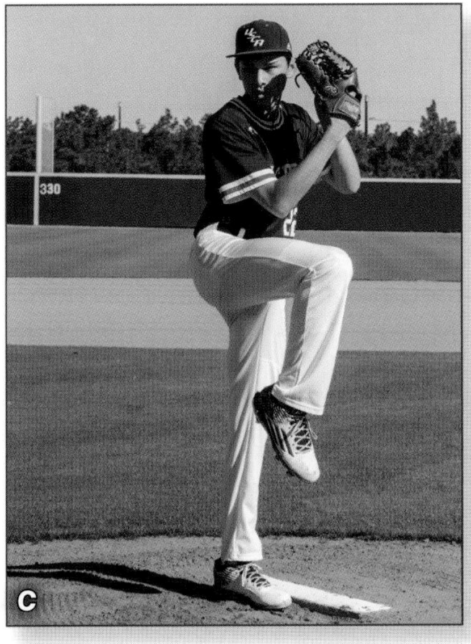

Address the Rubber and Get Your Sign

1. The back foot should be placed at the front edge of the rubber.
2. The feet should be spread slightly past shoulder-width.
3. The ball should be in the glove as you look in to get the sign from the catcher (figure 3.5*a*).

Set Position

1. After you get the sign, you move into the set position. The feet should be slightly past shoulder-width apart with the weight balanced or slightly on the back foot.
2. The throwing hand should be in the glove gripping the ball (figure 3.5*b*).
3. You need to hold this position for at least one full second so that you have an opportunity to focus on the target and create a complete stop.

Lift and Balance Point

1. After you have held the position for a moment, begin the delivery process.
2. Lift the front leg to waist height, creating the tabletop, or balance, position.
3. The front foot at the balance point should be relaxed.
4. Position your head over the back foot, putting the body in a tucked position.
5. Now let's incorporate the hands. From the set position with the hands in front of the body, pretend that a string is connecting your hands to your front knee. As your hands move up, your knee will lift. This simultaneous motion ensures that your arm is getting started in the delivery process (figure 3.5*c*).

(continued)

Figure 3.5 *(continued)*

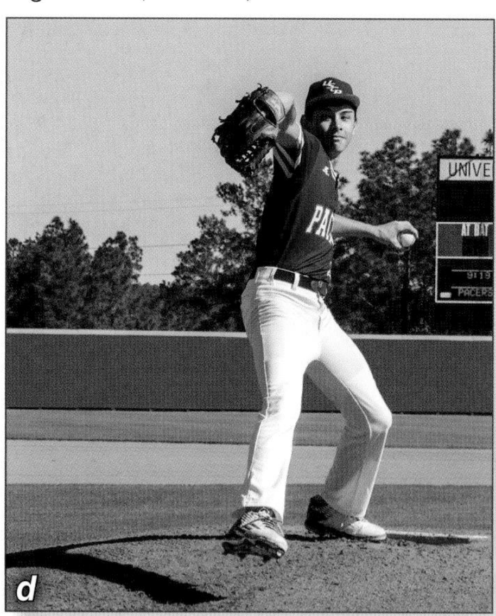

Power Position

1. From the balance point, the hands separate.
2. As the front leg starts toward the target, the throwing arm begins the arm swing.
3. You should drive your weight from the back foot down the mound and through the release.
4. As the front foot lands and the hips begin to rotate, the arm should be in the proper, natural throwing position, or natural arm slot.
5. The landing point should be on or near the center line.
6. The shoulders should have a slight upward tilt (figure 3.5*d*).

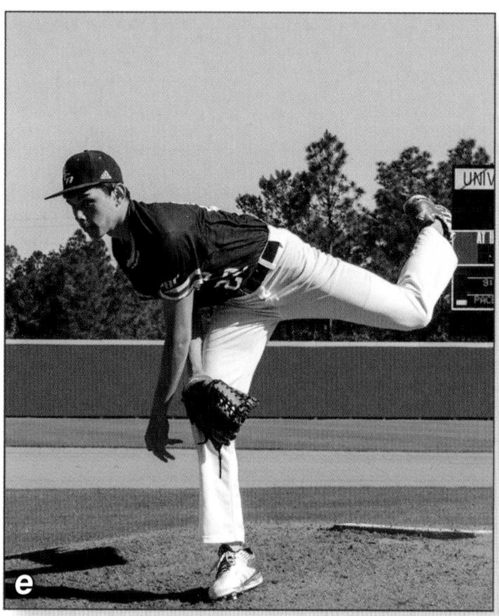

Release and Finish

1. If the body and the arm are in the proper power position, the release point should remain consistent.
2. As the ball is released, the back leg will follow through (figure 3.5*e*).
3. The glove-side arm should be in a tucked position near the body.
4. The finish will put you into a good fielding position.

WINDUP

The windup adds a couple of steps to the delivery process. In youth leagues, some may throw out of the windup at all times because of the rules regarding base runners. At the higher levels, the stretch position is used when a runner is on base. The windup at these levels is used when no one is on base and sometimes with a runner on third. Let's look at how the windup works (figure 3.6). Again, take it step by step, inserting a pause between steps. Add in the speed and rhythm as you feel comfortable.

As you create fluidity within the steps, you will find that your throwing motion will differ slightly from those around you. This dissimilarity is natural. At this point, you can evaluate each pitch to determine whether your release point is consistent. Consistent accuracy is derived from a consistent release point, and a consistent release point is derived from a consistent delivery. If your accuracy is not consistent, the timing within your delivery is flawed. Again, if you can feel it, you can fix it. With continued repetitions, you will be able to find the timing mechanisms that work for you and that help you make adjustments.

Figure 3.6 **WINDUP MECHANICS**

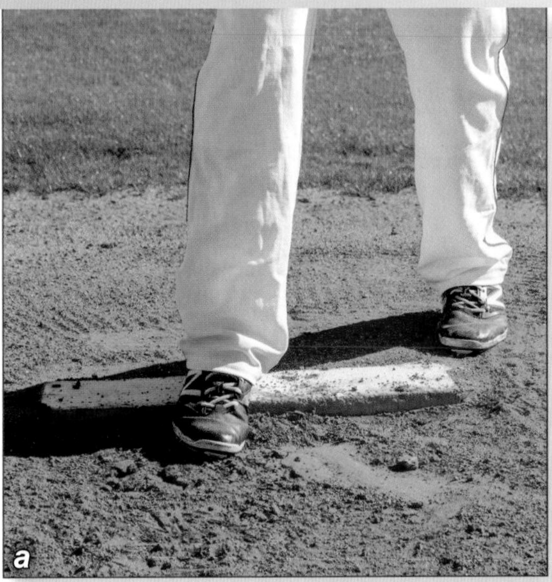

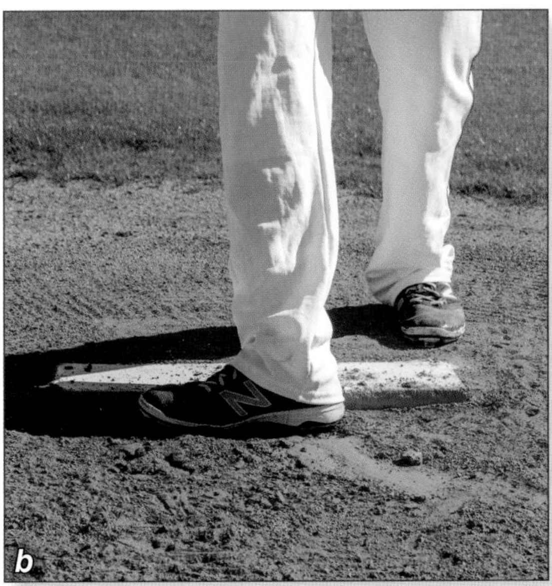

Addressing the Rubber and Rocker Step

1. The windup starts with you facing the catcher and addressing the rubber with your feet as shown (figure 3.6*a*). Notice the slight angle with the feet and the body. This angle should be at no more than 45 degrees toward your throwing side. The angle reduces error throughout the process of getting to the balance point.
2. The ball should be in the glove in a comfortable position. Unlike in the stretch, as you get the sign your hands may be separated or together; this is strictly personal preference.
3. As the windup begins, the throwing hand should grip the ball in the glove.
4. The rocker step is a slight step backward with the front foot, but your weight should shift only slightly.
5. As the step occurs, your head should remain centered or slightly toward the back foot. The hands should remain centered with the body.

Pivot

1. As the rocker step is completed, the back foot must pivot into the position that it is in during the stretch, addressing the mound as shown (see figure 3.6*b*).
2. You now lift the front foot into the balance position. Be sure to keep the weight transfer minimal throughout these steps so that the balance point is successful.

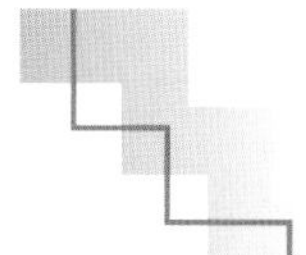

MISSTEP

The rocker step throws you off balance.

CORRECTION

Be sure to keep the "nose over toe" approach in mind as you take the step to keep the weight from overshifting.

STRIKE ZONE

Before we move forward, let's look at the target that all pitchers are throwing to—the strike zone. The strike zone consists of an area the width of home plate, which is 17 inches (43 cm) across. The top of the strike zone is at the chest of the hitter, and the bottom of the zone is at the hitter's knees.

Pitchers and pitching coaches often separate the zone into specific areas, as shown in figure 3.7. As we move into our pitching drills, the primary targets we will focus on are at the bottom of the zone. Pitches in this area are difficult to hit, so you need to be able to locate your pitches here consistently.

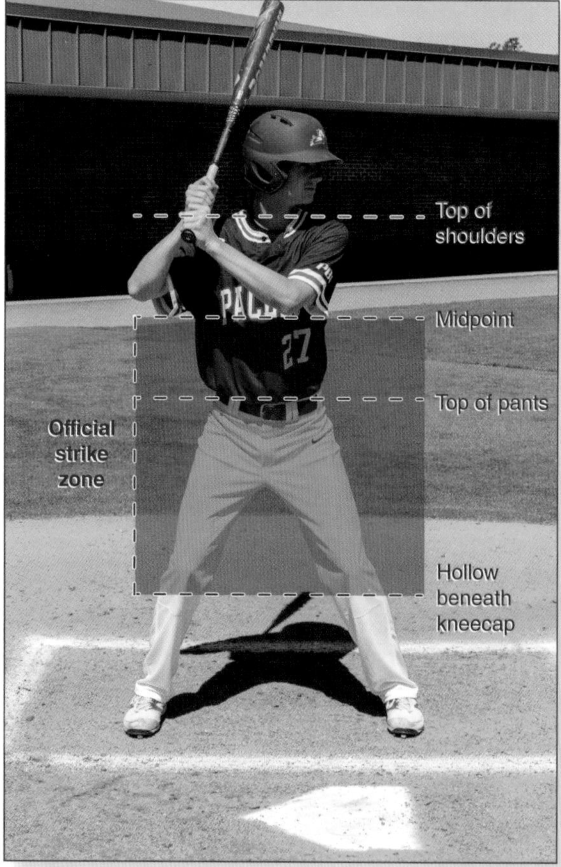

Figure 3.7 Strike zone.

Pitching Drill 1 **One-Knee**

The one-knee drill (figure 3.8) focuses on the arm action and movement of the upper body. From the one-knee position, the pitcher starts with the glove and ball centered on the chest. The partner should be 40 to 50 feet (12 to 15 m) away. The pitcher then separates and rotates, going through the throwing motion all the way through delivery. The throwing arm finishes across the front leg.

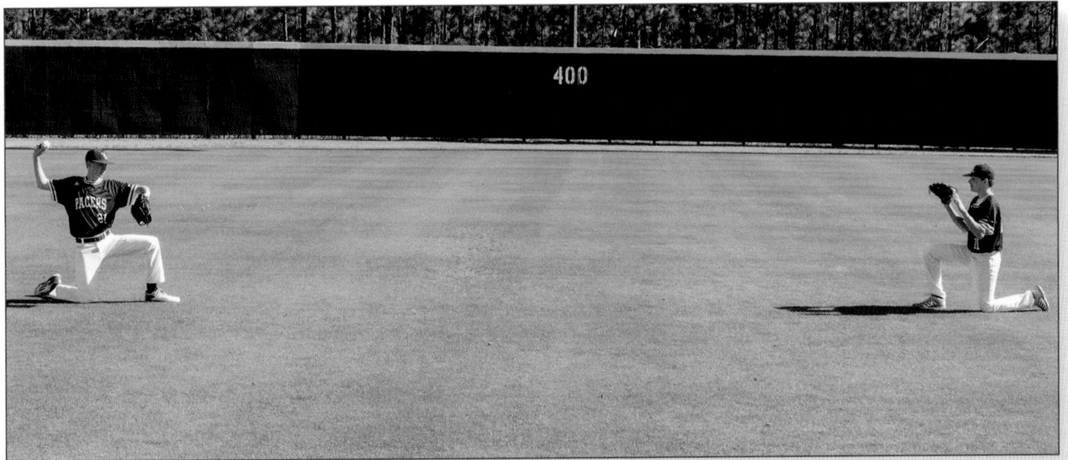

Figure 3.8 One-knee drill.

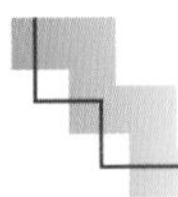

TO INCREASE DIFFICULTY

- Mix in different pitches.

TO DECREASE DIFFICULTY

- Shorten the distance between players.

Success Check

- The goal is to feel the proper release point.
- Can you feel a different release point or a difference in timing when you miss the target?
- The arm action and finish should become repeatable, building consistency with locating the baseball on target.

Score Your Success

You earn 1/2 point for every target hit within your partner's upper body.

You earn 1 point if your partner doesn't move the glove.

Your score ____ of 10

Pitching Drill 2 **Balance**

The balance drill is designed to teach proper timing and arm action from the balance point. From 40 to 50 feet (12 to 15 m) away, the pitcher is in the stretch position. To begin, the pitcher lifts the front leg into the balance position. A coach or partner should be behind the pitcher holding the ball (see figure 3.9). At the balance position, the coach hands the ball to the pitcher at the bottom of the arm circle. After receiving the ball, the pitcher continues through the delivery.

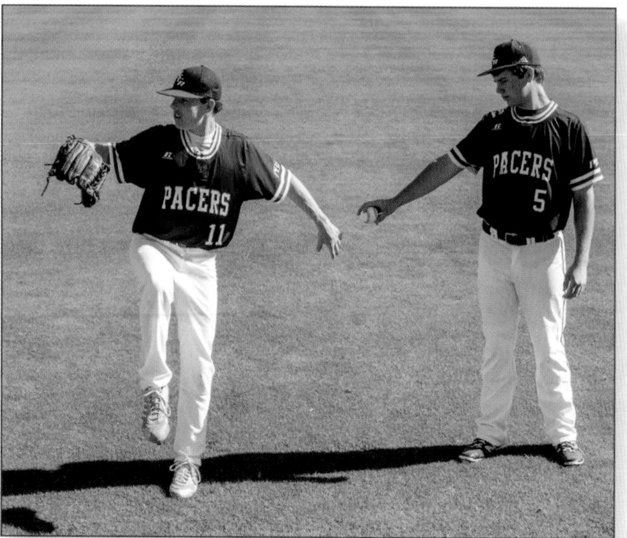

Figure 3.9 Balance drill.

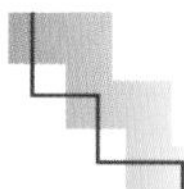

TO INCREASE DIFFICULTY

- Mix in different pitches.

TO DECREASE DIFFICULTY

- Shorten the distance between players.

Success Check

- You should be in the balance position for a full second before receiving the ball.
- The natural timing of the arm swing should connect with the lower half throughout the rest of the delivery.
- You should be able to repeat the delivery and hit your target consistently.
- Can you feel improper timing or a change in release point with a missed target?

Score Your Success

You earn 1/2 point for every target hit within your partner's upper body.

You earn 1 point if your partner doesn't move the glove.

Your score ____ of 10

Pitching Drill 3 **Flat Ground**

Flat-ground work is a common drill that many pitchers use regularly. The flat-ground drill is done from 45 to 60 feet (14 to 18 m) away. The partner is in a catching stance, and the pitcher is on an even plane, not on a raised mound (figure 3.10). The object of the flat-ground drill is to go through proper mechanics at a slower pace than game speed. Throwing on the flat surface ensures that the arm is getting to a good release point and that the finish of the delivery is being done properly.

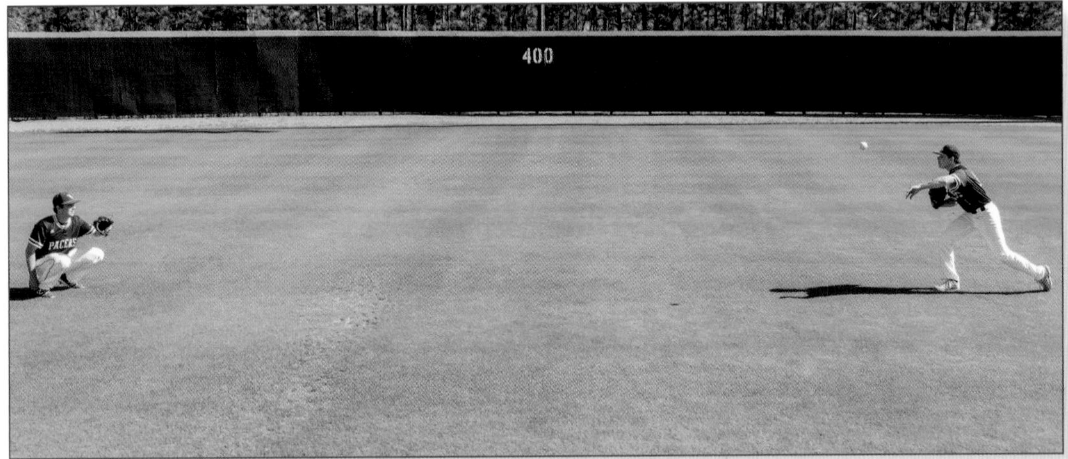

Figure 3.10 Flat ground drill.

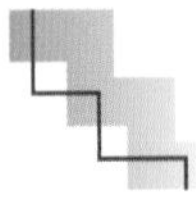

TO INCREASE DIFFICULTY

- Mix in different pitches.
- Have the catcher change the target position every pitch.

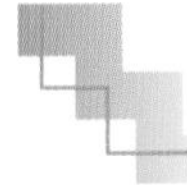

TO DECREASE DIFFICULTY

- Shorten the distance between players.
- Only one pitch is thrown to one location.

Success Check

- You should be able to repeat the proper mechanics and hit the target consistently.
- You should be able to feel the timing flaws, enabling you to make adjustments in your delivery as needed.

Score Your Success

You earn 1/2 point for every target hit within your partner's upper body.

You earn 1 point if your partner doesn't move the glove.

Your score ____ of 10

Pitching Drill 4 **Down the Mound and Transitions**

At this point in our drill set, we are ready to move to the mound. Our first drill from the mound is designed to get the body moving forward, creating momentum toward the target and getting the arm in the proper arm slot during the delivery. The pitcher starts from behind the rubber with the ball in hand, and the catcher stands 60 feet (18 m) away. The pitcher then takes a step behind or a modified crow hop, placing the back foot in front of the rubber (see figure 3.11) and throwing downhill to the catcher.

To add another element to the process, the coach can stand diagonally in front of the rubber to the pitcher's glove side. The pitcher can act as a shortstop turning a double play. As the pitcher steps toward the mound, the coach can flip a ball to him, causing the pitcher to transition into a throw down the mound as if he were turning a double play at second base. This fluid and natural arm action will coincide with the momentum of going down the mound.

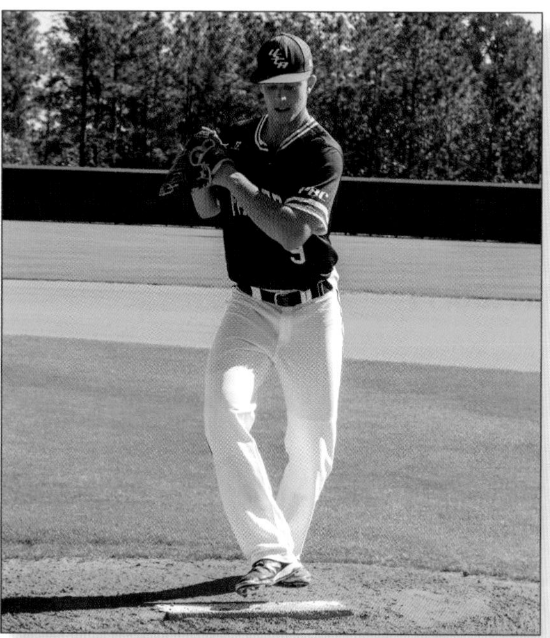

Figure 3.11 Down the mound and transitions drill.

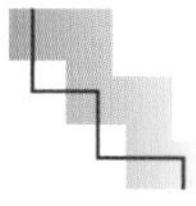

TO INCREASE DIFFICULTY

- Coach flips the ball.
- Increase the target distance.
- Move the target location.

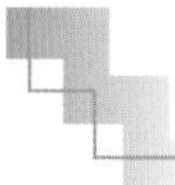

TO DECREASE DIFFICULTY

- Have the pitcher start with the ball in the glove.
- Shorten the distance to the target.

Success Check

- The timing of the arm action should correspond with the movement of the body. This movement should be at a faster rate than a normal pitching delivery.
- The finish should carry the pitcher a couple steps toward the catcher after the release.

Score Your Success

You earn 1/2 point for every target hit within your partner's upper body.

You earn 1 point if your partner doesn't move the glove.

Your score ____ of 10

Pitching Drill 5 **Short Box**

The short box is a drill designed to help the pitcher work on mechanics and accuracy at a distance shorter than 60 feet (18 m). Using the windup or the stretch, the pitcher works on locating all his pitches using proper mechanics. This drill allows the pitcher to see results from a shortened distance, giving him the ability to make mechanical adjustments at a slower pace. The number of pitches thrown in a short box will vary depending on the pitcher. A common short-box theme is to locate five pitches in a row in the same spot before moving on to a different pitch or different location. The following is a 25-pitch short-box breakdown.

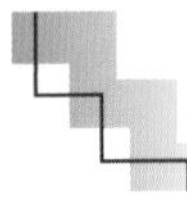

TO INCREASE DIFFICULTY

- Hit a specific spot before moving to the next.
- Rotate through each pitch and location in sequence rather than five at a time.

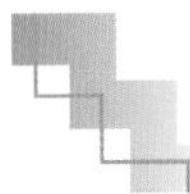

TO DECREASE DIFFICULTY

- Throw only one or two pitches.
- Focus on locating specific spots.

Success Check

- Repeat the spot five times before moving on.
- Make the proper mechanical adjustments as needed.

Score Your Success

Fastball outside—Your score ____ of 5

Fastball inside—Your score ____ of 5

Changeup outside—Your score ____ of 5

Curveball outside—Your score ____ of 5

Fastball middle—Your score ____ of 5

Total—Your score ____ of 25

Pitching Drill 6 **Bullpen**

Bullpens can be set up in a variety of ways, depending on the goal for the pitcher that day. For instance, a bullpen thrown during the season may consist of fewer pitches than one thrown in the off-season. The focus of each bullpen may vary as well; a midseason pen may focus on slight mechanical adjustments, whereas an off-season pen may focus on developing a new pitch. The general idea of throwing a pen is to create repetition with the delivery while finding mechanical or mental adjustments that you can carry with you to the field.

The most important tip that we can give is to be sure to have structure with your pen. Most pens can be designed similar to the short-box format, but to give you variety, the following is an alternative format to structuring a pen.

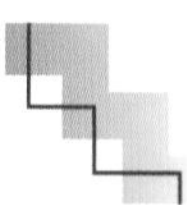

TO INCREASE DIFFICULTY

- Hit a specific spot before moving to the next.
- Rotate through each pitch and location in sequence rather than five at a time.

TO DECREASE DIFFICULTY

- Throw only one or two pitches.
- Focus on locating specific spots.

Success Check

- Simulate game at-bats by going through four sequences of pitches.
- Simulate a sequence of facing a right-handed hitter and then a left-handed hitter.

Score Your Success

You earn 20 points for every simulated strikeout.

You earn 10 points if you reach two strikes before walking the hitter.

You earn 0 points if you walk the hitter on four straight pitches.

Hitter 1—Your score ____ of 20

Hitter 2—Your score ____ of 20

Hitter 3—Your score ____ of 20

Hitter 4—Your score ____ of 20

Total—Your score ____ of 80

CAT AND MOUSE GAME

Now that you have a feel of some different pitches, we can take an advanced look at the game within the game. At higher levels of play, the cat and mouse game between pitcher and hitter is often a mental battle involving the hitter's approach and the pitcher's choice of what pitch to throw and what location to throw it to. From the pitcher's perspective, within this battle many other factors play a role in determining pitch and location. This section looks at the mental approach that a pitcher should develop to become more consistent and more successful.

Self-Awareness

Before you toe the rubber, you should ask yourself a few questions to help you understand what kind of pitcher you are. The key to becoming self-aware is to be honest with your answers. Take a look at the following questions.

1. Can I consistently locate my fastball?
2. What velocity and action do I have on my fastball?
3. What are my secondary pitches? Am I comfortable throwing them in any count?
4. What results do I want to get, and what results do I usually get with my secondary pitches?
5. Do I have an out pitch?
6. What mechanical adjustments can I feel?

These questions are designed to help you understand exactly what you are throwing. As you try to answer, consider the feedback you have received from coaches and other players. A pitcher who understands what he has can use his knowledge as a tool to get outs. A pitcher who is not self-aware typically struggles to find outs. Answering honestly, therefore, is important. If you think that you throw a 91-mile-per-hour (41 m/s) fastball, but the coaches tell you that the radar gun keeps reading 81 (36 m/s), maybe your mind-set should change. If you are honest with yourself, you will certainly change your approach when throwing to hitters.

Knowing the Situation

The pitcher must always be aware of the situation. For beginners, being aware of every situation is difficult. Teaching awareness really happens by trial and error. By reviewing actions that happened, good or bad, a player can more easily correct the action the next time. The difficulty for beginners is being able to process the amount of information that goes into every situation, all while trying to pitch to a hitter. So let's look at how a pitcher can filter the information and still be able to execute a pitch.

A pitcher must be aware of the following list of factors at all times. Although it may seem like a lot to filter, at the professional and higher collegiate levels, this list will grow even bigger. The question format is designed to illustrate the thought process that a pitcher may go through between pitches.

SURROUNDING FACTORS

- Who are the good runners and hitters in the opposing lineup?
- What inning are we in?
- What is the score?
- How many outs are there?
- What is the count?
- Are runners on base?
    - Is the runner a steal threat?
    - Is this a time they might bunt or try to create action?

- Where do I go with the ball if it is hit to me?
- Has a defensive play been called? What is our defensive setup?

HITTER

- Who is at bat, and where is he in the lineup?
    - Where are the outs?
- Is the hitter in a situational at-bat?
    - What is the hitter trying to do?
    - Has he adjusted his position in the batter's box?
- What pitch sequence have we used or are we using?
    - What pitch are we trying to get to based on my strengths and the hitter's weaknesses?

EXECUTING THE PITCH AND EVALUATING THE INFORMATION

- Is a runner on base?
    - How can I control the base runner from the set position?
- Did I execute the pitch to the location?
    - What reaction did the hitter have?
    - Was there action with the base runner?
    - Did I feel a mechanical adjustment that I can make to execute the next pitch better?
- Reset and refocus.
    - How has the situation changed?

For a beginner, this cycle has an abundance of information that can be difficult to process without slowing the tempo of the game. In time, many of these specific questions will become part of the pitcher's natural process between pitches. A pitcher who is capable of understanding the situation and can cycle through this information quickly will have a higher baseball IQ and a greater feel of the game and the way in which it is played.

For those who can do this, most of the answers to the questions in this breakdown will be stored subconsciously, thereby allowing the pitcher to focus on three major factors. The three major factors for a pitcher to focus on help determine the answers to the other questions in the breakdown. The advanced pitcher will quickly adjust the answers to the other questions. Here is how it works.

Mechanics

The first major factor that a pitcher focuses on is the delivery itself. Given all the other information that the pitcher must process, he must make only minimal mechanical adjustments during the game. One goal of practice, or throwing in the bullpen, is to find those minor mechanical adjustments that the pitcher can feel and that he can use during a game.

What Is the Count? Pitch Sequencing

The count on the batter determines many aspects of how a situation is played. The count affects the running game, the hitter's approach, and the decision on what pitch is called. In turn, it can affect the defensive setup. For the advanced pitcher who is self-aware, the count encompasses all of these factors and plays a big role in pitch selection.

The cat and mouse game for a starting pitcher begins with his looking at the entire lineup. Each hitter is different, and the pitcher must figure out what weaknesses he can exploit in the lineup by using his strengths. As the game is played, the pitcher should note the sequencing he used to get hitters out. The goal is to keep the offense off balance by creating soft contact. The pitcher can do this by establishing the fact that he can command the fastball.

Working off of the fastball, the pitcher can mix in secondary pitches. Throughout the course of a game, the sequencing of pitches within each at-bat will factor into the sequencing of the next at-bat for each hitter, but the pitcher must be conscious of not getting into a pattern with the sequencing. If the pitcher throws a first-pitch fastball to every hitter, the offense is likely to notice and make adjustments, so the pitcher must be able to throw secondary pitches in every count. This unpredictability will keep an offense from getting accustomed to a specific pitch sequence.

Controlling the Running Game

Pitch sequencing can also be affected when a runner is on base, although it is only part of what a pitcher can do to help control the running game. When facing an offense that likes to steal or put base runners in motion, a pitcher must be able to adjust his set and delivery to throw off the runner's timing. Stealing bases usually happens when a runner times the pitcher's set position and breaks at the moment the pitcher begins to deliver. Here are several things that a pitcher can work on to slow the running game:

- Vary the hold time from set to delivery.
  - Quick holds
  - Long holds
- Vary looks with a runner at second base.
- Pickoffs.
  - Snap picks
  - Picks before coming to the set position
  - Multiple picks in a row
- Be quick to the plate.
  - A time of 1.3 seconds or less from the start of the delivery until the ball hits the catcher's mitt

Holding runners and pickoffs are covered in Step 7: Playing the Infield.

FIELDING THE POSITION

After the pitch is delivered, the next aspect of the position becomes important—defense. Defending as a pitcher is a vital part of the game. Pitcher's fielding practice, or PFP, is the time for the pitcher to focus on proper technique for fielding the position. A typical PFP focuses on fielding a bunted ball, fielding a batted ball and throwing to a lead base, covering a base, and backing up a base. In this section we look at the main areas that you can work on to become a better defender on and around the mound.

Bunt Defense

A few guidelines apply to defending against the bunt. These guidelines will help you be in proper position and use proper technique while eliminating room for error. First, you need to know and understand the situation. Each situation determines the positions that the other defenders should be in, so you must know where you should be in case of a bunt.

Second, get an out. Errors often occur when the defender rushes the play to get a lead out. Typically, as a pitcher, unless the ball is bunted hard back to you, the only play you will have is to first base. With that being said, you must still be quick in getting to the baseball. Most of the time, you should take the out at first base that the opponent is giving you.

After you get to the baseball, the third point is to control your footwork. You should be in an athletic position as you field the ball and shuffle through the throw. Most throwing errors that occur when fielding a bunt stem from improper footwork. Let's look at how it should be done.

Batted Balls

The same guidelines used for bunt defense fielding are used for fielding a ball off the bat. The difference in the batted ball is the mound that you are standing on. Each mound is different, so you need to move your feet when you throw. Having good footwork will result in fewer throwing mistakes.

Covering First

Another common responsibility for pitchers is to cover first base on any batted ball toward the right side of the infield. In some scenarios, the first baseman may be in a deep position, or he may go after a ball, taking him away from the first-base bag. The pitcher must be able to get to the base in time to receive the throw for the force-out.

In this situation, the pitcher takes a banana-shaped angle, which allows him to get to the base without crossing the path of the base runner. Again, the footwork around the bag is important. From the time of contact, the pitcher should sprint at full speed. As the angle is approached, you need to control your strides so that you can safely step on the bag and continue through while receiving a flip or throw. The strides and feet must be in control so that you can break down at the bag and receive a throw as a first baseman would if you are going to get to the bag early.

Backing Up Bases

Backing up bases is a must as a pitcher. Backing up is a mental aspect of defending as a pitcher. Young pitchers often stand on the mound and watch a play unfold, especially on batted balls to the outfield. The rule that each pitcher must realize is that he always has a place on the field that he should move to during the course of a ball in play. Proper positioning when backing up will eliminate extra bases given to an offense in the event of a thrown ball getting past an infielder. At the higher levels, pitchers have no excuse for not moving to back up. Here is an overview of the proper positioning for backing up.

- For a hit to left or center field with no one on base, the pitcher backs up second base directly in line with the outfield throw.
- For a hit to the outfield with a runner on first base, the pitcher should back up third base in line with the throw from the outfield.
- For a hit to right field with no one on base, the pitcher should move to first base in case of a play there.
- For any play at home, the pitcher backs up home in direct line with the throw.
- For any extra base hit with no one on, the pitcher backs up the base where ball may be thrown.
- For an extra base hit with a runner on first base, the pitcher should move to a spot about halfway between third base and home plate. Once he sees where the throw will go, he should back up that base.

SUCCESS SUMMARY

Pitching is more than throwing a baseball at a target. On the field, this position requires the development of baseball IQ, physical development of mechanics, and total development to control a game with your ability and feel of the game. Off the field, this position requires extensive care of the throwing arm for maximum development. To take the steps to success as a pitcher, you must strategically develop the craft of the position over time.

This development should start by setting specific goals relative to your abilities. To reach these goals, you must realize the importance of daily arm care and preparation. Even if you are not pitching off a mound, you can prepare by practicing skills such as your pickoff moves and fielding bunts, or even by discussing pitch sequences and getting feedback. Pitching is a mental game, and the more information you can process, the better prepared you will be.

Pitching Drills

1. One-knee	_____ out of 10
2. Balance	_____ out of 10
3. Flat ground	_____ out of 10
4. Down the mound and transitions	_____ out of 10
5. Short Box	____ out of 25
6. Bullpen	____ out of 80
Total	____ **out of 145**

If you scored 100 or more points, congratulations! You have mastered the basic mechanics of pitching. If you scored fewer than 80 points, you may want to continue practicing your mechanical drills to ensure proper arm slot and continued arm health. By practicing these drills, you will develop the techniques needed to take the next step to success.

STEP

4

Catching

To follow up our discussion on pitching, we now look at the other side of the battery. Catching is a dirty, tireless, and thankless position that embodies physical and mental toughness while combining them with technique, savvy, and baseball IQ. This position is unlike any other in the game; the less a catcher is noticed during a game defensively, the better he likely performed his duties. A catcher is typically noticed defensively only if his performance costs the team. Catchers must understand this concept, especially those new to the position. By having a grasp of this concept, the player will be able to begin each day in the right mind-set knowing that his diligent efforts will likely go without thanks or credit.

The duties of the catcher involve a vast array of techniques, and the art of being a great catcher requires detailed knowledge of all aspects of the game. Step 4 breaks down the catching position, beginning with the fundamentals of setting up and receiving the baseball. Using this as our foundation, we show the proper technique for throwing, blocking, and fielding the position. We conclude by looking at the traits that define a successful catcher, and we show how you can learn to take charge as the quarterback of the defense. Now, get your gear on, and let's begin!

SETUP

The setup skill for a catcher involves the variation and sequence of squatting positions that he needs to understand and use. Each position is designed for specific purposes. Proper body positioning throughout the setup gives the catcher the ability to transition quickly into other movements such as blocking or throwing. The first position, primary, is designed so that the pitcher and catcher can communicate with hand signals, or signs (figure 4.1).

Figure 4.1 PRIMARY POSITION

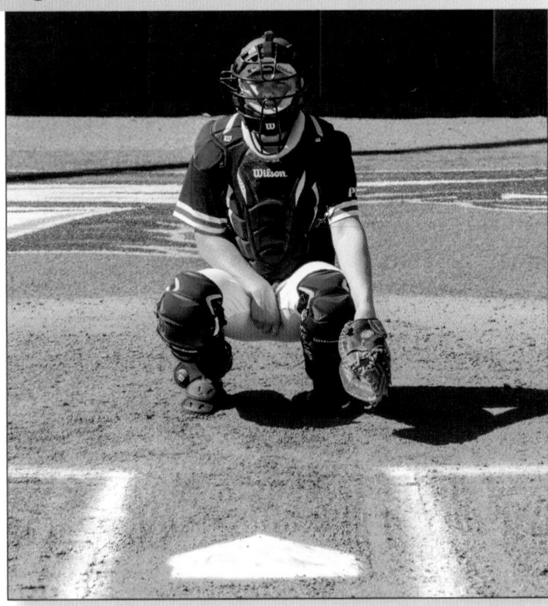

1. Face the pitcher from 5 to 7 feet (1.5 to 2 m) directly behind home plate.
2. Get into a relaxed squatting position and turn slightly toward the shortstop.
3. The feet should be under the buttocks with the knees pointed forward.
4. The chest should be upright.
5. The mitt should be placed outside the leg, below the shin.
6. The signs should be given tucked in between the legs.

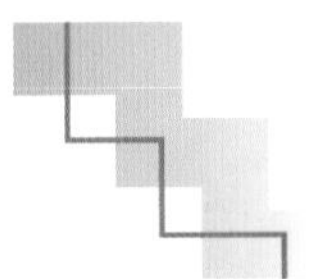

MISSTEP

Common missteps with the primary stance are the positioning of the glove and the angle of the knees. If your legs are open or your mitt is out of place, the base coaches for the other team can often see the signs.

CORRECTION

Practice giving your signs while having coaches check from both coach's boxes. Find a position where the signs are hidden and that is comfortable for you. Be conscious of this position at all times.

The secondary positions are the stances from which you block and throw. They are the most difficult stances for a catcher to be in. There are two occasions when the catcher needs to be in a secondary stance—when there are two strikes on the batter (figure 4.2), and when there are runners on base (figure 4.3). The stances differ slightly for each situation.

Figure 4.2 SECONDARY POSITION WITHOUT BASE RUNNERS AND TWO STRIKES

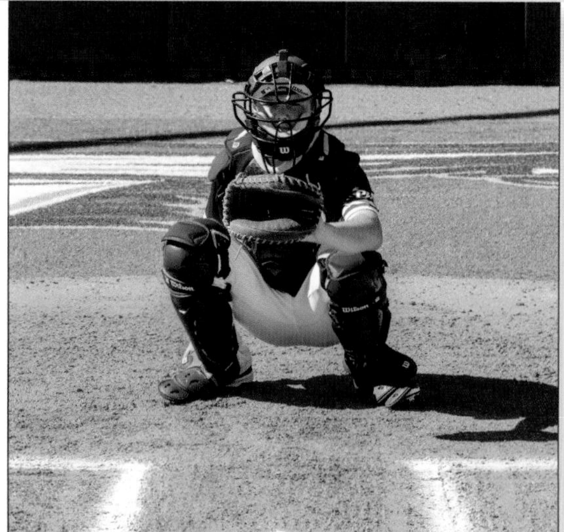

1. After you give the sign in primary, position your body behind the side of the plate the ball should be thrown to.
2. The feet should be spread so that the hips and butt can sink down into the squat.
3. The feet and body should angle slightly toward the second baseman, and the left foot should be slightly in front of the right. This position puts the glove-side arm in front, giving the catcher a wider range of motion to receive the pitch.
4. The chest should be low, close to between the knees.
5. The target (mitt) will show where the pitch should be located.
6. The throwing hand should be placed in a comfortable position beside the leg.

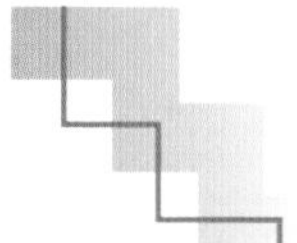

MISSTEP

A common misstep is a high stance. The ability to sink the hips between the feet while keeping the upper body in proper position requires hip and ankle mobility. Poor mobility creates poor positioning, often causing the left knee to obstruct the range of motion of the left arm.

CORRECTION

You must keep your range of motion with the glove; therefore, you have to dedicate time to stretching and performing mobility exercises. This mobility will translate to quickness while transitioning into secondary movements such as blocking or throwing.

Figure 4.3 **SECONDARY POSITION WITH BASE RUNNERS**

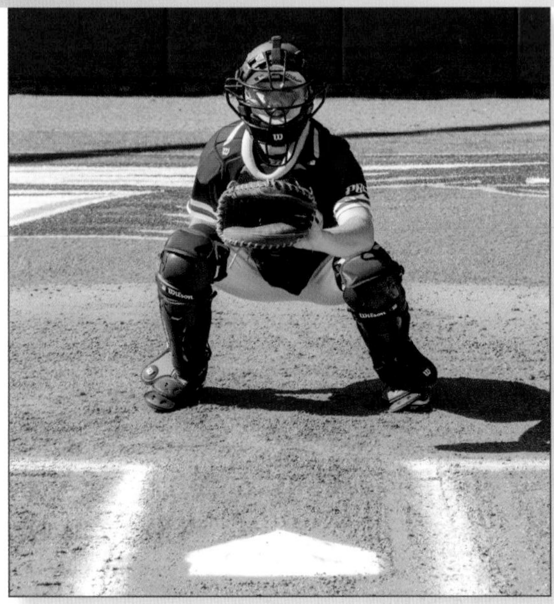

1. After you give the sign in primary position, position your body behind the side of the plate the ball should be thrown to.
2. The feet should be spread almost twice shoulder-width, and the left foot should be in front of the right foot, angling the body slightly more than in the previous position.
3. Weight should be positioned on the balls of the feet, allowing maximum mobility and quickness when reacting to the pitch.
4. The hips should be raised to the same plane as the knees.
5. The chest should be lowered between the knees.
6. The target should be given out front, giving you a full range of motion with the mitt.

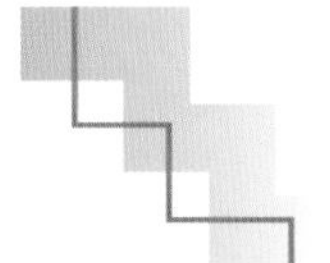

MISSTEP

A common mistake with catchers in this position is the hip height. You often let your hips sink between your feet, causing a decrease in mobility.

CORRECTION

Maintaining this position requires strength and athleticism. The lack of strength is often the cause of the problem, but you may just need subtle reminders to keep your hips up. To develop your mobility and the strength needed to maintain this position, you should do the majority of your drill work from this position.

RECEIVING THE BASEBALL

Receiving is an art. Of the many skills that a catcher must possess, the ability to receive the baseball stands alone above the rest, and it can differentiate a good catcher from a great one. Let's look at how catchers can paint a picture with the mitt for the umpire (see figure 4.4).

Figure 4.4 RECEIVING TECHNIQUE

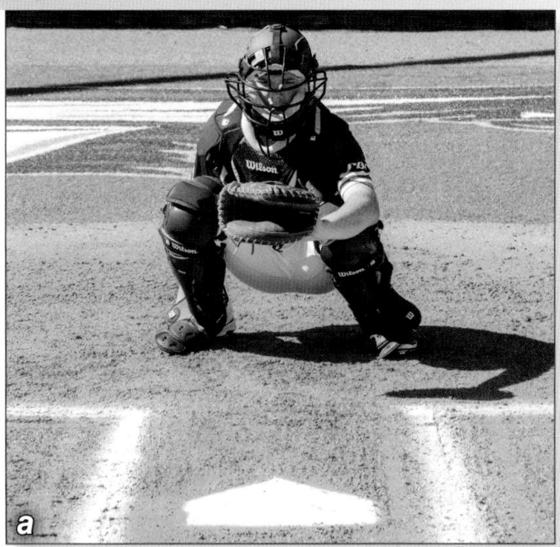

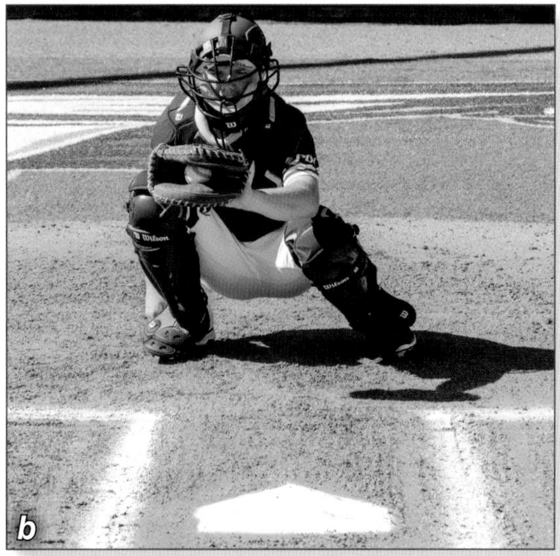

1. From the secondary position, give the target to the pitcher.
2. The wrist should be flexed upward, and the thumb should be angled up slightly as well (figure 4.4*a*).
3. The elbow should be flexed and firm, not locked.
4. The shoulder is the pivot for the arm, giving maximum range of motion.
5. As the pitch is delivered, sway the hips in the direction of the ball so that you can catch the ball inside your body (figure 4.4*b*).
6. For pitches outside your body, catch the ball and throw it back. For pitches inside your body, catch the ball firmly, or "stick it." The glove should pause for a second at the moment of impact, giving the umpire a look at where the pitch was located.
7. For pitches to the glove side, the stick should be made with the thumb up (figure 4.4*c*). For the opposite side, the thumb should be level or slightly down (figure 4.4*d*).

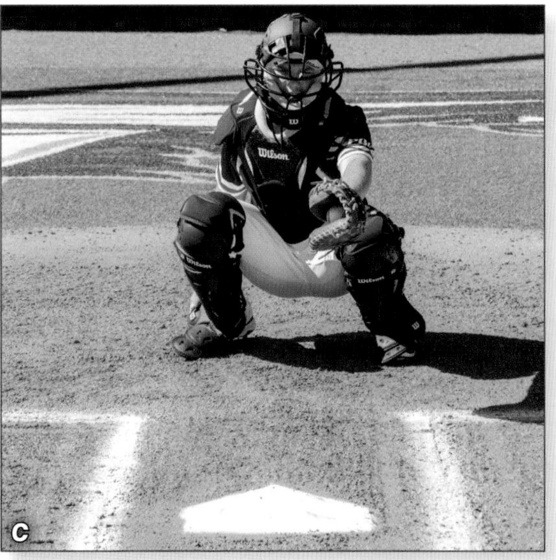

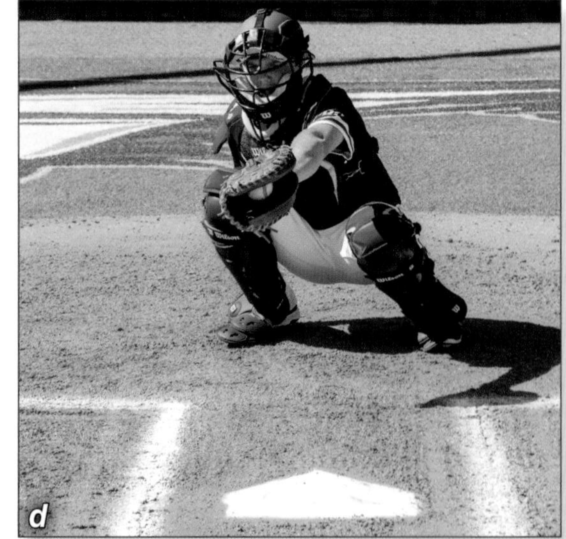

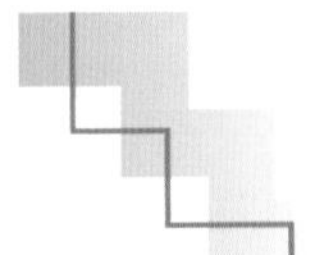

MISSTEP

The elbow should remain flexed and firm, giving you the ability to control the mitt at the impact of the catch. When the elbow is locked out at full extension, the range of motion is limited and the ability to control the mitt at impact is diminished. When the elbow is bent, the shoulder is no longer the pivot for the arm. This setup creates a smaller range of motion as well, but, more important, glove positioning at impact will be flawed.

CORRECTION

The goal is to get you to feel the proper technique so that you can repeat it. Let's look at a few drills that can help correct or improve your receiving technique. These drills are designed to be a repetitive tool for proper form and to help you build the strength and agility needed to maintain proper body positioning.

Receiving Drill 1 **Receiving Bare-Handed**

Bare-handed drills are a good tool to use on a daily basis as a constant reminder of proper technique and body movements. With most of the drills, the catcher will be in the secondary position simulating runners on base, but drills such as this one allow the catcher to be in a more relaxed secondary position, simulating no runners on base. To perform the bare-handed drill, the coach or partner is on a knee 10 feet (3 m) away. With the catcher in the secondary position of choice, the partner flips the ball underhand to a given spot. The catcher sways his hips and sticks the ball, catching it with the thumb, ring finger, and middle finger (figure 4.5).

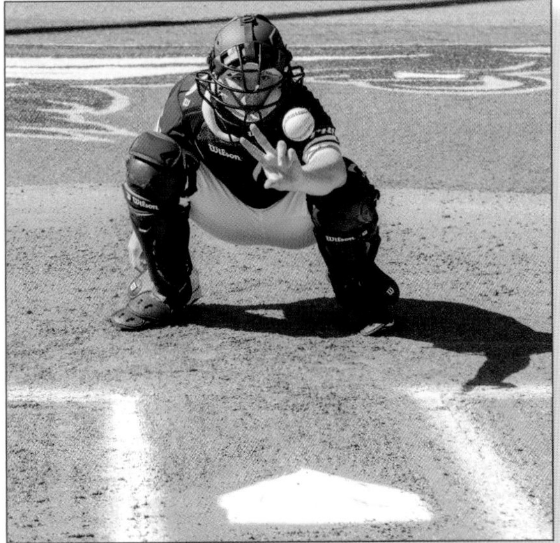

Figure 4.5 Receiving bare-handed drill.

(continued)

Receiving Drill 1 *(continued)*

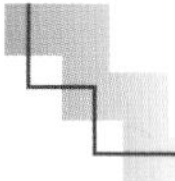

TO INCREASE DIFFICULTY

- Use only the index finger and thumb for reception.
- Have the coach stand and throw ping-pong balls.
- Speed up the time between pitches so that it becomes a rapid-fire drill.

TO DECREASE DIFFICULTY

- Allow the use of the whole hand for reception.
- Use tennis balls instead of baseballs.

Success Check

- Check the movement of the shoulder and elbow. Did the elbow remain flexed and firm while pivoting the arm on the shoulder?
- Did the hips sway, if needed, so that the ball was caught inside the body?
- Did the fingers get around and secure the ball in either the thumb-up or the thumb-down position?

Score Your Success

You earn 1 point for every ball received with good technique and hip sway.

You earn 1/2 point if the technique is good but the ball drops.

You earn 0 points for bad technique.

Your score ____ of 10

Receiving Drill 2 **Receiving With Mitt**

Now that the glove is on, the catcher can do numerous drills to work on receiving the baseball. First, the coach can stand 30 feet (9 m) away and feed pitches to the catcher, working on the same technique used with the bare-handed drill (figure 4.6). Remember, if the coach throws a ball that the catcher cannot catch inside the body with the hip sway, he should catch it and return it without the stick. In this way, the catcher practices showing the umpire what pitches the catcher thinks are strikes and what pitches the catcher thinks are balls, thereby earning the umpire's respect and trust by showing that he will stick and show only quality, well-located pitches. If the catcher attempts to stick a pitch blatantly out of the strike zone, some umpires might lose trust and think that the catcher either doesn't know where the strike zone is or is trying to show him up. By earning the umpire's trust early, the catcher can sometimes expand the umpire's strike zone later in the game. This drill is a great way to work on the technique of what some call framing.

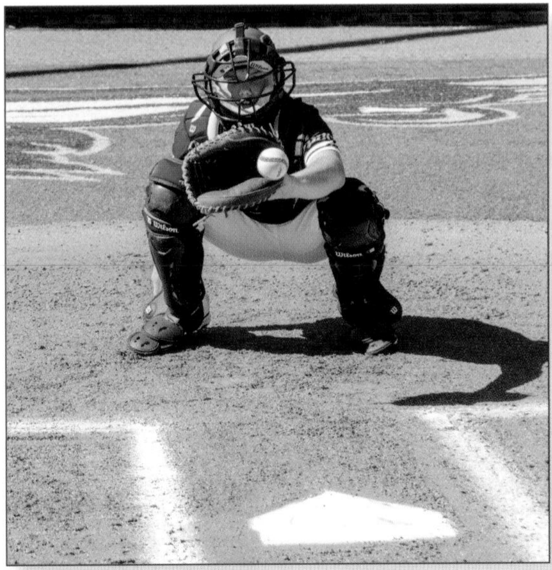

Figure 4.6 Receiving with mitt drill.

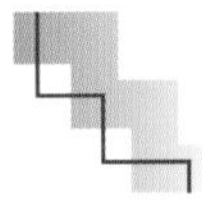

TO INCREASE DIFFICULTY

- Have two coaches each hold five balls. Have coach 1 stand 30 to 45 feet (9 to 14 m) away from the plate, angled at the first baseman. Have coach 2 at the same distance, angled at the third baseman. Starting with coach 1, the coaches alternately and rapidly feed pitches from both sides of the field. This rapid-fire drill is great for developing eye-hand coordination and glove work.
- Use the time catching bullpens with the pitchers to work on your technique.

Success Check

- Check the movement of the shoulder and elbow. Did the elbow remain flexed and firm while pivoting the arm on the shoulder?
- If the catcher cannot catch a pitch inside the body with the hip sway, he should catch it and return it without the stick.

Score Your Success

- You earn 1 point for every ball received with good technique and hip sway.
- You earn 0 points if the technique is good but the ball drops.
- You earn 0 points for bad technique or framing a ball out of the zone.

Your score ____of 10

TRANSFER, FOOTWORK, AND THROWING TO BASES

The technique of throwing out potential base stealers (figure 4.7) is unique enough for some to consider it an art form. "Throwing down" is a distinct part of the game in that it embodies a group of skills that few excel at, especially when you consider the enormous number of people who play the game. Coaches heavily evaluate this skill to determine level of play for each catcher. The term *pop time* refers to how long it takes a catcher to throw the ball to a base. When being evaluated, the catcher is timed throwing the ball to second base from the secondary position. The time begins at the moment the ball hits the catcher's mitt and ends at the moment the ball is caught at the second-base bag. The average major league pop time is 2.0 seconds.

Having a good pop time requires multiple skills and talents to come together into one fluid and repetitive motion. A common misconception is that pop time is directly correlated with arm strength. This is not the case. Arm strength is a factor, but so are footwork, transitioning, timing, body positioning, and quickness. The step-by-step breakdown in figure 4.7 shows how the transition and throwing motion works.

Figure 4.7 **THROWING TO SECOND BASE**

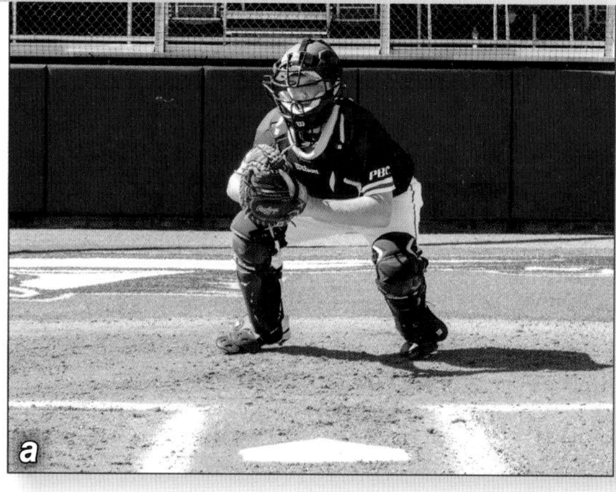

a

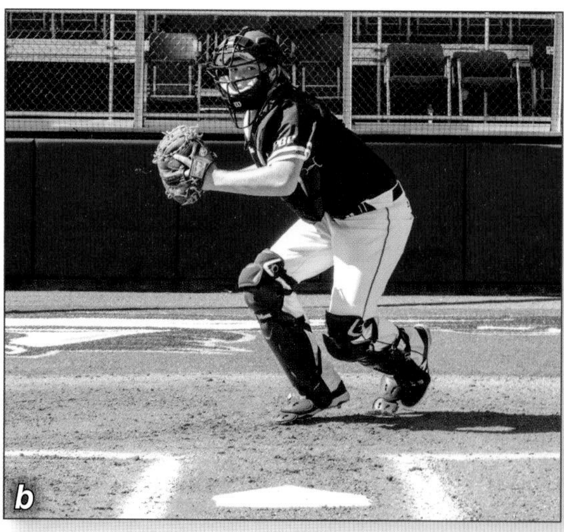

b

1. The catcher should be in the secondary position with runners on base.
2. As the ball is in flight, the right foot should move toward the ball, turning so that the instep faces second base when it plants (figure 4.7*a*). The catch should be made simultaneously as the back foot lands.
3. As the pitch is caught, the left foot should be in transition toward second base (figure 4.7*b*).
4. As the left foot lands, the hips and shoulders should rotate with the feet so that the catcher is in line to throw to second.
5. During this rotation, the ball should transfer from glove to hand.

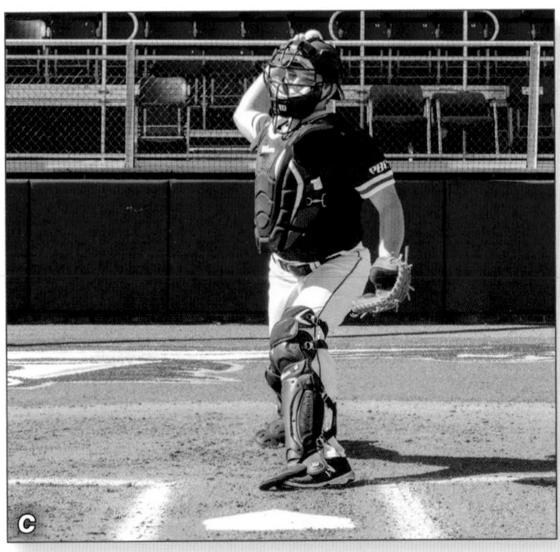

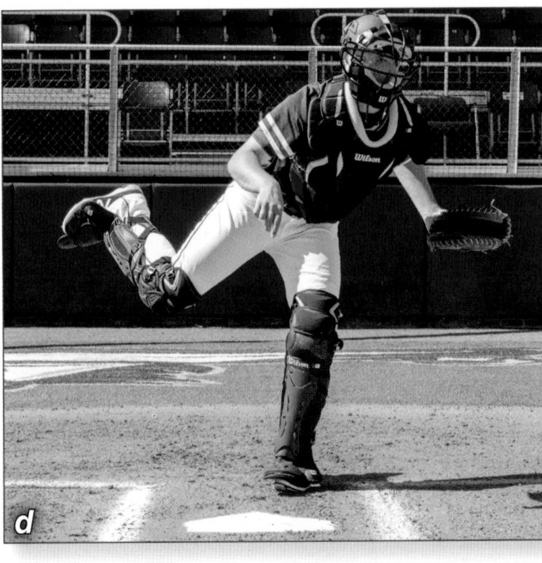

6. As the front foot lands, the throwing elbow should be up and the ball should be ready to be released (figure 4.7*c*).
7. The hips and upper body should not rise up during the transition. At the time the front foot lands, the catcher should be in the power position of the throwing motion.
8. Follow through and finish the throw (figure 4.7*d*).

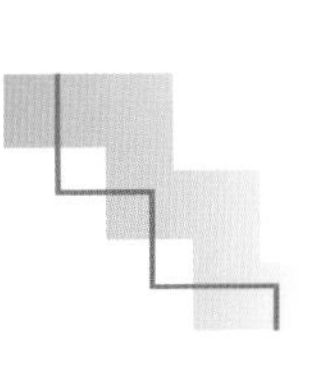

MISSTEP

Rhythm and timing are the keys to the transition. If you wait to catch the ball before gaining ground to second, the transition will be slow and the throw will rely heavily on arm strength. If you start too soon, the timing with the reception will be off, throwing the rhythm of the transition out of sync.

CORRECTION

After learning the technique, you should be able to determine whether you can speed up the transition process based on your ability, quickness, and timing. Repetition is extremely important for continued development. The following drill set breaks down the transition process and helps correct timing issues with your transition. The goal is to create one quick, fluid motion that gives direction and momentum to each throw.

Transfer, Footwork, and Throwing Drill 1
Step-by-Step Transitioning

The catcher starts in the secondary position with runners on base, and the coach stands 45 feet (14 m) away, holding five baseballs. Each time the ball is thrown, the catcher steps with the back foot and lands simultaneously with the catch (figure 4.8). The catcher must be sure to keep the hips down. He resets after every catch.

For the next five pitches, the catcher again steps and lands with the catch. After the catch, the catcher pauses for two seconds to ensure good form. After two seconds, the catcher simultaneously transfers the ball from glove to hand while rotating the feet and body into the power throwing position. He resets after holding and examining the proper position.

For the next five pitches, the catcher eliminates the pause between steps, but the speed of the process should remain slow and fluid, ensuring proper form throughout the motion.

The last five pitches speed up the process to simulate game speed. The catcher should hold the power throwing position to ensure that the feet and body placement are correct.

Practicing form and technique can be done during bullpens. This is a good way to focus on timing of the transition at game speed.

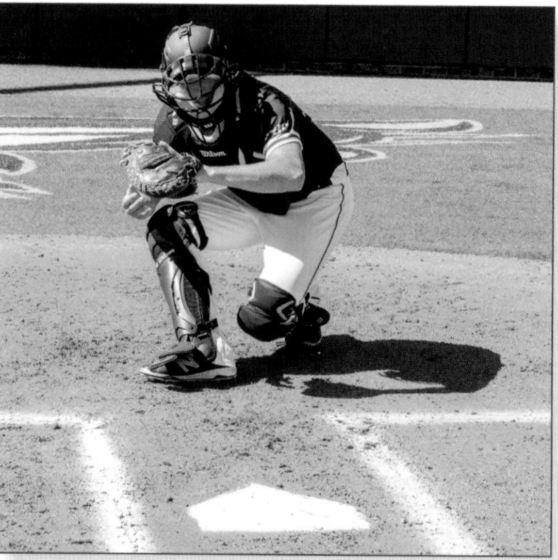

Figure 4.8 Step-by-step transitioning drill.

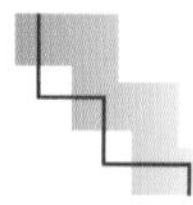

TO INCREASE DIFFICULTY

- Have a pitcher deliver the ball at full speed.
- Mix the pitches for the catcher to receive.

TO DECREASE DIFFICULTY

- Start with the ball in the catcher's mitt.

Success Check

- Does the catcher have the ability to stay low with the hips after the speed is picked up?
- Is the ball ready to be released as the front foot lands?
- After the speed is picked up, the initial step with the back foot is minor. At this point both feet should work in sync, gaining ground and creating one quick, fluid motion.

Score Your Success

You earn 1 point for each step using proper technique ending in good form.

You earn 0 points for standing up during the transition.

Your score ____ of 20

Transfer, Footwork, and Throwing Drill 2
Ball in Glove With Throw

Have the catcher start in the secondary position with the ball in the glove (figure 4.9). He goes through the transition process at full speed and completes the process by throwing to second base.

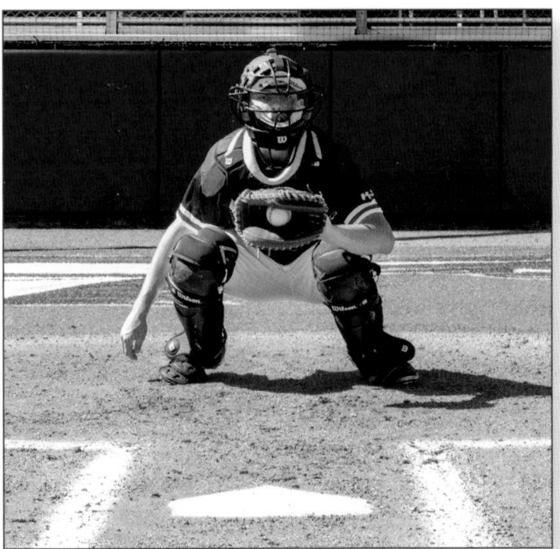

Figure 4.9 Ball in glove with throw drill.

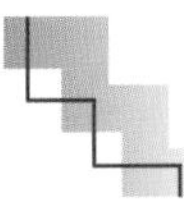

TO INCREASE DIFFICULTY

- Have the catcher throw to a small target such as a hat on the ground.
- Have the catcher throw blindfolded or with his eyes closed.

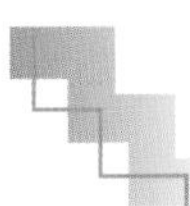

TO DECREASE DIFFICULTY

- Move the target closer to the catcher
- Have the catcher go through the step-by-step transition before the throw.

(continued)

Transfer, Footwork, and Throwing Drill 2 *(continued)*

Success Check

- Was the transition done with proper form?
- Was the transition fluid?
- Did the catcher gain ground and make a quality throw?

Score Your Success

You earn 1 point for a quality throw with good form.

You earn 1/2 point if the throw bounces but is on line.

You earn 0 points for an overthrow.

You earn 0 points if the form is lost in transition.

Your score ____ of 10

Transfer, Footwork, and Throwing Drill 3
Full-Speed Transition and Throw

At this point, the catcher is ready to throw down at full speed, putting the entire process together into one motion. Have a coach stand 45 feet (14 m) in front of the plate and feed the catcher 10 pitches. The catcher should go through the transition process at full speed in making throws to the second-base bag (figure 4.10).

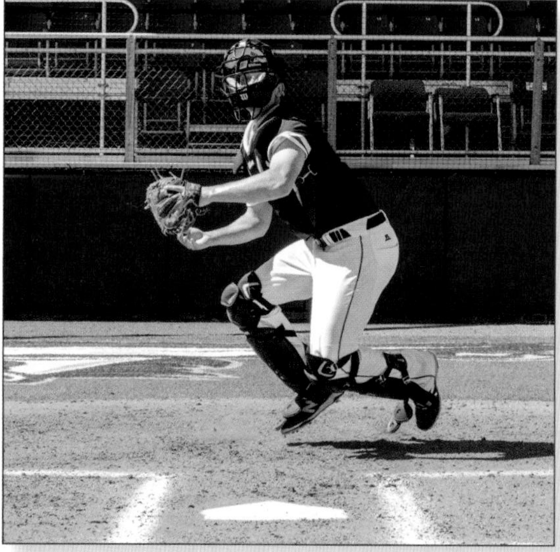

Figure 4.10 Full-speed transition and throw drill.

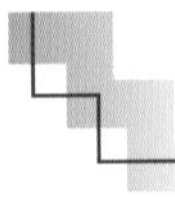

TO INCREASE DIFFICULTY

- Have a pitcher deliver the ball at full speed.
- Mix pitches.

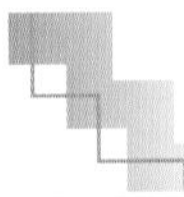

TO DECREASE DIFFICULTY

- Deliver the ball slower.
- Start with the ball in the mitt.

Success Check

- How was the timing and fluidity of the transition?
- What was the pop time?

Score Your Success

You earn 1 point for every throw with proper form that hits the target.

You earn 1/2 point for a throw that is on line but bounces.

You earn 0 points for an overthrow.

You earn 0 points for poor technique.

Your score ____ of 10

BLOCKING

Blocking is a skill that requires technique, athleticism, and toughness. Whenever there is a close play at home plate, meaning the ball and runner arrive at the plate at about the same time, the catcher will squat in front of the plate to "block" the runner's path. The catcher may not block the plate unless he already has possession of the baseball. When the catcher blocks the plate, the runner can either slide around the catcher to avoid being tagged out, or collide with the catcher in an attempt to make him drop the ball. Proper blocking technique (figure 4.11), along with drills to practice blocking, are covered here.

Figure 4.11 BLOCKING TECHNIQUE

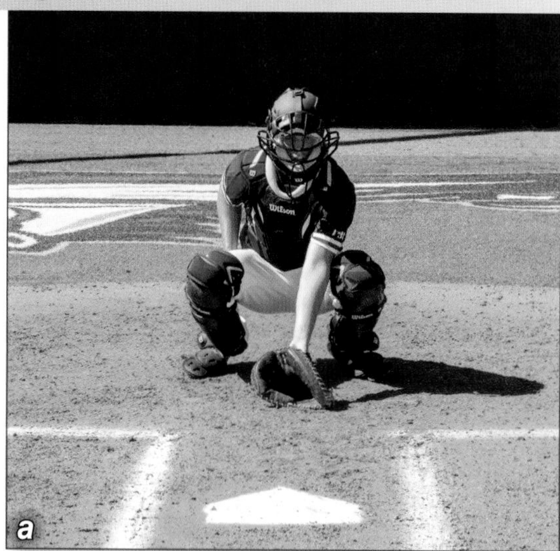

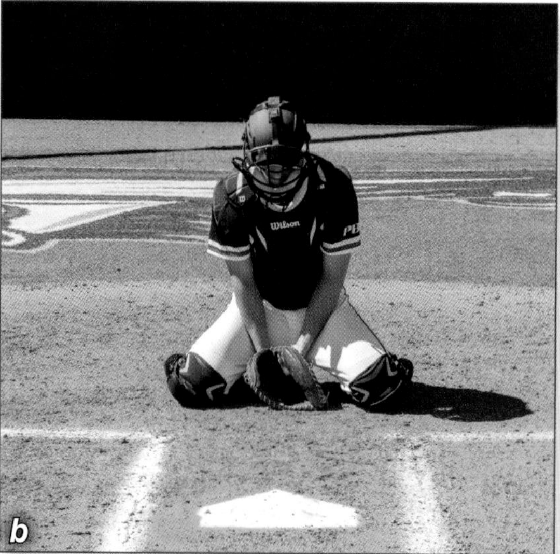

1. From either secondary position (figure 4.11*a*), the catcher drives the knees into the ground.
2. The glove should turn over so that it prevents the ball from going between the legs.
3. The throwing hand should be placed behind the glove.
4. The chin should be tucked into the chest.
5. The shoulders should roll forward, and the chest should be used to redirect the ball straight down (figure 4.11*b*).

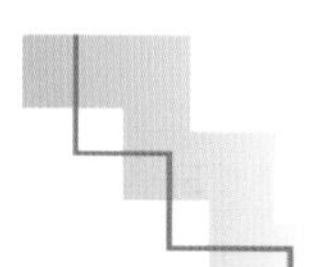

MISSTEP

Your chest is upright as the ball hits your body, causing the ball to be redirected to the side.

CORRECTION

Try to bury the ball into the ground.

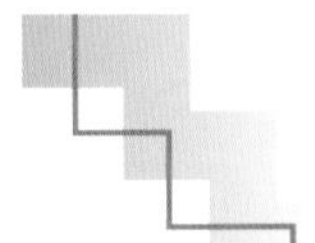

MISSTEP

You raise your glove and the ball goes between your legs.

CORRECTION

Lead with your glove first and let your body get in position behind it.

Blocking Drill 1 **Mental Toughness**

Blocking drills are well known and often thought of as a difficult part of the life of a catcher. The fact is that a catcher can practice technique only so much, and it will get him only so far when he is attempting to block a pitch. Mental toughness, focus, anticipation, and will are the primary factors that contribute to blocking. Therefore, the drills for developing this aspect of the game are directed at testing and strengthening the intangibles that make up the mentality of the catcher.

From the distance of 45 feet (14 m), the catcher is in the secondary position with runners on base. As the coach delivers the pitch, one of three things can happen.

The coach says, "Runner," as he throws, simulating a base runner attempting to steal second base. The catcher goes through the throwing transition, stopping at the power position and checking form.

1. The coach says nothing, and the pitch is delivered in the dirt, forcing the catcher to block the baseball.
2. The coach says nothing, and a pitch is delivered for the catcher to stick.

From this distance, the catcher must react to the pitch rather than guess and cheat (slightly move but not so much that it's noticed by the opposing team) toward one of the possible scenarios. This drill focuses on the mental toughness required to play the position.

Success Check

- Was the pitch handled properly, or did the catcher get caught guessing?
- Was the pitch handled with proper form and good timing?

Score Your Success

You earn 1 point for handling the pitch with proper form and good timing.

You earn 1/2 point if the timing is off but you still handled the pitch.

You earn 0 points for guessing wrong.

You earn −1 point if a dirt ball goes between your legs.

Your score ____ of 10

Blocking Drill 2 **Standard Blocking**

As with throwing down, the coach is 45 feet (14 m) in front of the plate, throwing dirt balls to the catcher (figure 4.12).

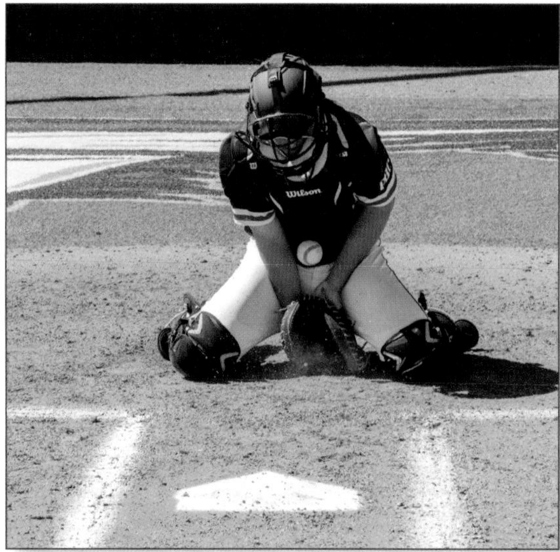

Figure 4.12 Standard blocking drill.

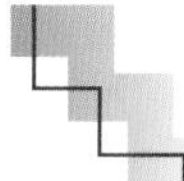

TO INCREASE DIFFICULTY

- Speed up the process with rapid-fire block and recover.
- Have two coaches hold five balls each. Have coach 1 stand 30 to 45 feet (9 to 14 m) away from the plate, angled at the first baseman. Have coach 2 at the same distance, angled at the third baseman. Starting with coach 1, the coaches alternately feed dirt balls from both sides of the field.

TO DECREASE DIFFICULTY

- Use a pitching machine to feed the balls to the catcher.
- Use tennis balls instead of baseballs.

Success Check

- Did the catcher get the glove down?
- Was the proper form reached in time, or was the chest up?
- Where was the ball redirected?

Score Your Success

You earn 1 point for every ball blocked in front with good form.

You earn 1/2 point if the ball is kept in front regardless of form.

You earn 0 points if the ball kicks beyond 10 feet (3 m) away.

You earn −1 point if the ball goes between the legs.

Your score ____ of 10

TAKING CHARGE

Catching has three primary technical areas to focus on—receiving, throwing, and blocking. Being competent in these areas is important, but more is required to be a great catcher. The catcher is the quarterback of the defense. As coaches, we look for intangibles in each catcher that go beyond technical ability. Baseball IQ is a key aspect of the position. Knowing the game goes a long way in communicating with the coaching staff about the opposing team. It is also necessary for communicating with the pitching staff and for directing defense during the course of a play. Vocalization goes hand in hand with knowledge of the game. A catcher who has confidence in what he's doing will be vocal and loud when communicating with the defense, establishing with the defense that he is in charge.

Another intangible is effort. A catcher who can put out effort daily, a high-energy guy who can control his emotions, is a catcher who will be a leader not only for the defense but also for the pitching staff. When a pitching staff has trust and confidence in the guy behind the plate, the entire team will reap benefits in the long run.

SUCCESS SUMMARY

Catching is not for the weak. It is a daily challenge of mental toughness and physical endurance. These drills are designed to develop and maintain the primary skills you need to play this position. How did you do?

Receiving Drills

1. Receiving bare-handed ____ out of 10
2. Receiving with mitt ____ out of 10

Transfer, Footwork, and Throwing Drills

1. Step-by-step transitioning ____ out of 20
2. Ball in glove with throw ____ out of 10
3. Full-speed transition and throw ____ out of 10

Blocking Drills

1. Mental toughness ____ out of 10
2. Standard blocking ____ out of 10

Total ____ **out of 80**

If you scored 65 or above, congratulations! You have taken the next step to success with your ability as the quarterback of the defense. If your score was less than 60, keep repeating the drills that are giving you trouble. Lower the difficulty as needed to ensure proper form, good timing, and a successful technique.

STEP

5

Hitting

The next step to success is hitting. Hitting a baseball is considered by many to be the single hardest skill to perform in all of professional sports. The act of hitting a baseball may appear simple, and it can be easy when the entire process is understood and performed at a high level. But the ability to develop consistency is extremely tough. The first thing you must understand is that as a hitter, you must define consistency as the ability to repeat your swing and make adjustments. Consistency should not be defined by results such as batting average, RBIs, home runs, or any other statistical measurement. Your statistics will reflect consistency in your swing and approach, not the other way around.

As you are probably aware, there are many different ways to hit a baseball. Throughout the game you will see many different batting stances, swings, finishes, and approaches. For us to elaborate on every factor would be impossible. Our goal in step 5 is to focus on several key elements within the stance, the swing, the finish, and the approach that all successful hitters have in common. Building on these key points, we will give you several drills to help you find a swing that works for you. So, grab your bat and let's begin!

BATTING GRIP AND STANCE

Baseball players use many different batting stances. The stance may be open or closed, wide or narrow, upright or crouched, and the hands might even be spread apart on the bat. Our goal in discussing the batting stance is to get you in a position that is comfortable for you. A proper grip allows the player to make contact with the bottom hand palm down and the top hand palm up (figures 5.1*a-b*). And by finding a comfortable stance, you can have a repeatable starting position to revert to when adjusting your swing (figure 5.1*c*).

Figure 5.1 **GRIP AND STANCE**

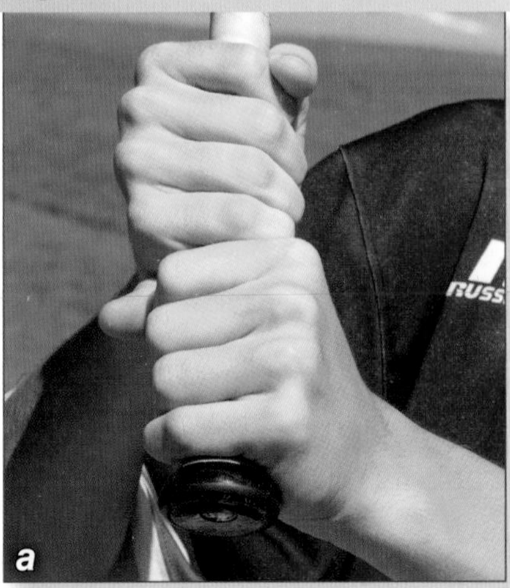

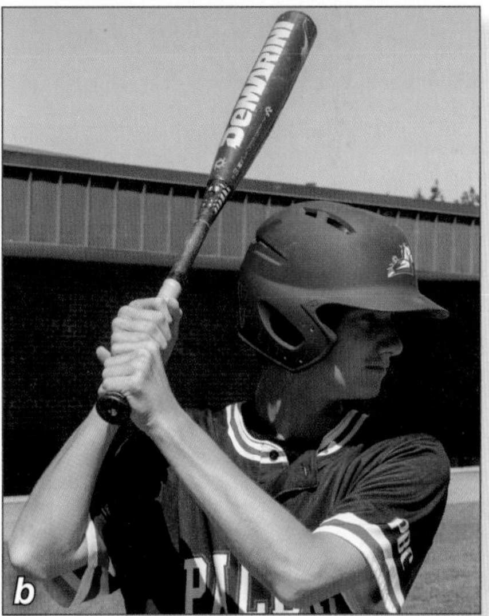

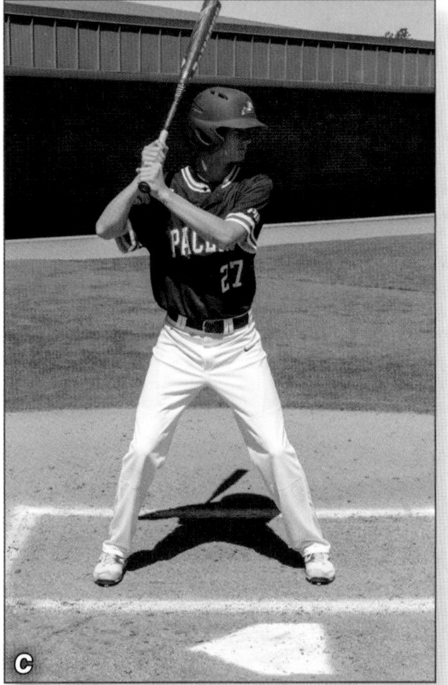

Grip

1. For left-handed hitters, the right hand should grip the bottom of the bat. For right-handed hitters, the left hand should grip the bottom of the bat.
2. The opposite hand grips the bat, stacking up next to the bottom hand.
3. Having the bottom hand over the knob or raised above the knob, that is, choked up, is a preference for each hitter.
4. The bottom hand should have a firm grip in the palm, and the top hand should be slightly flexed at the wrist and gripped to preference (figure 5.1*a*).

Hand placement

1. The hands should be in a comfortable position behind the head.
2. The front arm should be bent, not barred or straight out.
3. The back arm should be in position to control the barrel (figure 5.1*b*).

Lower body

1. For advanced players, feet placement will vary, but we recommend that the feet be placed perpendicular to the plate, slightly wider than shoulder-width.
2. The weight should be evenly distributed inside the two feet. The knees should be slightly bent in a comfortable, athletic position (figure 5.1*c*).

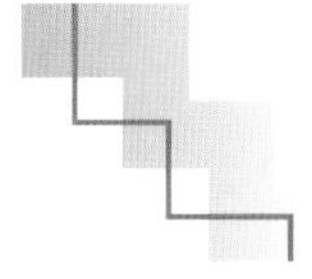

MISSTEP

Your grip should allow barrel control, meaning that you should be able to feel and control the movement of the barrel at all times. Lining up the knuckles so that the bat is held in the fingers or gripping the bat too tightly in the palms will cause you to lose feel of the barrel as the swing begins and lose control of the barrel as the bat nears the contact point.

CORRECTION

A good correction technique is to simulate gripping an axe while holding the bat. Now, flick the barrel in front of your body, keeping it parallel with the ground. A raised barrel shows that the grip is too deep in the palm, whereas a low barrel shows a grip that is too far in the fingers.

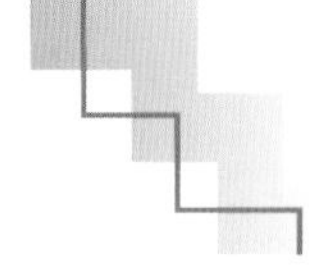

MISSTEP

We often hear coaches say, "Elbow up" or "Elbow down," but the placement of the elbow is simply a personal preference. The misstep that we often see is a lack of consistency in hand placement from swing to swing.

CORRECTION

You should have your hands in a position that allows complete barrel control, regardless of the position of your elbow. This position should be a consistent starting point for the load. Varying this starting position often means that you do not have complete barrel control in the swing. To correct this issue, repeat the stance, load, and swing during a soft toss or tee drill and video or take pictures from various angles. Often, if you can explain what you feel while pointing out specifics on video, you will be able to make corrections easier than when you are just being told what to do.

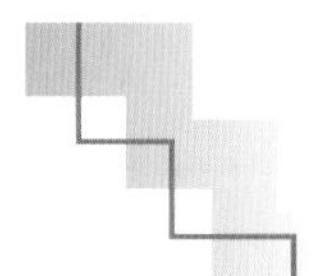

MISSTEP

Weight distribution can be an overlooked misstep when trying to make adjustments to the swing. If the weight is shifted outside the back foot, the ability to shift the weight forward during the swing will be compromised.

CORRECTION

The mental correction for weight distribution is always to keep the weight inside the feet. If too much weight is shifted over your back foot, you should reset. Video is a great tool to see this action if you cannot feel it.

SWING

Now that you are in a comfortable stance, let's diagnose the swing. Swings vary widely among baseball players, but several common traits are seen with all successful hitters. The swing consists of the load (figure 5.2*a*), the bat path and contact point (figure 5.2*b*), and the extension and finish (figure 5.2*c*).

Figure 5.2 THE SWING

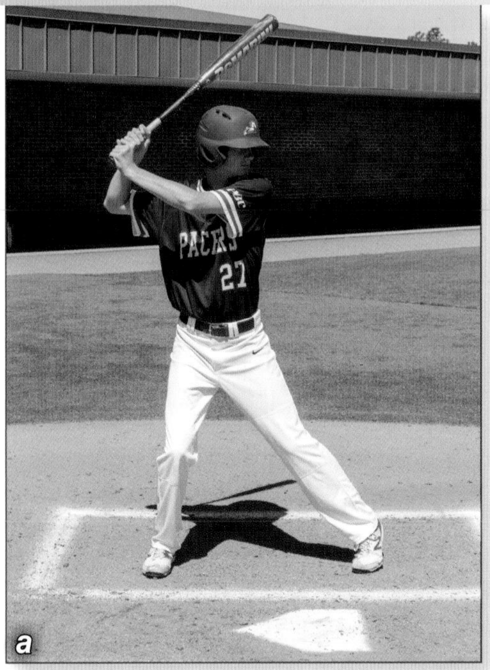

Load

1. The hands load by moving slightly backward but not fully extending the front arm.
2. The hands cock, allowing maximum feel and control of the barrel.
3. The weight shifts to the inside of the back foot as the hips cock slightly inward.
4. The front foot can raise, lift, or remain in place, depending on the preference of each hitter.
5. The head remains in the same position, but the chin tucks into the front shoulder as the hands load (figure 5.2*a*).

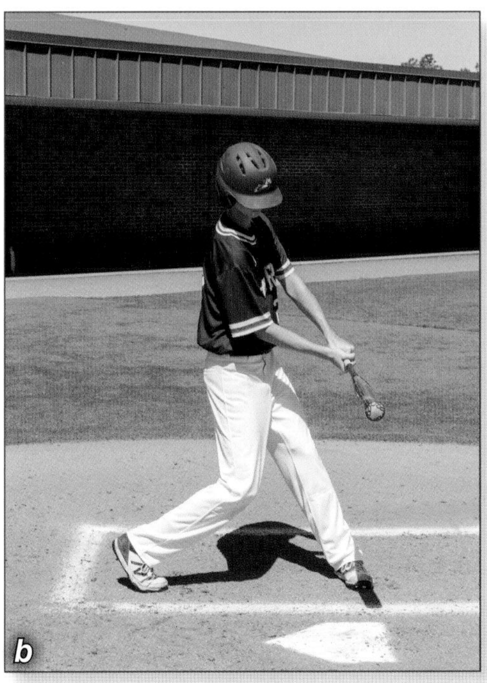

Bat Path and Contact Point

1. From the load, the eyes should track the ball out of the pitcher's hands, causing the chin to stay tucked.
2. As the front foot lands, the hands start the swing.
3. The hands drive the barrel from the load to the contact point as quickly as possible, attacking the inside of the baseball.
4. As the hands begin to drive the barrel, the hips rotate as the weight shifts from inside of the back foot to inside of the front foot.
5. The front leg is stiff and firm. This firm front side, along with the hip rotation, causes the energy from the weight transition to be expelled through the barrel at contact.
6. At the contact point, the back leg will be pivoted, creating an L-shape.
7. The back arm will be in the same shape with the hands in the palm up, palm down position.
8. The head, back shoulder, and knee should be centered between the feet (figure 5.2*b*).

(continued)

Figure 5.2 *(continued)*

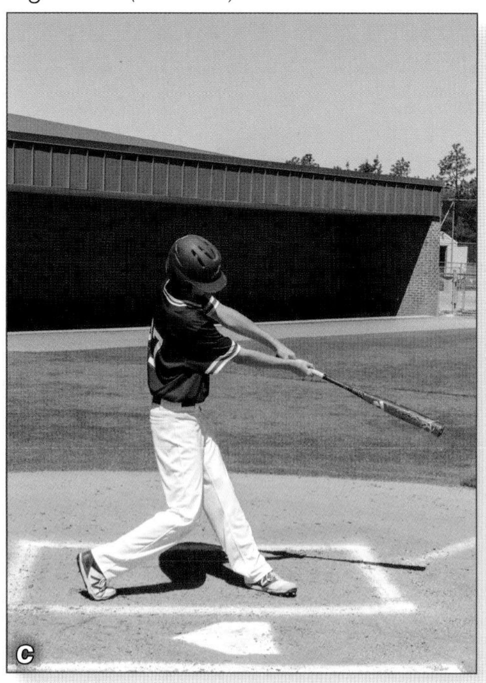

Extension and Finish

1. From the contact point extension, the hands should extend through the baseball.
2. The arms extend fully forward as the hips continue to rotate, in what is called the second extension. This action releases the maximum amount of energy through the baseball as it releases from the barrel.
3. As the ball leaves the bat, the shoulders continue to rotate. The top hand may release, depending on the height of the finish and the preference of the hitter (figure 5.2*c*).
4. If the head remains in the center of the body, the chin should be tucked into the back shoulder as the body finishes the rotation. This swivel action of the head allows the eyes to remain still throughout the swing, while also allowing more fluidity with the upper body.

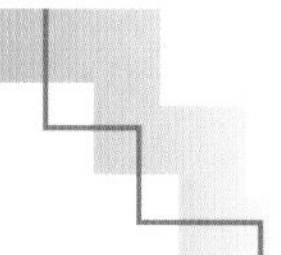

MISSTEP

Sometimes, your hands may overload, causing the barrel to fall, or wrap around your head. This causes the barrel to drag, creating a delay in getting to the contact point.

CORRECTION

Try to keep the barrel tall but do not allow the barrel to point back or too far forward. Keeping the barrel tall will give you maximum control as the swing begins, eliminating the wrap while speeding up your hands to the point of contact.

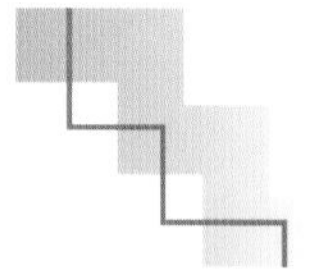

MISSTEP

We need to address a couple of missteps. First, the barrel needs to be on time. Lag in the barrel often results from a poor load. Second, this process revolves heavily around timing and rhythm. Poor timing or rhythm will cause inconsistency in the fluidity of the swing.

CORRECTION

Timing is a constant issue among players at every level. You must figure out timing mechanisms in your swing that you can use when you need to make adjustments. The more common timing mechanisms are the slot in which the hands load to, the height of the leg kick in the load, and the timing of when the front foot plants. These mechanisms are all triggers to begin your swing on time and in rhythm.

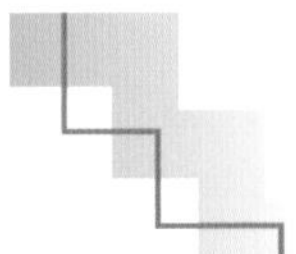

MISSTEP

If the head moves, such as a forward dive or a pull away from the body, the eyes will move as well. Moving your head in this way will give you the impression of additional ball movement. This head movement will also cause the entire swing to be flawed.

CORRECTION

Keeping your head in place is a difficult habit to establish. Tee drills and video feedback are good tools to use to establish this habit. The best mental approach to breaking the habit of moving your head is to focus on watching the ball hit the bat.

TRAINING THE SWING

The baseball swing is complex, to say the least. The swing is a mental and physical series of actions that must work through the total body in precise harmony. Training these actions can be done in a variety of ways such as tee drills, soft toss, front toss, and batting practice, all of which have multiple variations that cater to specific needs. Our approach for training the swing will remain consistent throughout these drills.

"Squaring up" the baseball, or perfect contact, can be defined as hitting the ball on the same trajectory as it was delivered. You will be hitting on a line straight through the pitcher's release point. With this in mind, the following drills are designed to create a repeatable swing so that you can consistently square up the ball at contact.

Each swing has a result called ball flight. The trajectory of the ball off the bat will help you determine the quality of the swing, giving you immediate feedback regarding flaws in your timing or mechanics. Using the ball flight as a tool, you should be able to make minor adjustments to correct the issue.

Hitting Drill 1 **Tee Work**

Tee drills eliminate the movement of the baseball. The object is to place the ball at the exact point where you want to make contact. From your batting stance, our first drill will have the ball placed at belt height, even with the front leg, and centered on the plate (figure 5.3). This contact point is the neutral reference for perfect contact, resulting in a line drive through the middle of the field. Take 10 swings, driving the ball through the center of the field.

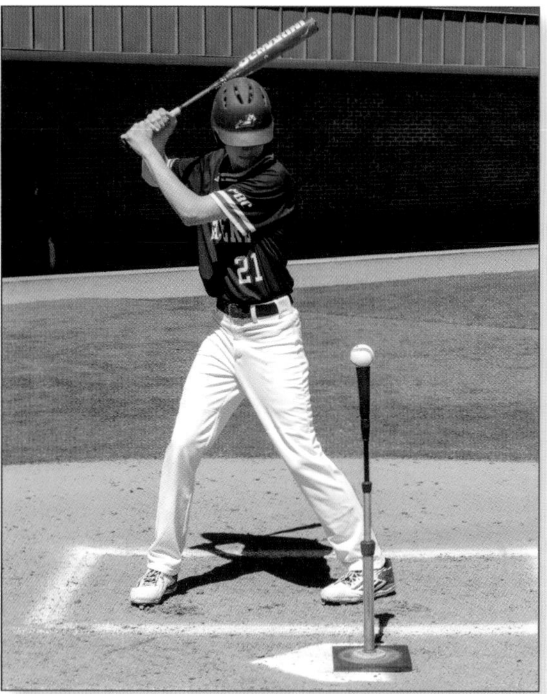

Figure 5.3 Tee work drill.

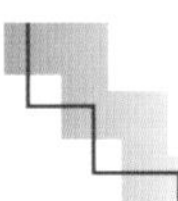

TO INCREASE DIFFICULTY

- The tee drill has many variations. Each variation focuses on certain skill elements that the hitter can single out. These variations are:
  - The outside or inside pitch
  - High tee or low tee
  - Blind swings
  - Step through and swing
  - Top hand or bottom hand swings with a smaller bat.

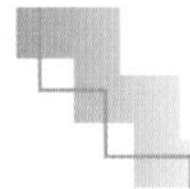

TO DECREASE DIFFICULTY

- Place the tee at a single contact point in the center of the plate.

Success Check

- What was the flight path of the ball after contact? Did it slice away from you? Did it topspin to the ground?
- What did you feel that was different when you squared up the ball versus when the ball had a different flight path?
- Were you able to make adjustments from swing to swing?
- Did your results remain consistent throughout the drill?

Score Your Success

You earn 1 point for every line drive between the second baseman and the shortstop.

You earn 1/2 point for a hard-hit ground ball in the same region.

You earn 0 points for a ball hit above 20 feet (6 m) or outside the given area.

Your score ____ of 10

Hitting Drill 2 **Soft Toss**

Soft toss adds the element of timing the body movement and the swing with the ball in flight. With a coach or partner on a knee in the opposite batter's box, have the hitter in the batting stance. The ball should be shown to the hitter. The coach lowers the ball, triggering the load of the hitter. The coach then raises the arm, flipping the ball to a given contact point, thus triggering the hitter to swing (figure 5.4). For this drill, let's take three rounds of eight swings.

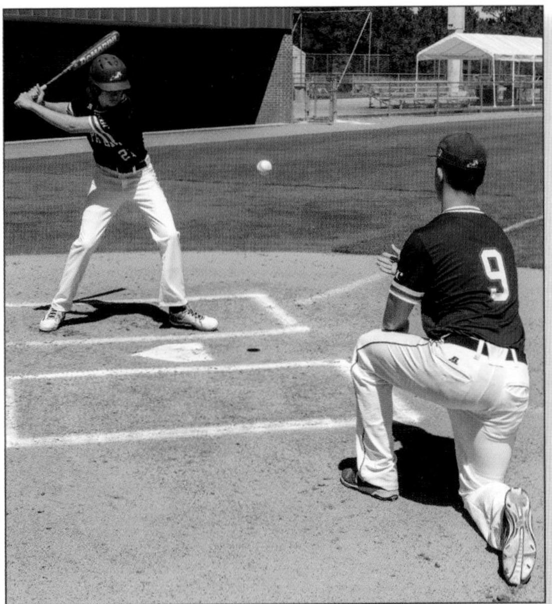

Figure 5.4 Soft toss drill.

(continued)

Hitting Drill 2 *(continued)*

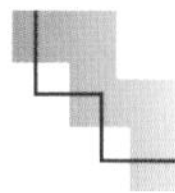

TO INCREASE DIFFICULTY

- Have the partner toss the ball from the catcher's box.
- Speed up the pace between flips.
- Challenge the hitter's various contact points (in, out, up, down).
- Use the top hand or bottom hand only with a smaller bat.

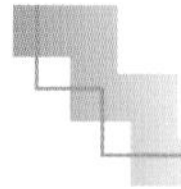

TO DECREASE DIFFICULTY

- Slow down the rhythm of the flip.
- Flip to the same spot every time.

Success Check

- The success checks remain virtually the same as those for the tee drills.
- Because the ball is in flight, your timing and rhythm may be affected.
- Can you still repeat your swing, getting successful results, as you did with the tee drill?

Score Your Success

You earn 1 point for every line drive between the second baseman and the shortstop.

You earn 1/2 point for a hard-hit ground ball in the same region.

You earn 0 points for a ball hit above 20 feet (6 m) or outside the given area.

Round 1 ____ of 8

Round 2 ____ of 8

Round 3 ____ of 8

Your score ____ of 24

Hitting Drill 3 **Front Toss**

Front toss is the next variation of soft toss. It is done from 20 to 30 feet (6 to 9 m) in front of a hitter with the coach behind a screen (figure 5.5). The flips should give the hitter a better perspective of a ball traveling from the pitcher, only at reduced speed. This slower pace allows the hitter to get his timing mechanisms within the swing in sync. It also gives a more realistic result of the flight path of the ball given the angle of the drill. For this drill, let's take three rounds of eight swings.

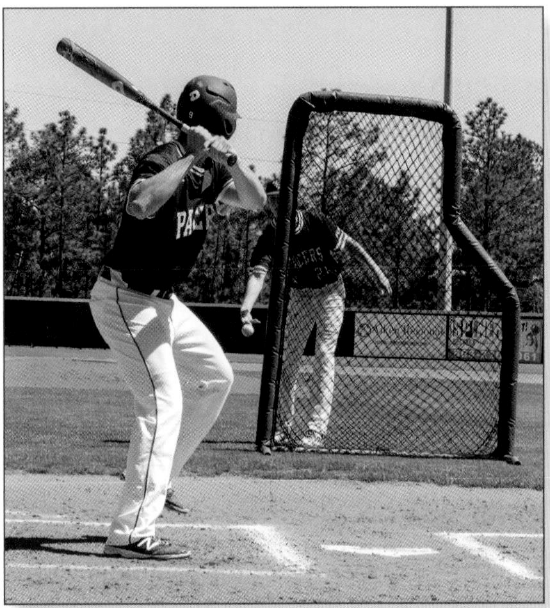

Figure 5.5 Front toss drill.

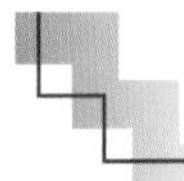

TO INCREASE DIFFICULTY

- The drill can also be done at an angle toward the opposite field, forcing the hitter to keep the front side from rotating too soon.
- Instead of flipping the ball underhand, the coach can bounce the ball into the zone, creating another timing element for the hitter to overcome. This variation teaches the hitter to keep the hands back, or barrel control.
- The speed at which the ball is flipped can be varied pitch to pitch.

Success Check

- Did you consistently square up the baseball?
- What adjustments do you find yourself making pitch to pitch?

Score Your Success

You earn 1 point for every line drive between the second baseman and the shortstop.

You earn 1/2 point for a hard-hit ground ball in the same region.

You earn 0 points given for a ball hit above 20 feet (6 m) or outside the given area.

Round 1 ____ of 8

Round 2 ____ of 8

Round 3 ____ of 8

Your score ____ of 24

Hitting Drill 4 **Standard Batting Practice**

Batting practice (BP) is done with a coach throwing from behind a screen at a preferred distance between the mound and the plate. We could write an entire book about the many variations on BP. The standard BP is done by the coach throwing balls into the hitter's strike zone. The pitches should be firm yet at a rate that allows the hitter to focus on his timing. Throwing harder or softer may seem like the obvious way to change the difficulty, but the goal is to get the hitter to repeat his swing and consistently find the barrel at contact. For this drill, let's take four rounds of eight swings.

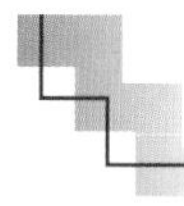

TO INCREASE DIFFICULTY

- Focus the BP round on the hitter's weaknesses with the strike zone.
- Change the area where the ball should be hit, regardless of pitch location.
- Mix in a round of breaking balls.

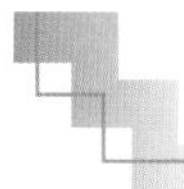

TO DECREASE DIFFICULTY

- Shorten the distance that the coach is throwing from so that the ball can be thrown to a specific spot.
- Throw to the hitter's strengths so that he can reiterate the proper swing before increasing the difficulty.

Success Check

- Did you consistently square up the baseball?
- What adjustments do you find yourself making pitch to pitch?
- What adjustments did you make round to round?

Score Your Success

You earn 1 point for every hard-hit line drive or ground ball.

You earn 1/2 point for a hard-hit fly ball.

You earn 0 points for a pop-up.

Round 1 ____ of 8

Round 2 ____ of 8

Round 3 ____ of 8

Round 4 ____ of 8

Your score ____ of 32

BUNTING

Bunting is an integral part of every offense. No matter what team you are playing on or what your skill level is, you must be able to perform a sacrifice bunt successfully. Figure 5.6 describes the best techniques to execute a sacrifice bunt.

Figure 5.6 **BUNTING TECHNIQUE**

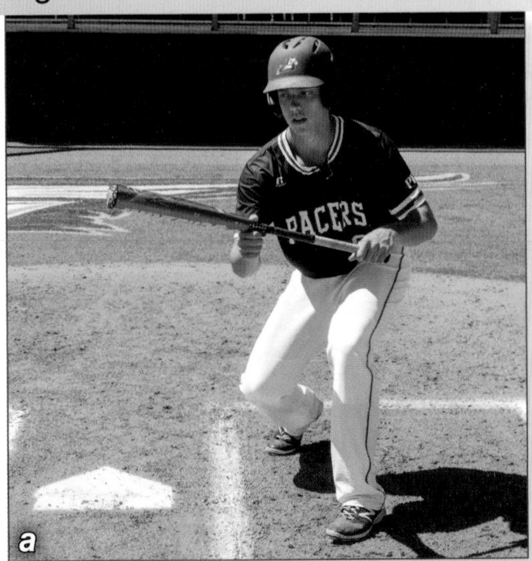

a

Grip and Hand Placement

1. The top hand should be down the barrel of the bat and holding the bat at its balance point between the pointer finger and thumb.
2. The bat should be pinched so that no fingers are around the bat.
3. The bottom hand should be positioned slightly up from the knob and used as a pivot point to direct the bunt.
4. Make sure to hold the bat out away from your body and keep the barrel of the bat above the knob to ensure that you bunt the ball to the ground rather than up in the air (figure 5.6*a*).

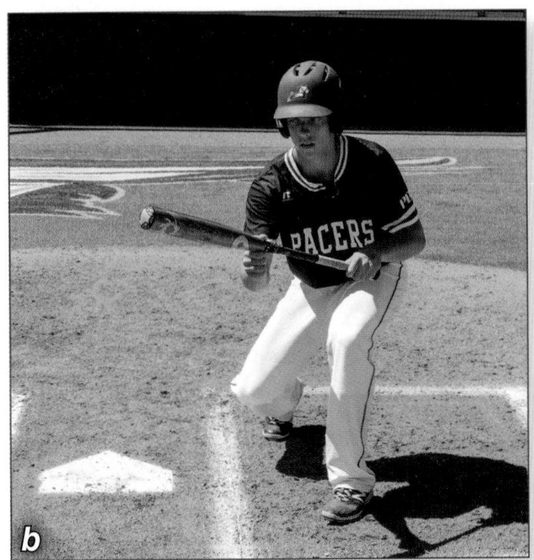

b

Lower Body

1. During a sacrifice bunt, the lower body should be much like it is in the normal batting stance.
2. The only thing that changes is that both feet are turned so that the toes are facing the pitcher and the batter's center of gravity is lowered.
3. The feet should remain close to parallel so that you are in an athletic stance and able to move in case the pitch is thrown at you (figure 5.6*b*).

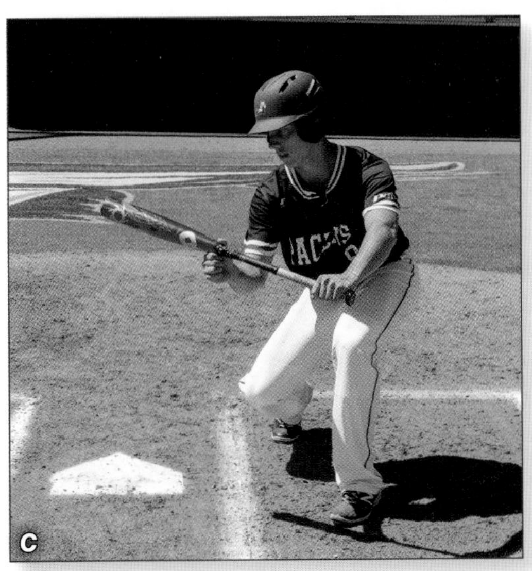

c

Contact Point

1. When you bunt the ball, you want the barrel of the bat out in front of the plate to ensure that you will place the ball in fair territory.
2. You also want to make contact with the ball out in front of your body so that you can use your arms to soften the bunt and not hit the ball too hard.
3. You should start in the front of the batter's box with the barrel of the bat at the top of the strike zone. This positioning allows you to determine quickly whether the pitch is going to be a strike; if it is above your bat, it is clearly a ball (figure 5.6*c*).

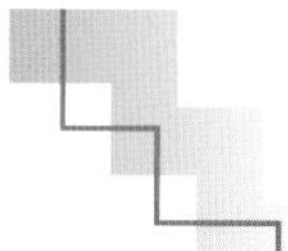

MISSTEP

Your top hand is either too far up or down the bat, making the bat unbalanced in your hands.

CORRECTION

Make sure that the top hand is at the balance point of the bat so that the bat could be held perpendicular to the ground with only one hand.

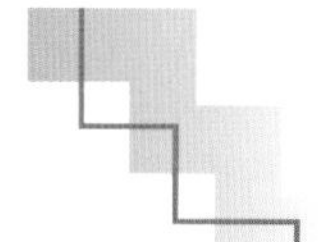

MISSTEP

The feet are shoulder-width apart facing the pitcher (square to the pitcher).

CORRECTION

Make sure that your feet are parallel so that you can easily move to avoid being hit by an errant pitch.

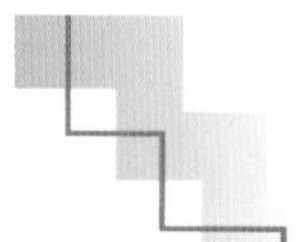

MISSTEP

Balls are being bunted into foul territory.

CORRECTION

Make sure that you are standing in the front of the batter's box and that the barrel is in front of the plate. This positioning gives you the maximum amount of area to get the sacrifice bunt down in fair territory.

HAVE AN APPROACH

The mental approach to hitting is arguably as important as the mechanics of the swing. At the higher levels, where players are capable of repeating their swing and making proper adjustments, the mental approach is vital to taking the next step to success. Looking back at the drills we have discussed, each drill should be done with a more specific purpose as you begin to grow and learn as a hitter. For instance, as you advance to higher levels, the pitching will become more advanced as well. Therefore, pitches will be located more consistently in zones that are more difficult to hit. Knowing this, your drills should focus on hitting balls in these zones.

You should have a purpose for each swing you take. You should mentally prepare yourself before each swing, before each round, and before each day so that you take quality swings. Each swing taken without a purpose creates bad habits. Given the amount of body movement and timing required for each swing, lack of mental focus and bad preparation will create bad habits that can knock you off the steps to success.

SUCCESS SUMMARY

Hitting a baseball is not easy. It never will be. These drills are designed as a foundation for you to use to find your swing and your adjustments. To be honest, the number of repetitions that we have suggested is not even the bare minimum of what college and pro hitters do daily, but they do give you a way to grade yourself in regard to repeating your swing. This foundation will not only help you develop into a successful hitter but also will allow you to coach yourself based on your honest results and your feel of your swing.

Hitting Drills

1. Tee work	____ of 10
2. Soft toss	____ of 24
3. Front toss	____of 24
4. Standard batting practice	____ of 32
Total	____ **out of 90**

If you scored 70 or above, congratulations! You have taken the next step to success with your ability to hit the baseball. If your score was less than 60, keep repeating the drills that are giving you trouble. Lower the difficulty as needed to ensure proper form, good timing, and successful technique.

STEP

6

Baserunning

Chapters 1 through 5 covered individual skills and drills to help each player develop his game. As we transition into the second half of our steps to success, we begin looking at the game from a team perspective. Although baserunning is an individual skill, it is often taught in a team setting. Therefore, we begin looking at our drill sets both in a team format and in the way in which they can be used in a practice.

Chapter 6 begins with the finish of the swing. The transition of hitter into base runner happens as soon as the ball leaves the bat. Therefore, the first topic we will discuss is getting out of the batter's box and running down the first-base line. From there, we look at getting a lead, stealing bases, sliding, and situational baserunning.

Running the bases is often an overlooked, undercoached part of the game that can cost an unprepared team significantly. Those who take the practice time to focus on baserunning often see more success in their offensive production. In this chapter, our goal is to demonstrate proper baserunning techniques and show you how they can be implemented in a practice setting. So, get your legs loose, and let's begin!

GETTING OUT OF THE BATTER'S BOX

Running the bases properly requires the player to give maximum effort while remaining under control. Remaining under control means that the runner must understand the situation, anticipate what will happen, and know where the ball is at all times. Being a base runner begins as soon as the ball leaves the hitter's bat. With that in mind, we begin with the process of running from home plate to first base (figure 6.1). We'll then cover making turns around the base (figure 6.2) and extra-base hits (figure 6.3).

Figure 6.1 RUNNING THROUGH FIRST BASE

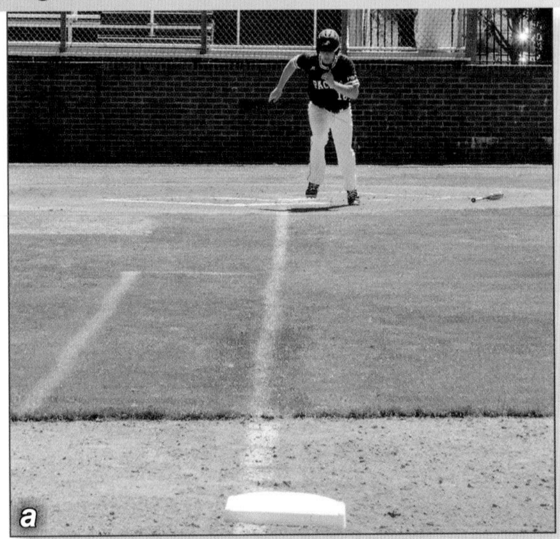
a

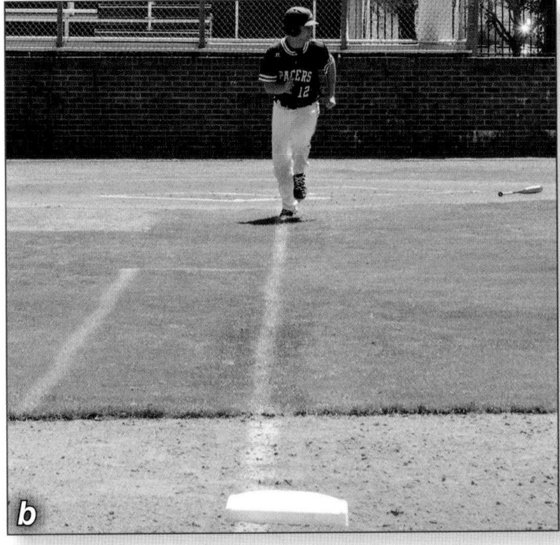
b

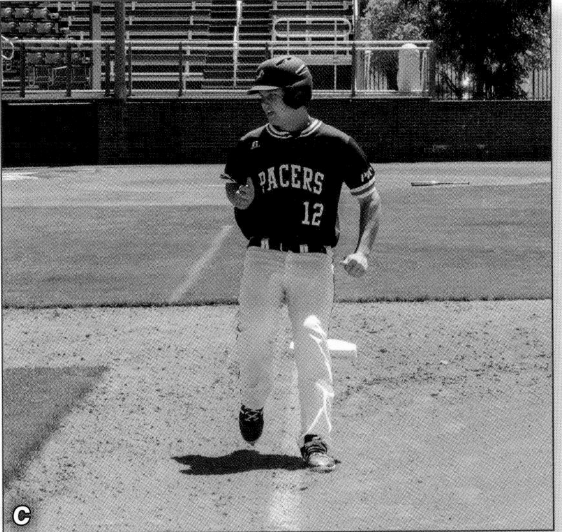
c

1. After hitting the ball, the hitter should drop the bat (figure 6.1*a*). The hitter is now a base runner.
2. The runner should run as hard as possible toward first base.
3. At the 30-foot (9 m) mark, the runner should glance to see whether the defender fielded the ball cleanly (figure 6.1*b*).
4. The runner's stride should not change as he approaches the bag.
5. The runner should step on the front of the bag, in stride, and continue full speed through first base.
6. After two strides past the bag, the runner should break down into an athletic position and look right to check for an overthrow (figure 6.1*c*).

Figure 6.2 MAKING A TURN

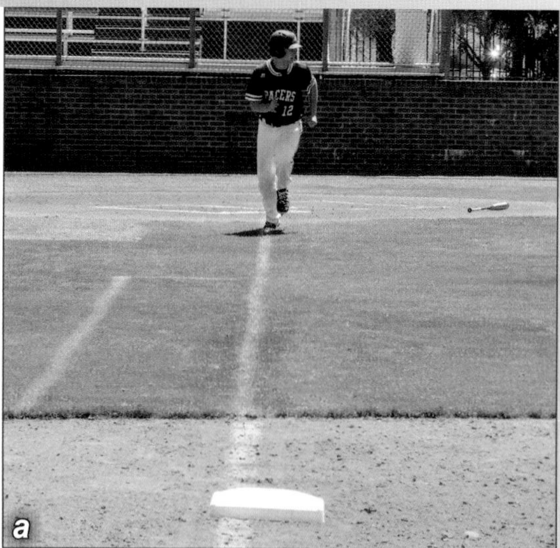

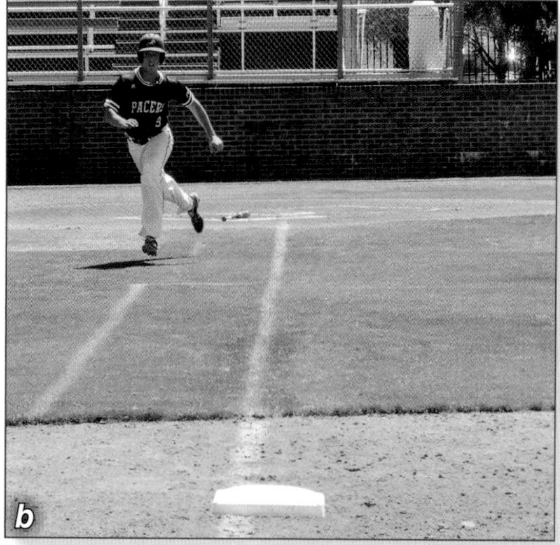

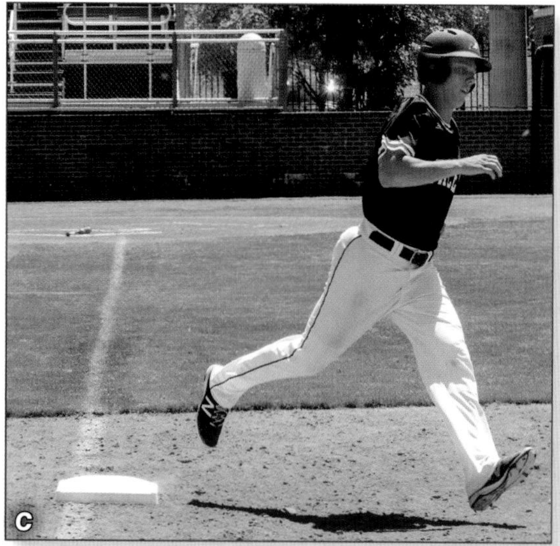

1. After the ball is hit, the runner should sprint toward first base.
2. At the halfway point, the runner should look to find the baseball (figure 6.2*a*).
3. After finding the ball, the runner should be slightly past halfway to first base. At this point, he will begin to take a turn to round the bag (figure 6.2*b*). This turn is often referred to as the banana because of the shape of the turn being made.
4. The runner peels away from the line and then lowers his left shoulder as he approaches the bag.
5. The runner should hit the inside of the bag with the left foot, which drives him toward second base.
6. He should make several hard steps toward second while reading the outfielder and the throw back to the infield (figure 6.2*c*).
7. After making the read, the runner should turn and hustle back to the first-base bag.

Figure 6.3 **EXTRA-BASE HIT**

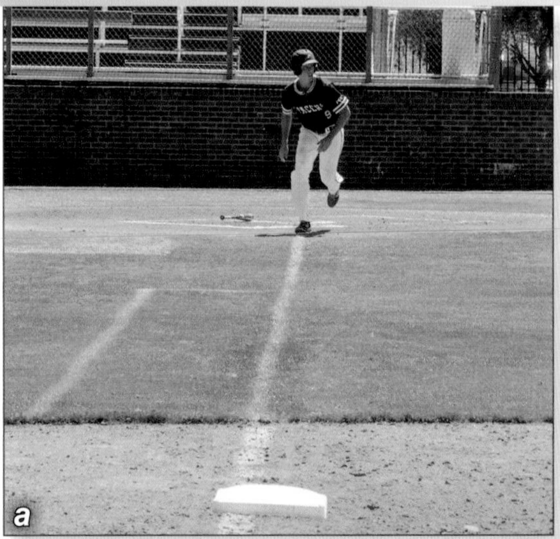

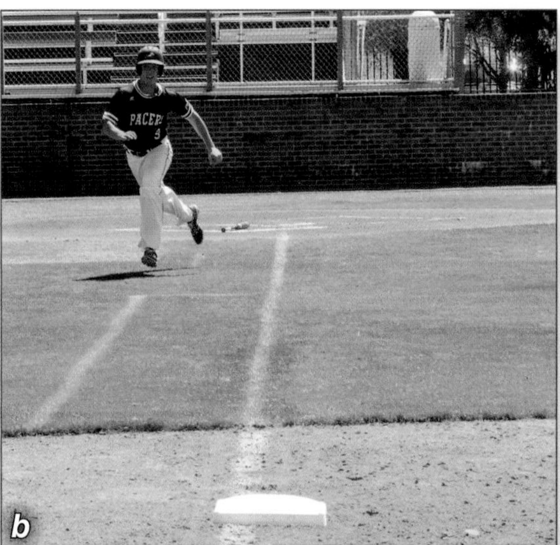

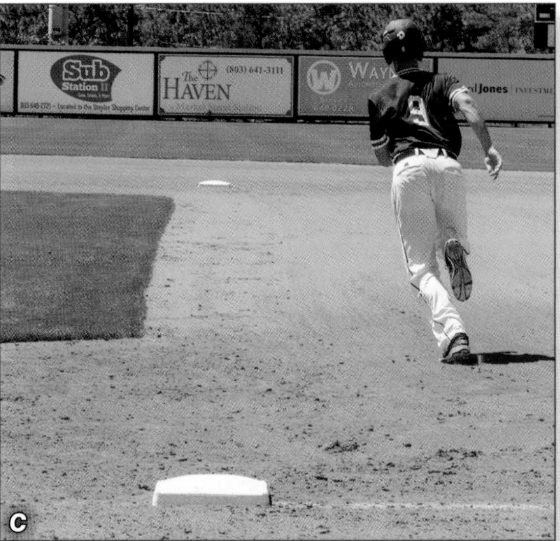

1. The runner makes the same banana turn that he made in the previous step (figure 6.3*a-b*).
2. After the runner hits the bag, he should be in full stride toward second base (figure 6.3*c*).
3. At the halfway point to second base, the runner should be aware of the location of the baseball.
4. If the ball is being thrown to second, he should be prepared to slide into the base. If the ball is not thrown to second, the runner should pick up the third-base coach for further instruction.

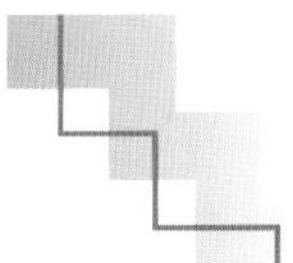

MISSTEP

Breaking stride to step on the bag properly will slow you down, as will lunging at the bag.

CORRECTION

Run full speed straight through the bag, stepping on the front part of the base. Do not slow down until you are several steps past the base.

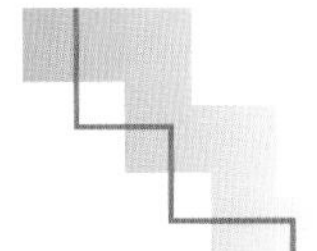

MISSTEP

A common mistake is lack of hustle down the line on a single. This habit will lead to a nonaggressive turn and the inability to advance to second on a slight error by the defense.

CORRECTION

The first-base coach should always be giving the runner direction. Lack of hustle is a mental mistake that should not be tolerated and should be corrected as soon as possible. You should always be mentally prepared to advance to second base, holding up only if the defense forces you back to the bag.

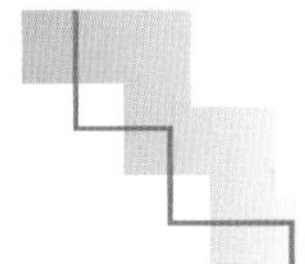

MISSTEP

Taking too wide a turn around the bag will cause a delay in getting to second base.

CORRECTION

You should focus on making a sharp turn around first base and getting in line with second as soon as possible without losing stride.

Baserunning Drill 1 **Getting Out of the Box**

The first baserunning drill involves the communication between the first-base coach and the base runner. With the team lined up at home plate, each player takes a turn simulating hitting the ball and running to first. Without a ball actually in play, the first-base coach is the guide for the runner. The instructions should be for the runner to run straight through the base, take a turn, or run out a double. This drill tests the player's ability to get instruction while at full speed and builds communication and trust between player and coach. For this drill, each player completes five repetitions.

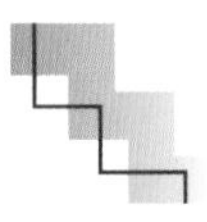

TO INCREASE DIFFICULTY

- The drill can be done using a live defense with a coach throwing batting practice.

TO DECREASE DIFFICULTY

- The drill can be done one at a time (i.e., all repetitions running straight through the base).

Success Check

- Each player should be graded on hustle and technique.
- Be sure that the runners are hitting the front of the base, taking hard turns, and challenging themselves on turn angles for doubles.
- Timing each runner is a good way to give immediate feedback.

Score Your Success

You earn 1 point for running full speed and giving maximum effort in each repetition. (You should never earn less than 5 points in five reps.)

You earn 1 point for every successful touch of the inside or front part of the bag while remaining in stride.

You earn 1/2 point for chopping steps on approach.

You earn 1/2 point for a wide turn around first base.

You earn 0 points for lunging to the bag.

You earn 0 points for not stepping on the front of the bag.

You earn 0 points if you do not break down and look right when running straight through.

Your score ____ of 10

LEADING OFF

Getting a lead may seem like part of the game that doesn't need to be coached or practiced, but each step in the process is vital to putting the base runner in proper position when the pitcher comes set. In all honesty, leading off is one of the most practiced aspects of every championship team at the collegiate level, and it should be part of your daily routine. A good lead can be the difference between advancing the base runner and an out. Here, we'll discuss leads at first (figure 6.4), leads at second (figure 6.5), and leads at third (figure 6.6).

Figure 6.4 **LEADS AT FIRST BASE**

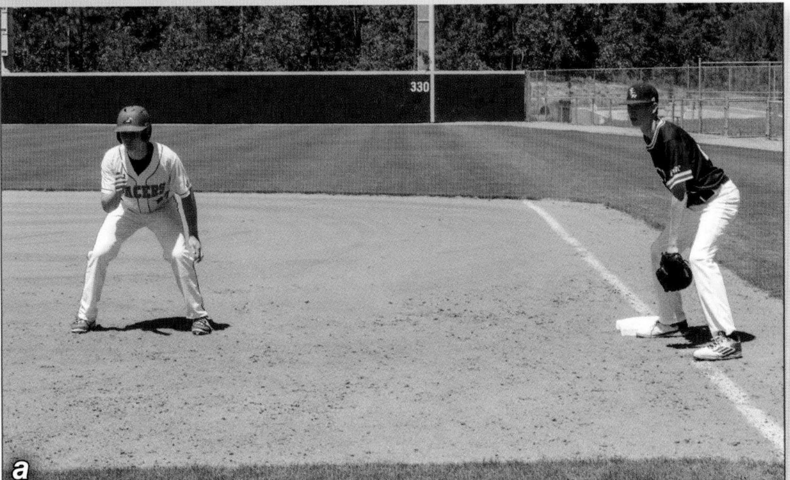

(continued)

Figure 6.4 *(continued)*

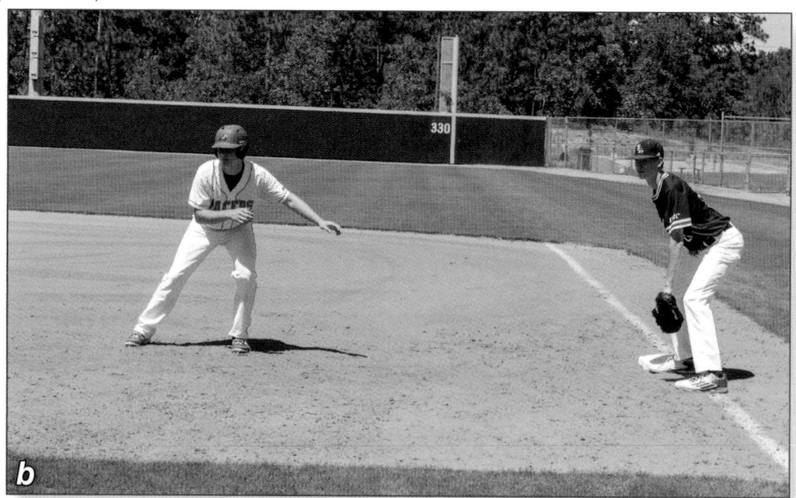

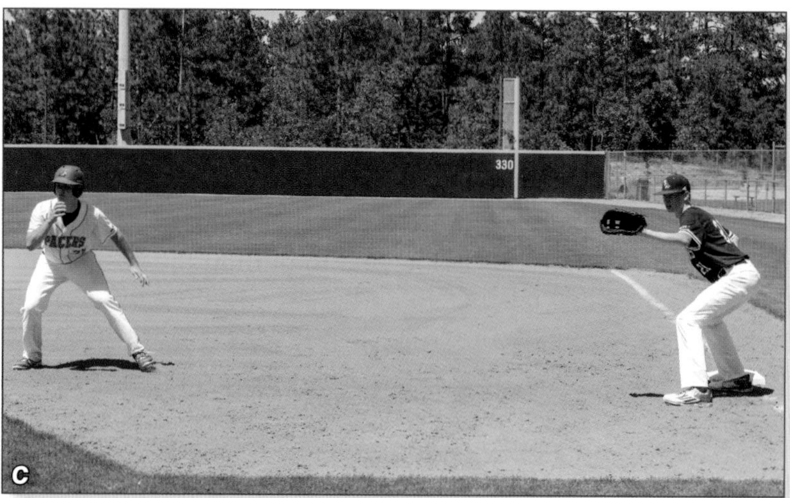

1. The player should stand facing second base with his heels on the bag.
2. The player should take two or three steps toward second, turn in line with the base path, and add one or two shuffles. He should be at a comfortable distance so he can turn and dive back into first base on a pickoff—that is, when the pitcher or catcher throws to an infielder at an occupied base to try to get the base runner out.
3. When he is at this distance, the runner should get into an athletic position with the feet spread one and one-half times shoulder-width. His hips should be low, and his head should be centered over the body (figure 6.4*a*).
4. If the runner is not stealing, he should be in a one-way lead, meaning that his weight should be shifted slightly toward first base as he anticipates a pickoff (figure 6.4*b*).
5. After the pitcher delivers the ball, the runner takes a secondary lead by shuffling twice toward second base and reading the action of the ball (figure 6.4*c*).
6. As the ball enters the zone, the runner's weight should be neutral, allowing him to break either way, depending on the outcome of the pitch.

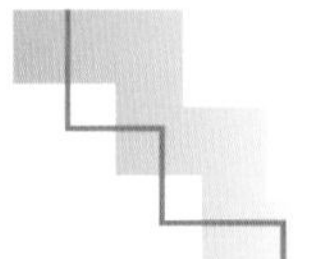

MISSTEP

Leading off too far or not far enough is common among those who do not practice baserunning enough.

CORRECTION

Find a lead that is comfortable by taking a step and a dive back into the bag. For the slower player, this lead may be shorter than the lead of those who are a little quicker.

Figure 6.5 LEADS AT SECOND BASE

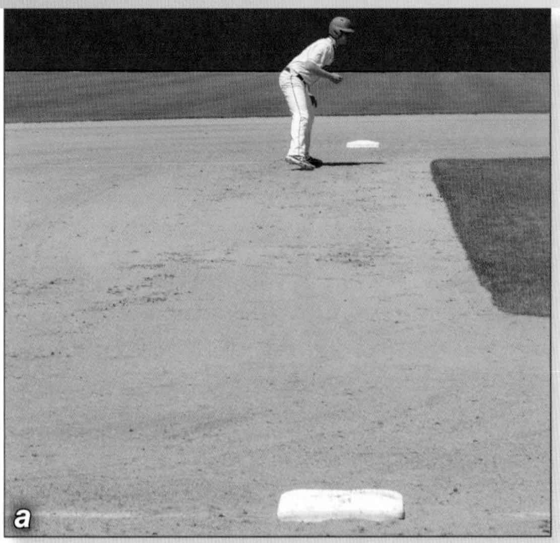

a

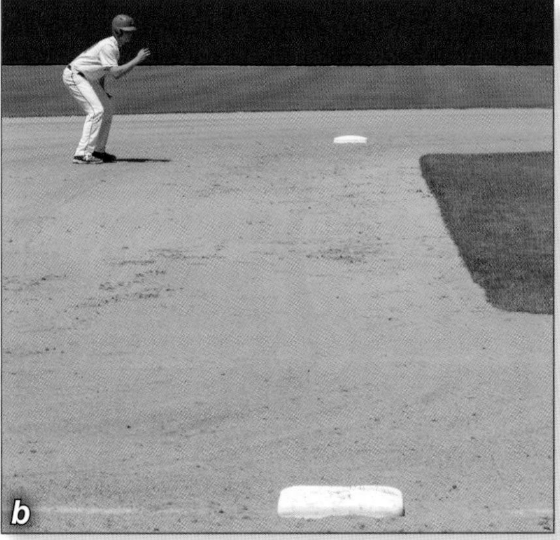

b

1. As with leads at first, the runner should remain in the baseline when getting the lead (figure 6.5*a*).
2. The lead at second base can be another step or shuffle bigger than the lead at first base because the runner will have more time to retreat on a pickoff than he will at first.
3. Some runners prefer to start a step or two behind the base path in the primary lead (figure 6.5*b*) and work into or parallel with the base path in the secondary lead. This approach is a coaching preference and is used to cut down the turn at third base if the runner is to score.

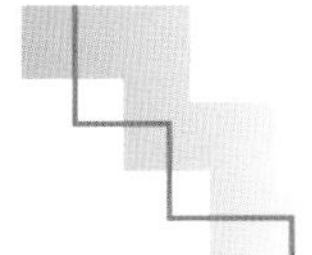

MISSTEP

Be cautious of getting too deep in the primary lead, which may open a window for a pickoff move from the pitcher.

CORRECTION

We recommend staying as close to the baseline as possible.

Figure 6.6 **LEADS AT THIRD BASE**

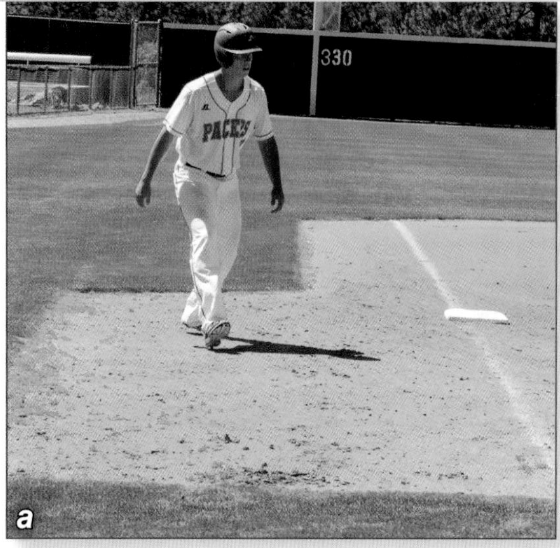

a

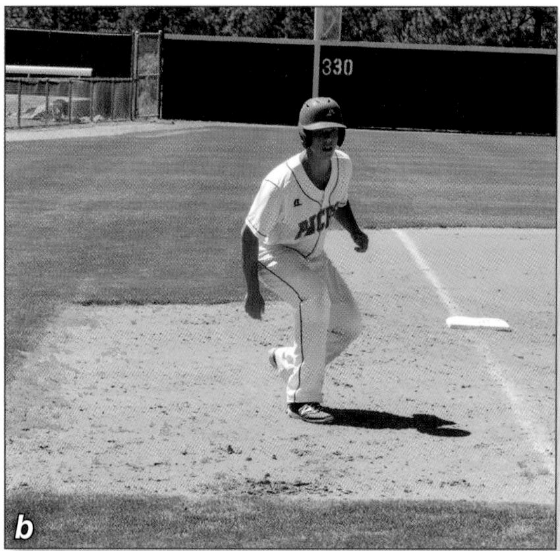

b

1. The lead at third is similar to the lead at second, given the fact that the third baseman will not be holding the runner on as the first baseman would.
2. When the pitcher delivers the ball, the runner should walk down the line instead of shuffling (figure 6.6*a*). This way, the runner does not advance too far off the bag in the event the catcher throws behind him.
3. As the pitch gets into the zone, the runner should be angled with the weight balanced and the right foot in front of the left (figure 6.6*b*).

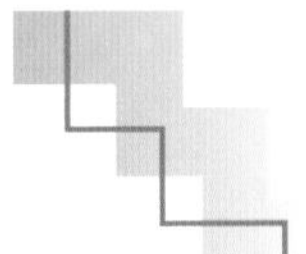

MISSTEP

If you square your shoulders to the catcher, retreating will be difficult if the catcher throws to third.

CORRECTION

You should remain balanced and always ready to get back to the bag.

Baserunning Drill 2 **Leads and Reads**

Next, here is a useful team drill can be done during batting practice. Have runners at each base, rotating after each repetition. The coach simulates a pitcher coming set and either delivering the pitch or picking off. The runners work on their leads and their ability to get back on a pickoff. Each player should go through five repetitions at each base.

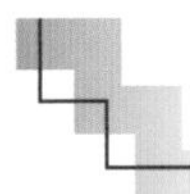

TO INCREASE DIFFICULTY

- Mix picks and pitches.
- Change tempo between pitches.

TO DECREASE DIFFICULTY

- Focus only on the pick or the pitch.
- Use the same technique each time so that the runner can become familiar with what to look for.

Success Check

- Did the runner get a quality lead?
- Was anyone picked off?
- Did the runner take a good, balanced secondary?

Score Your Success

You earn 1 point for every successful lead and read at each base.

You earn 0 points if you are picked off.

Your first-base score ____ of 5

Your second-base score ____ of 5

Your third-base score ____ of 15

Your total score ____ of 15

THE ART OF STEALING BASES

Stealing bases is more an art of technique than a skill based only on speed. Our next section focuses on the technique of stealing second (figure 6.7) and third (figure 6.8), giving the runner the ability to use tools other than pure speed. Granted, speed is a factor in stealing bases, but the average runner can use these techniques to gain an extra step or two.

When facing a right-handed pitcher, the runner can use a timing mechanism by counting the seconds that the pitcher holds in the set position. If the pitcher holds the set position for the same amount of time for every pitch, the runner can take advantage by breaking to second as the pitcher begins his delivery.

The runner also needs to be aware of the time the pitcher takes to deliver the baseball to the plate. From the beginning of the delivery to the reception of the pitch by the catcher, the time should be around 1.3 seconds. Anything quicker than 1.3 seconds will make stealing second base more difficult. By combining this time with the catcher's pop time, the runner will have a good idea of how long he has to get the bag. For instance, a catcher pop of 2.0 seconds with a pitcher's time of 1.3 allows 3.3 seconds to steal the base. Doing this is difficult for the average runner. Knowing this, what is your time from break to bag? How long do you need to steal the base?

Figure 6.7 **STEALING SECOND**

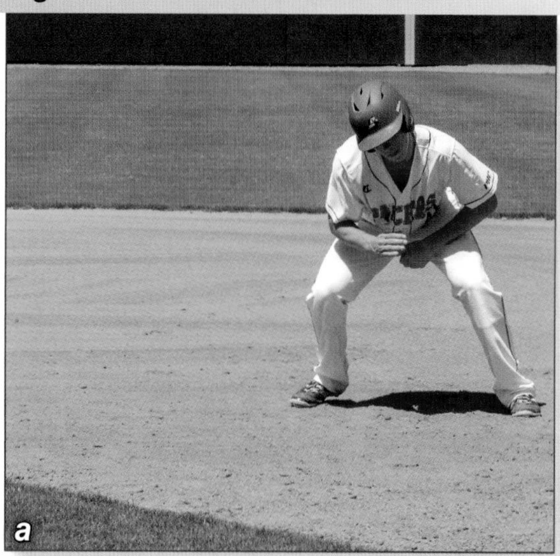

1. From the primary lead at first base, the runner's weight should be balanced (figure 6.7*a*).
2. With a right-handed pitcher, the runner should focus on the back heel. If the back heel lifts from the set position, the pitcher will be picking off, triggering the runner to get back to first.

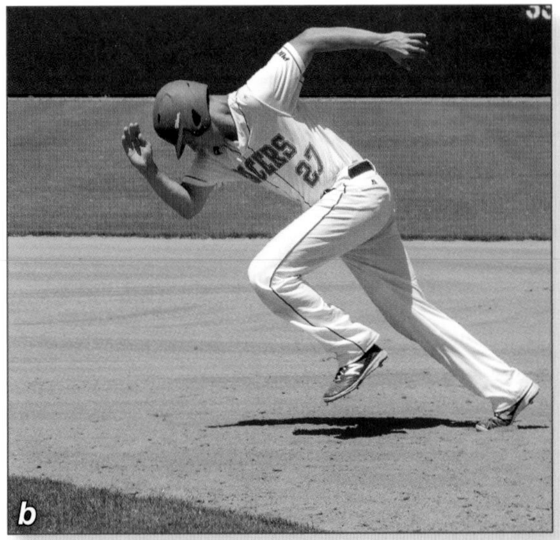

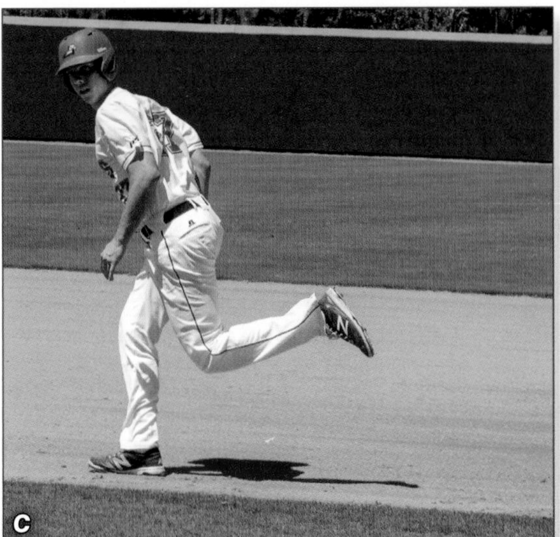

3. If the front foot lifts, the runner should use a crossover step and explode the lower body and hips toward second base. The head should stay level, not rising up (figure 6.7*b*).
4. With a left-handed pitcher, the runner often steals on the first movement of the pitcher from the set position, again using the crossover step.
5. After the runner takes several steps, he should peek in to see whether the hitter swings and makes contact or the catcher receives the pitch (figure 6.7*c*).

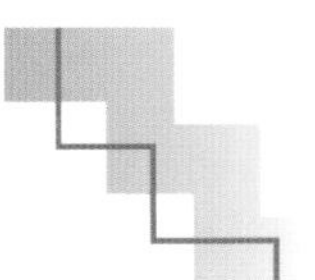

MISSTEP

If the runner gets a bigger lead or changes his body when he is about to steal, the defense often signals the pitcher to pick or step off.

CORRECTION

Always get the same lead so that you do not tip off your attempt to steal.

Figure 6.8 STEALING THIRD

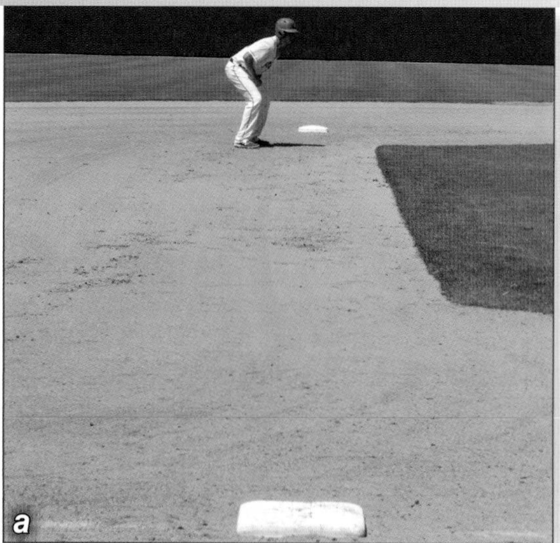

a

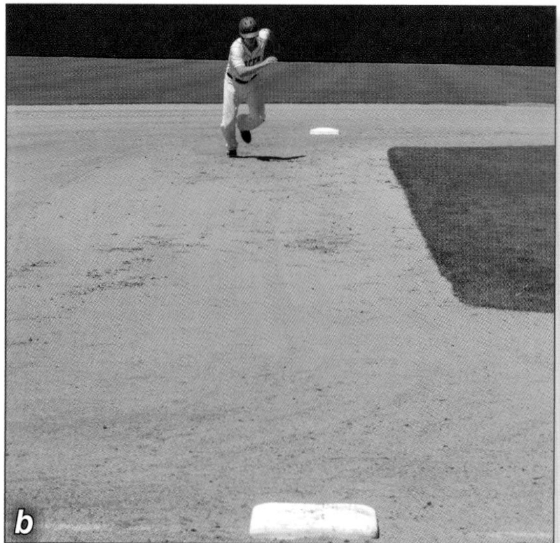

b

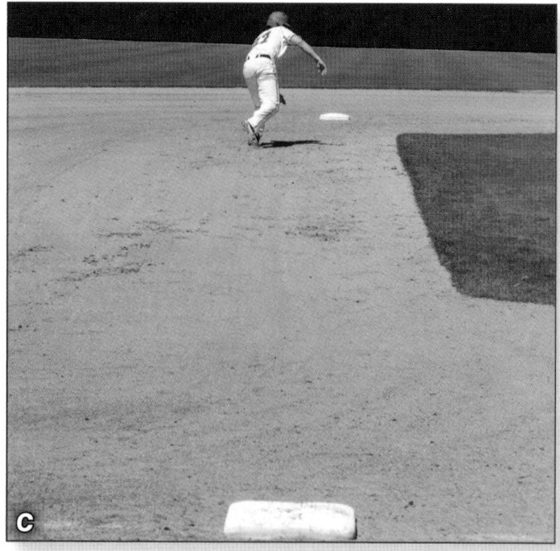

c

1. From the primary lead at second, the runner should be in the baseline (figure 6.8*a*).
2. As the pitcher sets, the runner watches the head of the pitcher. If the pitcher looks back, the runner keeps his feet still. As the pitcher looks home, the runner slowly creeps toward third.
3. Pitchers usually get in rhythm with looks to second. For a pitcher who always looks twice, the runner should hold his ground until the second look.
4. As the pitcher's head turns to home, after the given number of looks he usually takes (two looks in this scenario), the runner takes a big shuffle toward third. If the pitcher lifts to deliver home, the runner breaks from the shuffle into a steal (figure 6.8*b*).
5. If the pitcher does not deliver, the shuffle allows the runner to break down and retreat to the bag (figure 6.8*c*).

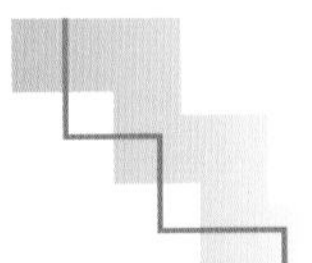

MISSTEP

If you attempt to steal from a standstill, an average throw will often catch you.

CORRECTION

Your feet must be moving and you must time the delivery on breaking to third.

Baserunning Drill 3 **Stealing Second and Third**

A good drill for working on stealing second is to have a coach or pitcher on the mound. Have your base runners at first and second. Each runner gets five steal breaks from each base. The pitcher alternately holds runners at first and then second. Have the pitcher simulate game speed, occasionally mixing in pickoffs at each base. The base runners should work on timing and a good crossover step.

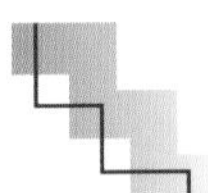

TO INCREASE DIFFICULTY

- Have a pitcher and defense playing live.

TO DECREASE DIFFICULTY

- Have a coach act as the pitcher.
- Work at a slower tempo and talk through what should be happening.

Success Check

- Could you time the pitcher's delivery?
- Did you get picked off?
- Were you conscious about keeping your leads the same?

Score Your Success

You earn 1 point for every successful steal break.

You earn 1/2 point if you had the proper lead but did not get a good jump.

You earn 0 points if you are picked off.

Your first-base score ____ of 5

Your second-base score ____ of 5

Your total score ____ of 10

SLIDING

Many young players consider sliding fun, although parents seem to disagree when they've spent countless hours trying to get red clay out of white pants. We should probably save that conversation for another book. Sliding is fun. It's a rush. The downside is that many players are not taught how to slide correctly. Let's look at the various ways to slide and the circumstances in which each should be used (see figures 6.9 and 6.10).

Figure 6.9 SLIDING FEETFIRST

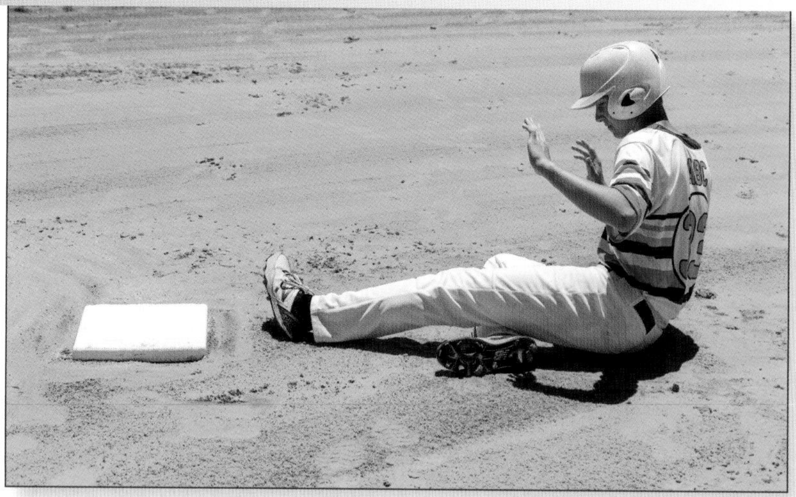

1. The runner should be running at full speed toward the base.
2. As the runner gets within 15 feet (5 m), he should be preparing to slide.
3. When the runner gets 5 to 10 feet (1.5 to 3 m) from the base, he slides with one foot extended toward the base.
4. The other foot should bend to an L-shape under the extended leg.
5. The weight of the body should land on the bent leg and buttocks.
6. The extended foot should touch the base and continue over the top. The bent leg stops the runner. For a pop-up slide, the extended foot should plant into the front of the base, and the runner can use the momentum to stand back up.

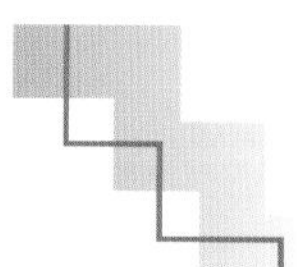

MISSTEP

You slide on the extended leg, which opens up the body to the baseball.

CORRECTION

Sliding on the bent leg protects the front of the body from the ball while allowing you to see an overthrow from the infield.

Figure 6.10 **SLIDING HEADFIRST**

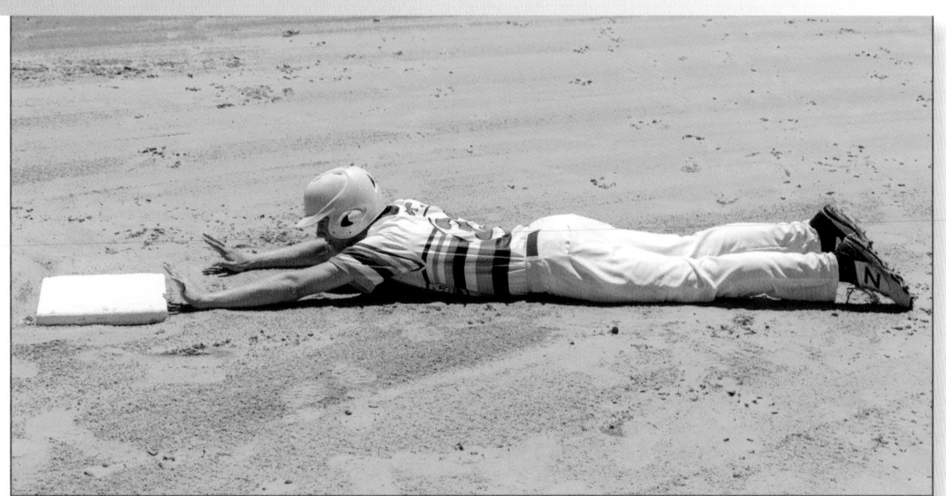

1. Players should usually slide headfirst only when diving back into a base, but base runners can use the headfirst slide at their discretion.
2. Two rules apply to sliding headfirst: (1) Never slide headfirst into home and (2) never slide headfirst when running to first base.
3. When diving into a base, remember to keep the palm up so that the fingers do not jam into the base.
4. Always keep the head up when sliding headfirst.

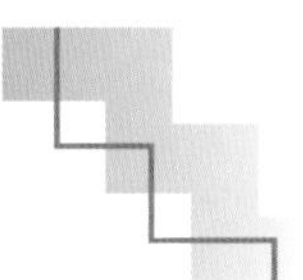

MISSTEP

Diving headfirst into home puts you at high risk of injury if contact is made with the catcher.

CORRECTION

Always use caution when sliding into a base; go feetfirst when possible.

Baserunning Drill 4 **Sliding**

A favorite drill for players is the slip and slide. Place a 15- to 25-foot-long (5 to 8 m) piece of plastic on a grass surface and wet it with a water hose and perhaps some baby oil. At the end of the plastic, you can use a throw-down base. Let the runners take turns running full speed and sliding on the plastic into the base (figure 6.11). Have them do five reps sliding feetfirst and five sliding headfirst.

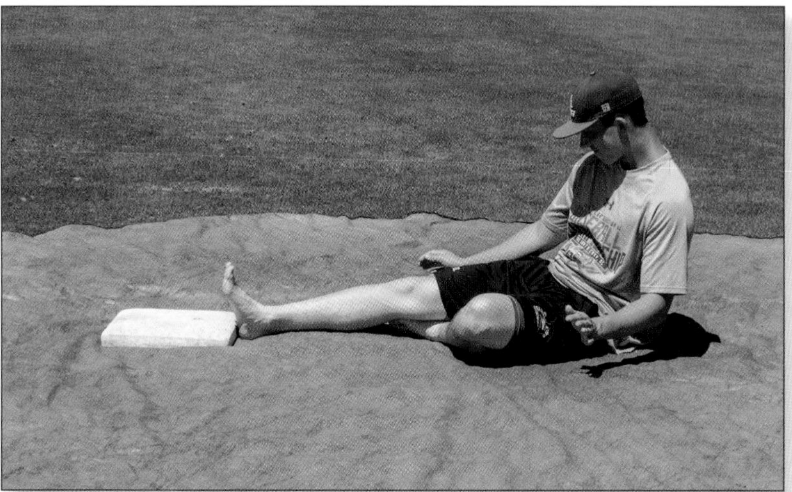

Figure 6.11 Sliding drill.

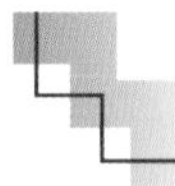

TO INCREASE DIFFICULTY

- Instead of sliding on the slip and slide, use the actual infield.

Success Check

- Did the player slide on the extended leg?
- Did the player dive with the head and palms up?

Score Your Success

You earn 1 point for every slide using the correct technique.

You earn 0 points for sliding on the wrong leg.

Your score ____ of 10

SUCCESS SUMMARY

As you move forward in your steps to success, we will take another look at baserunning in step 10, building on the foundation we have set in this chapter. We will discuss situational offense, giving us the proper setting to discuss tagging up, taking the extra base, being a trail runner, and applying baserunning to hit and runs, moving runners, and scoring. You need to have the right techniques built into your skill set from this chapter so that you can move forward in your next step to success.

Baserunning Drills

1.	Getting out of the box	____ out of 10
2.	Leads and reads	____ out of 15
3.	Stealing second and third	____ out of 10
4.	Sliding	____ out of 10
	Total	____ **out of 45**

If your score is greater than 40 points, you have taken the next step to success. If you have a score of less than 40, you likely had trouble with a minor part of your game that you can easily correct with more repetitions. Keep up the hard work and get ready to take your next step to success!

STEP 7

Playing the Infield

In the first six steps to success, we discussed the fundamentals of being a baseball player. In the next two steps to success, you will apply the fundamental skills you have developed as we begin to concentrate on the specific duties of each position on the field. Step 7 focuses on playing the infield. In this section, we break down the key elements of playing first base, second base, shortstop, and third base.

Our goal for the remaining steps to success is to show you how to use your skills within a team concept. By doing this, you will continue to enhance your baseball IQ, which was our mission from step 1. Again, baseball is an individual sport played within a team concept, so you need to understand individual responsibilities when playing team defense.

Every infielder must understand a few key points—rules of thumb, so to speak. The first point is to get an out. The main objective of playing defense is to get three outs, so when an out presents itself, take it. This rule leads to our next point, which is to make the routine plays. Now that you have made it to step 7, fielding a ground ball right at you should be routine because of the number of repetitions you did. Often, routine plays turn into errors because of a lack of concentration. We consider these errors mental mistakes. An infielder, especially the shortstop, should not make mental mistakes when it comes to team defense.

Building on the mental aspect of playing the infield, every infielder needs to know the situation. With every ball put in play, each defender has a specific responsibility. Each defender must know what he is supposed to do if the ball is hit to him and where he must be if it is not. Knowing the situation encompasses all aspects of the game, such as the inning, the score, the number of outs, the count, the hitter's and pitcher's tendencies, the speed of the hitter and base runners, where the base runners are located, and so on. All of these factors combined control how the defense should react as a unit to each situation. Therefore, the first element of the defense affected by the situation is the prepitch positioning of each defender.

PREPITCH POSITIONING

Prepitch positioning is standard among infielders at every level, although some may vary their positioning based on personal reasons such as lateral range and comfort, or even in-game situations that demand a defensive adjustment. The following is a look at the standard placements for every infielder in a variety of situations (figures 7.1-7.3).

Figure 7.1 STANDARD DEPTH

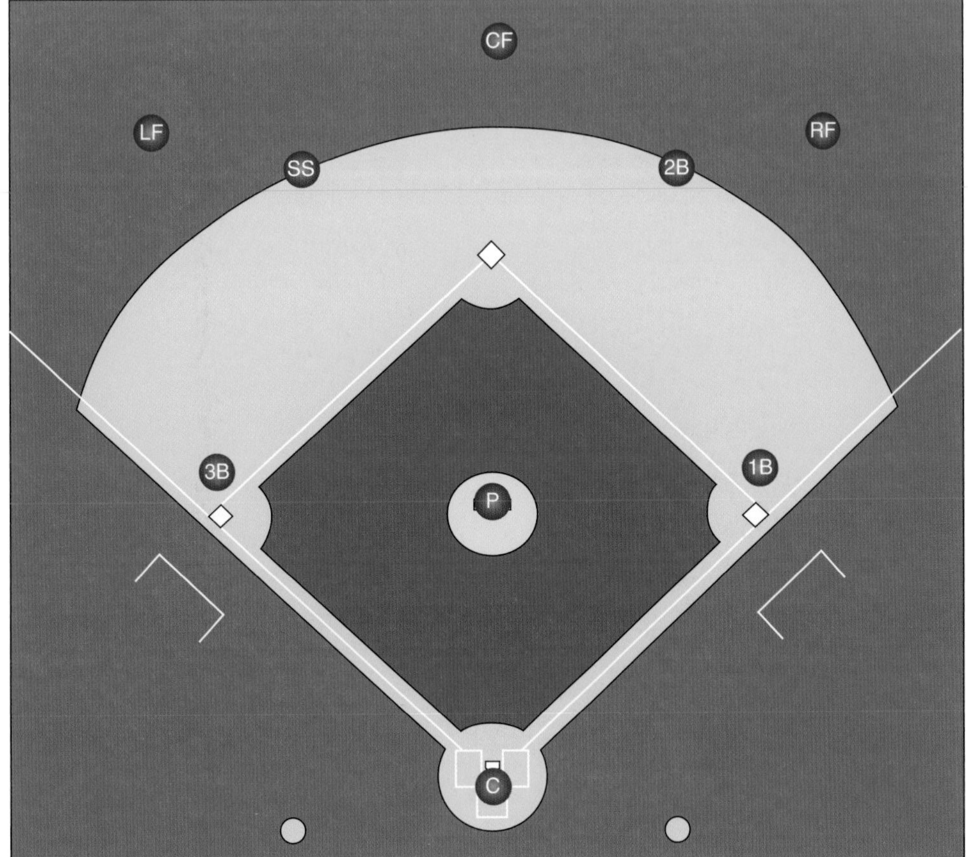

1. The first baseman and third baseman will be at a depth even with the base and 10 to 15 feet (3 to 4.5 m) off the line.
2. The shortstop and second baseman will be positioned on the back edge of the infield, approximately a third of the distance of the baseline away from the second-base bag.
3. Depending on game variables, the infielders may shift their positioning slightly in any direction.
4. The infielders may also choose to shift slightly in any direction for personal preference or field conditions.

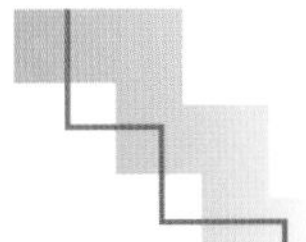

MISSTEP

Not knowing the situation can lead to poor positioning. One example of this would be when a fast runner who has a tendency to bunt for a hit is at bat and the corner infielders (the first baseman and the third baseman) remain at standard depth.

CORRECTION

Communicating with other infielders and coaches should help you shift according to each situation.

Figure 7.2 **DOUBLE-PLAY DEPTH**

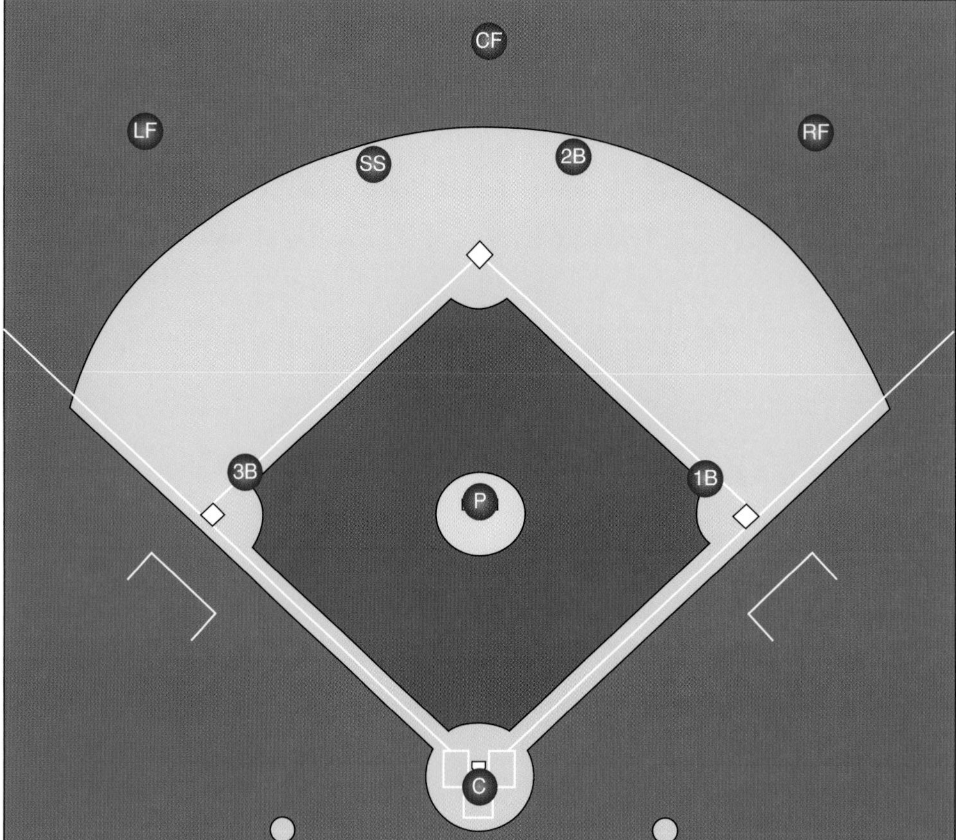

1. With a runner on first base or with runners on first and third, the first baseman will be holding the runner on base. With runners on first and second or with the bases loaded, the first baseman will be at standard depth.
2. The third baseman will be at standard depth.
3. The middle infielders will be positioned closer to the second-base bag than they are when at standard depth, approximately 15 to 20 feet (4.5 to 6 m) away from the base, but at the same angle.

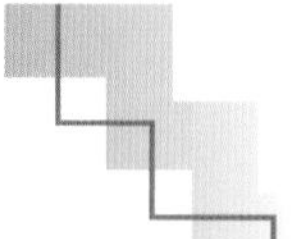

MISSTEP

Depending on the situation, the middle infielders must communicate to each other who is covering second base. Coverage miscommunication by middle infielders gives away potential outs and usually places one or both players out of position.

CORRECTION

You are responsible for knowing your assignment. To ensure that all players are on the same page, continuous communication is imperative.

Figure 7.3 **INFIELD IN**

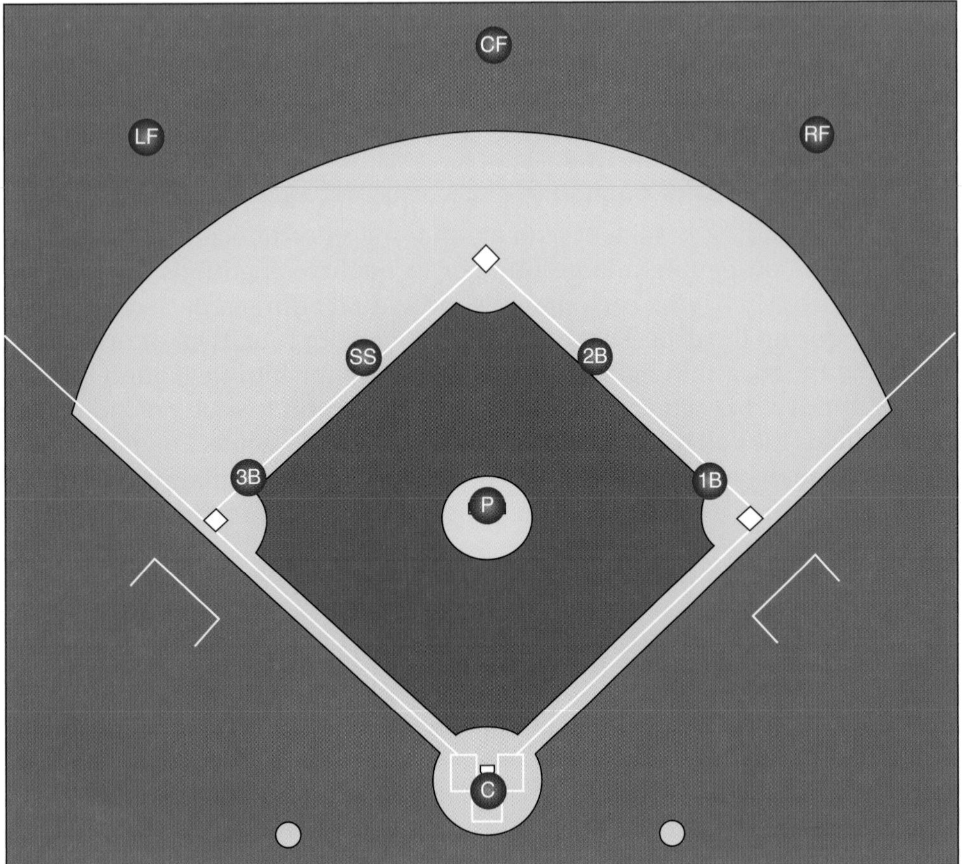

1. When trying to stop a runner on third base from scoring on a routine ground ball, the four infielders will be positioned on the front edge of the infield.
2. The corner infielders should be several feet (a meter or so) in front of the baseline. The middle infielders shift over, pinching the gaps between the first baseman and second baseman and between the shortstop and third baseman.

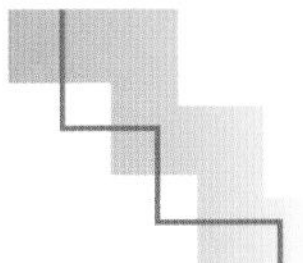

MISSTEP

If the gaps between fielders are not pinched, the hitter has a better chance of hitting a ground ball through the infield.

CORRECTION

The distance between the corner infielders and the middle infielders on each side should be a step and a dive away from the midpoint.

SQUARE DRILL

Each player's individual defensive success can be graded by fielding percentage. This statistic reflects the player's ability to make routine plays consistently. In a practice setting, each infielder must be given a number of ground balls on a daily basis. Each repetition must be performed with quality effort and technique so that the functional movements for successful execution become second nature to each defender.

The square drill is an individual defensive practice within a team setting: The team is the surrounding infielders who are moving in conjunction with each other. This drill focuses on getting a large number of quality repetitions for each player while simultaneously having each player's individual efforts reflected in the team's performance during the drill. The drill can be done with four, two, or one of the hitters using the fungo, a thin bat used during practice for hitting ground or fly balls that are not thrown. In each variation, ground balls are hit to each position and each player who fields the ball has a specific game situation to execute. For example, every ground ball hit may be fielded and thrown to second base, simulating a double play. As we move forward, we will detail the proper focus of the square drill as it relates to each position.

PLAYING FIRST BASE

The first baseman is the cornerstone of the infield. His efforts defensively can have a major impact throughout the course of a game. Infielders are not always perfect, but a first baseman who can work well around the bag and consistently dig out dirt balls (balls thrown in the dirt in front of him) thrown his way can improve the infield as a whole by covering up would-be errors. Here we discuss the techniques of footwork around first base (figure 7.4), picks (catching a short hopped thrown ball) (figure 7.5), and holding runners (figure 7.6).

Figure 7.4 **FOOTWORK AROUND THE BASE**

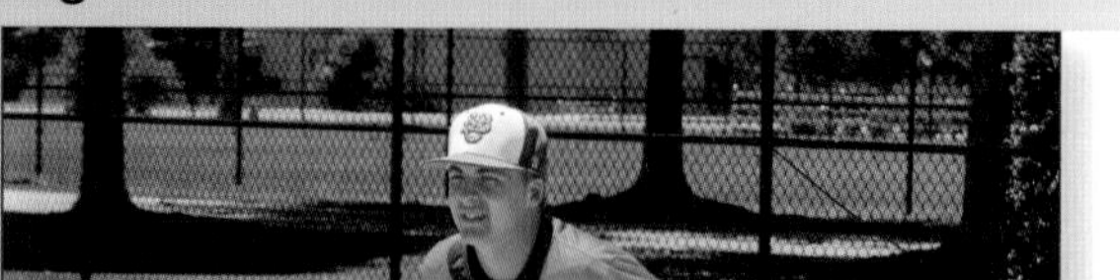

1. When the ball is put into play, the first baseman should get to the first-base bag and then position his throwing-side foot on the inside corner (figure 7.4*a*).
2. As the throw is made to him, the first baseman should read the flight of the ball.

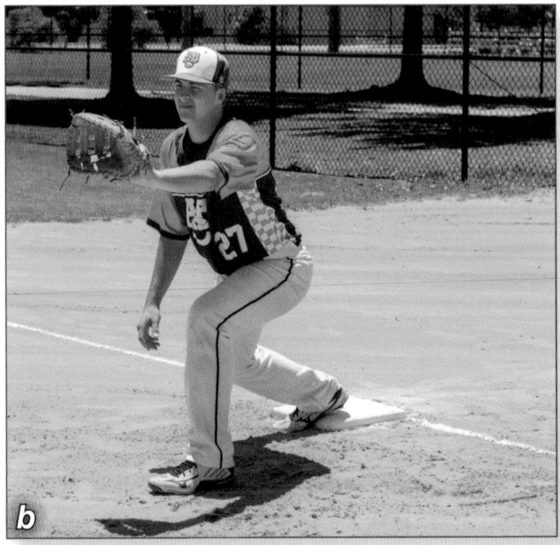

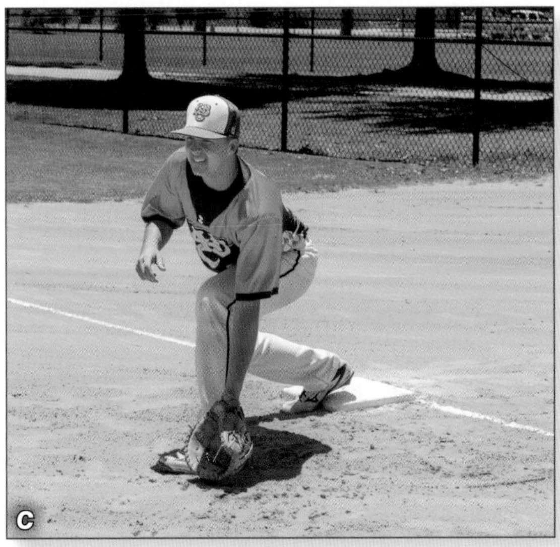

3. For a ball traveling to him in the air, the first baseman should stretch his glove-side leg out to the ball, plant the foot, and make the reception (figure 7.4*b*).
4. If the throw is low, the footwork should position the first baseman so that he can pick the baseball as it bounces (figure 7.4*c*).
5. For a throw that takes the first baseman toward the runner or across the base path, the first baseman should adjust his feet and position himself out of the running lane so that he can make the catch safely (figure 7.4*d*). If his footwork is correct, the first baseman will either remain in contact with the bag or be in position to make the catch and tag the runner before he gets to first base.

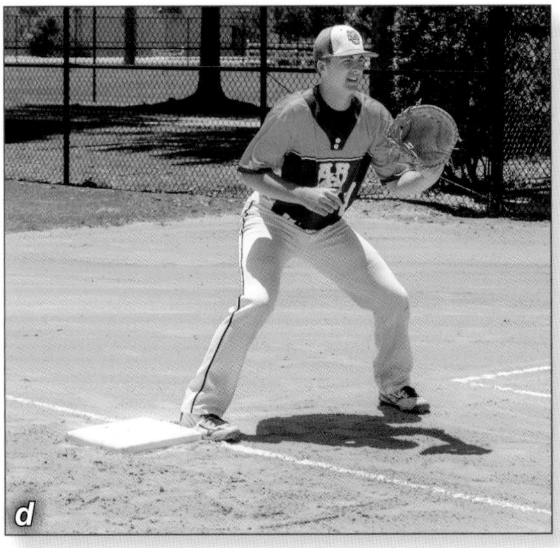

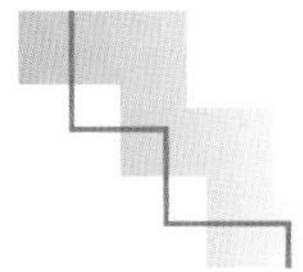

MISSTEP

Positioning the feet on top of or in front of the base places you in an unsafe area where the runner may step on you.

CORRECTION

The feet should start on the inside corner of the base and in position to shift in any direction as the ball is thrown.

Figure 7.5 **PICKS**

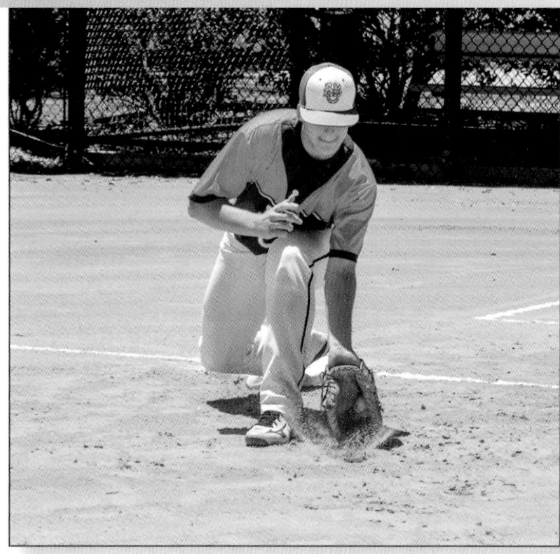

1. The ability to pick balls that are thrown in the dirt is a skill that an outstanding first baseman should possess.
2. The first baseman must be able to read the throw. He must also judge the hop of the ball—long hop (a thrown ball that hits the ground and bounces once smoothly to the defender), short hop, or no hop—time his stretch to the ball, and catch the ball as it bounces.
3. The glove work may vary depending on the condition of the field and the preference of the first baseman. We recommend working the glove through the ball on short hops. Working through the ball with the glove should correspond with the timing of the stretch.

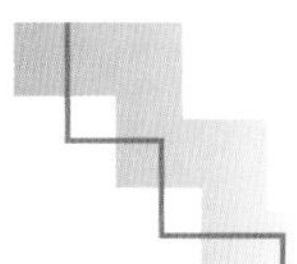

MISSTEP

Stretching too late or too soon will put you out of position for the hop.

CORRECTION

Proper reads of the flight of the ball will determine stride length, stride timing, and therefore proper positioning for making a short hop dig (catching a thrown ball that bounces near the fielder's feet out of the dirt).

Figure 7.6 HOLDING RUNNERS

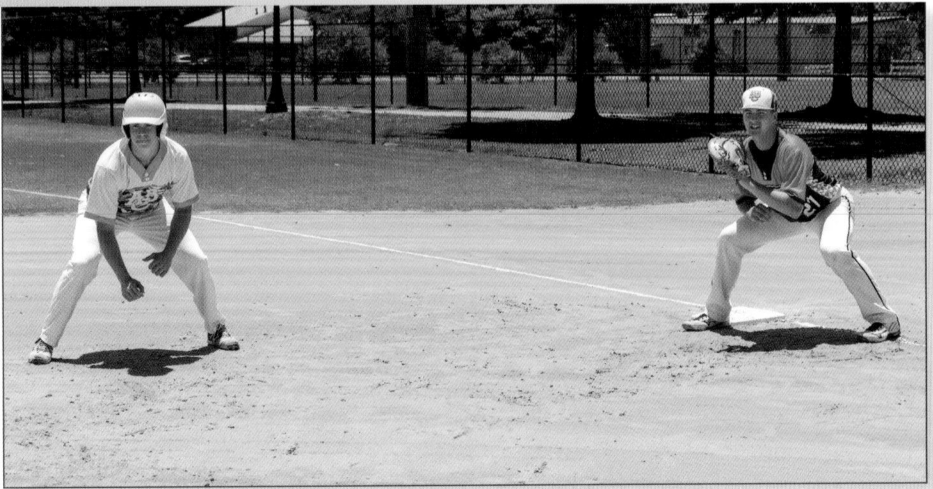

1. The first baseman holds a base runner on if a runner is on first base only or if runners are on first and third.
2. The feet should be positioned with the right foot at the front, inside corner of the base and the left foot near the first-base line in front of first base.
3. The feet positioning should angle the first baseman toward the pitcher, allowing the first baseman to make a catch and place a tag on the runner returning to the base.
4. The feet should also be in position so that the first baseman is capable of moving laterally quickly in case of a poor throw. From this position, he can move off the base and into fielding position as the pitch is delivered.

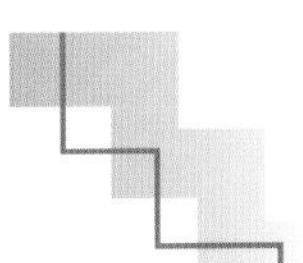

MISSTEP

If the left foot is too far toward second base, the body will be improperly angled, thus cutting you off from any throw to your left. This slows the process of getting into fielding position.

CORRECTION

When playing first base, you should always face the pitcher, making sure that your chest and shoulders are not cut off from home plate.

First-Base Drill 1 **Angle Throws and Picks**

The first baseman starts in the standard prepitch position. A coach or partner is at the standard second-base position with a ball in hand. The first baseman breaks to the bag. As he reaches first base, the coach throws the ball to him, forcing him to have correct footwork and timing with the stretch and reception (see figure 7.7). After the catch is made, the first baseman resets his position and repeats the drill, totaling five repetitions from the second baseman.

After the first five repetitions are completed, the coach remains at the second-base position for five more repetitions. The first baseman repeats the process, but the coach now throws the ball in the dirt, giving the first baseman repetitions on timing and glove work for picking balls thrown from the second baseman.

After the 10 throws are made from the second-base position, the coach shifts to shortstop and then third base and does the same at each position. The coach then moves to the catcher position and simulates a throw inside the running lane and then a throw outside the running lane. Five regular receptions and five picks should be done from each position.

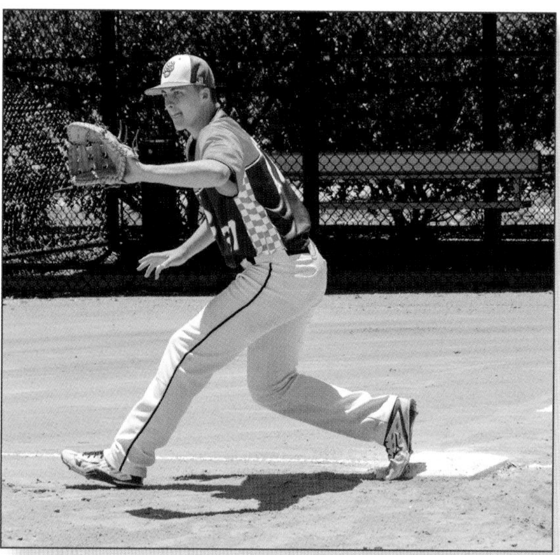

Figure 7.7 Angle throws and picks drill.

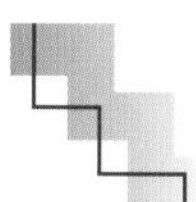

TO INCREASE DIFFICULTY

- Instead of throwing, the coach hits fungoes, balls hit using the fungo bat, to force the player to be quicker with his footwork and timing.

TO DECREASE DIFFICULTY

- Have the first baseman start on the bag while the coach remains stationary. The throws should repeat the angles of specific hops, helping the player to develop timing.

Success Check

- Are the feet properly positioned at the base?
- Is the stretch timed properly so that the positioning of the body is consistent and properly aligned with the throw?
- Did you pick the dirt balls cleanly?

Score Your Success

You earn 1 point for a catch with proper timing and correct positioning with the stretch.

You earn 1 point for every dirt ball that you pick while remaining in contact with the base.

You earn 1/2 point for a dirt ball that you do not catch but keep in front of you.

You earn 0 points if you miss a ball.

Second base ____ out of 5

Second base picks ____ out of 5

Shortstop ____ out of 5

Shortstop picks ____ out of 5

Third base ____ out of 5

Third base picks _____ out of 5

Catcher inside ____ out of 5

Catcher inside picks ____ out of 5

Catcher outside ____ out of 5

Catcher outside picks ____ out of 5

Your score ________ out of 50

First-Base Drill 2 **Square Drill Focus**

The square drill has three focus points for the first baseman, the first of which is fielding ground balls properly. As the drill progresses, the fielding of the ball expands into throwing to second base for double plays. In a standard drill, the first baseman performs 10 of each.

The square drill not only allows the first baseman to field ground balls but also gives him the opportunity to work on footwork, receiving throws, and picks. In the average drill, the first baseman typically receives 25 throws and 5 dirt balls to pick.

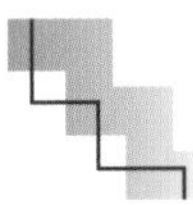

TO INCREASE DIFFICULTY

- Increase the tempo between reps.
- Apply different spin to each ground ball.

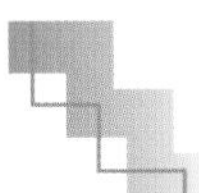

TO DECREASE DIFFICULTY

- Roll the balls instead of hitting them.

Success Check

- Did you consistently execute the routine play and get an out?
- Were your feeds to second base accurate?
- Did you pick the balls that were thrown in the dirt?
- How was your footwork around the bag?

Score Your Success

Ground balls ____ out of 10

Double plays ____ out of 10

Throws received _______ out of 25

Picks _______ out of 5

Your score _______ out of 50

PLAYING THIRD BASE

Third base is known as the hot corner. With little time to react to hard-hit balls from roughly 90 feet (27 m) away, playing third base requires great reflexes and quick reaction times. A common saying is, "Knock it down and throw him out," to encourage those who play here to keep the ball in front any way possible. Because the ball gets to the third baseman quickly, the player can knock it down and still have time to throw out a base runner. With the importance of quick reaction times in mind, the third baseman must always be in a good prepitch position that allows movement in any direction. Here we discuss reads and the third baseman's first steps (figure 7.8) and fielding slow rollers (figure 7.9).

Figure 7.8 READS AND FIRST STEPS

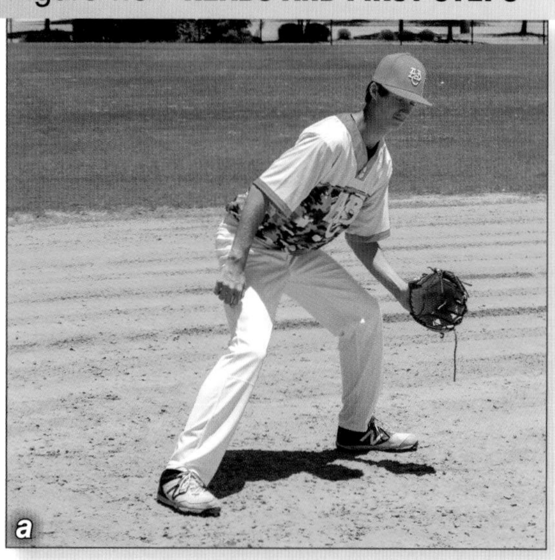

1. React and keep the ball in front when it is hit straight at you.
2. Use the X diagram for balls away from you. The X diagram illustrates the four angles you can step that cover any direction a ball might be hit.
3. The two backward angles are to step back left (figure 7.8*a*) and to step back right (figure 7.8*b*).

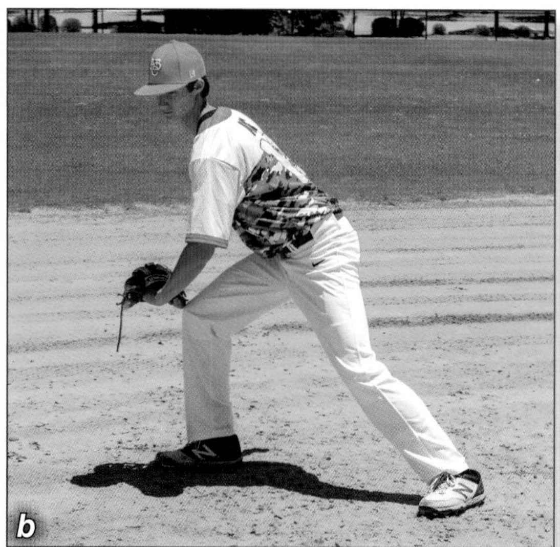

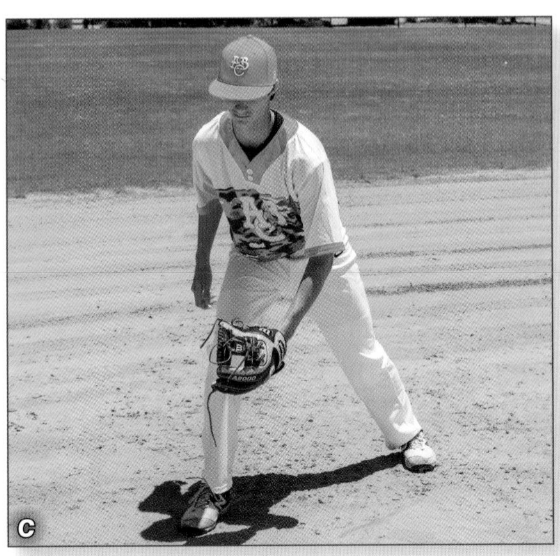

4. The two forward angles are to step front right (figure 7.8*c*), and to step front left (figure 7.8*d*).
5. By following the X diagram, you will take an angle to any ball hit away from you. These angles allow for added range and better positioning for the transfer.

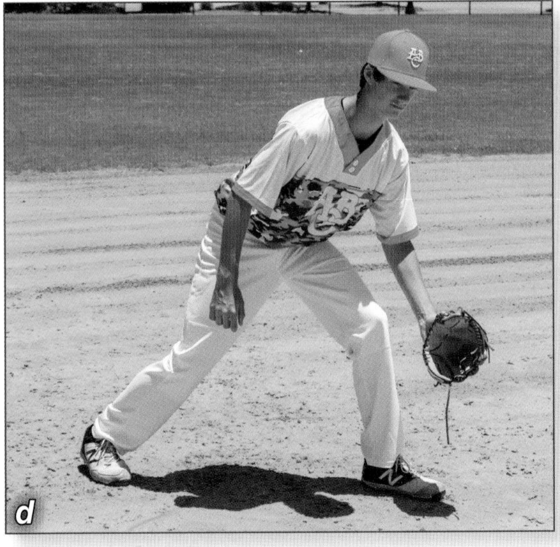

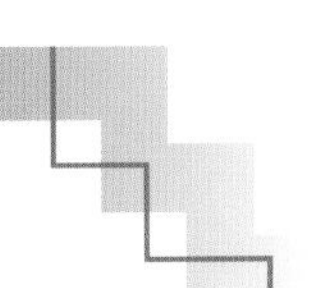

MISSTEP

Lack of focus can lead to improper positioning. In turn, your reaction times will diminish because of complacency within the prepitch setup.

CORRECTION

You must be on high alert and ready to react with every pitch. You should use the reset and refocus drill between pitches.

Figure 7.9 SLOW ROLLERS AND BUNTS

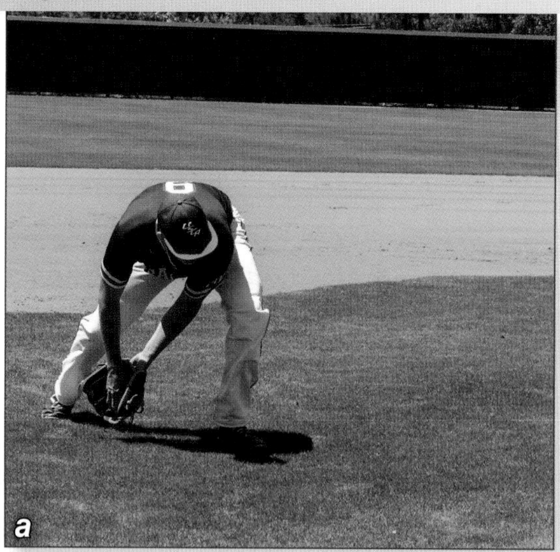

a

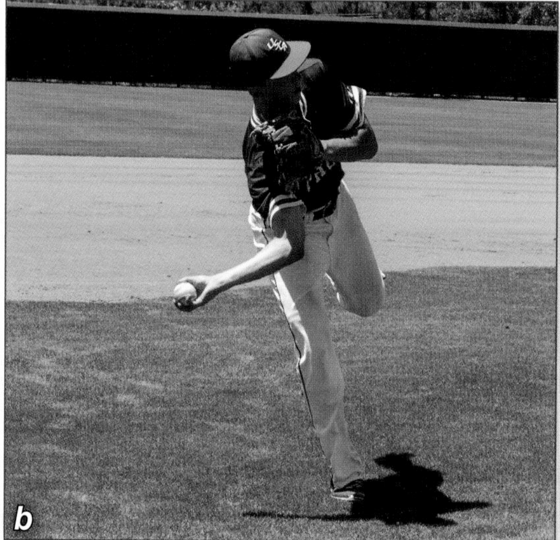

b

1. For balls bunted or chopped in front of him, the third baseman must charge the ball as quickly as possible.
2. The ball should be fielded with two hands, inside the right foot (figure 7.9*a*).
3. The transfer should be immediate. The upper body stays down, and the release of the throw should happen as the right foot lands (figure 7.9*b*).

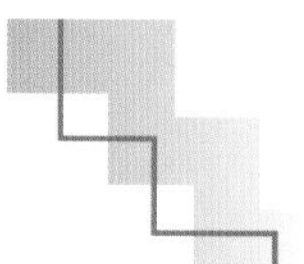

MISSTEP

Chopping the feet, or setting the feet to throw, takes too much time and causes the upper body to rise up.

CORRECTION

You should develop a rhythm that correlates your steps with your transfer and release. This synchronization comes with repetition.

Third-Base Drill **Square Drill Focus**

Square drill practice is the third baseman's primary time to get repetitions. In these reps, the focus should be on getting a quality first step, keeping the ball in front or fielding it cleanly, and making quality throws and feeds around the diamond. In a normal square drill, a third baseman should field and throw 10 balls straight at him to first and 10 straight at him for double plays. The same goes for forehands and backhands. To finish, he should field 10 slow rollers and throw to first base.

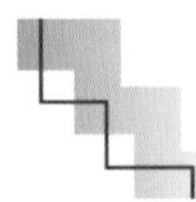

TO INCREASE DIFFICULTY

- Apply different spin on each ball.
- Challenge lateral range by delivering the ball to different areas.

TO DECREASE DIFFICULTY

- Deliver all the balls to the same spot for the fielder to field.
- Roll the ball.

Success Check

- Did any balls get past you?
- Did you use the X diagram for your first steps?
- Did you make accurate throws and feeds?

Score Your Success

You earn 1 point for every ball you field cleanly (or knock down) and follow with an accurate throw or feed.

You earn 1/2 point for using proper techniques but making a flawed throw on slow rollers.

You earn 0 points if you make an error.

Straight up ____ out of 10

Double plays ____ out of 10

Forehand ____ out of 10

Forehand double plays ____ out of 10

Backhand ____ out of 10

Backhand double plays ____ out of 10

Slow rollers _______ out of 10

Total _______ out of 70

PLAYING MIDDLE INFIELD

The shortstop and second baseman together are the heart of the defense. When they work in unison, communicate, and consistently make routine plays, the entire defense becomes stronger. The middle infielders, primarily the shortstop, have the greatest defensive responsibility for several reasons. The primary factor is the high volume of action that the middle infielders handle, including batted balls, double plays, cutoffs, relays, and situational team defense. This high workload demands that the middle infielders communicate, know and understand each situation, and control the baseball when they are given the chance. We cover holding runners (figures 7.10 and 7.11), double-play feeds (figure 7.12), turning double plays from second base (figure 7.13), and turning double plays from shortstop (figure 7.14).

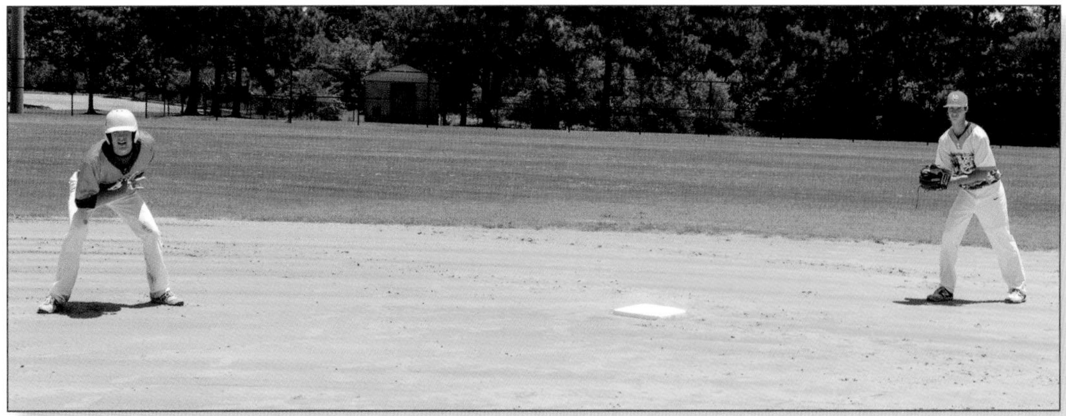

Figure 7.10 Holding Runners

The responsibility of holding a runner at second base mostly rests with the pitcher. There are a variety of things a pitcher can do to hold a runner (see figure 7.11, "Middle Infield Drill 1: Picks With Pitchers" for details). However, the middle infielders do have their own roles. The key for the shortstop and second baseman is to vary their approaches to holding the runner on each pitch—for example, sometimes they can be aggressive and sometimes they can ignore the runner. The idea is to switch things up to keep the runner guessing. Middle infielder positioning will vary depending on the pitcher, batter, runner, and game situation. For example, a fast runner will need to be covered closely. Also, remember that only one middle infielder should hold the runner at any given time. Either the shortstop or the second baseman will creep toward second in the ready position (see figure 7.10). As the throw from the pitcher is made, the left foot is placed on the back of the base, and the glove should be held so that it is ready to receive the pitcher's throw. Here are some other things to keep in mind.

1. Double holds mean that valuable prepitch positioning is being sacrificed.
2. Communicate with the pitcher. Let him know whether he is in a rhythm with his sets, and be on the same page with him with his pickoff moves.
3. Communicate with the other middle infielder. Know who is holding, and switch the hold if the situation stipulates. Know the situation. Weak holds and tight holds will vary with the situation and the base runner's speed. In a tight hold, the infielder plays closer to the base (see figure 7.10). He will give up a little fielding position, but for a fast runner or for certain game situations, this is necessary. With a tight hold, added movement from the infielder is wasted energy. Positioning in relation to the bag determines the strength of the hold, not how much you can jump back and forth and kick dirt.

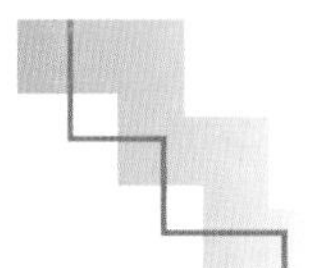

MISSTEP

Double holds with infielders are caused by lack of communication or lack of baseball savvy.

CORRECTION

If you notice that your partner is holding the runner as well, call time-out and communicate.

Middle Infield Drill 1 **Picks With Pitchers**

Pitchers can use various pickoffs at second base—an inside move (figure 7.11*a*), a daylight spin move working off the infielder holding (figure 7.11*b*), or a timing spin move signaled from the catcher (figure 7.11*c*). The inside move is a simple way to keep the runner on second base honest. A pitcher won't usually be able to pick off a runner using the inside move, but it's very useful for keeping him close to the base. To perform the inside move, the pitcher starts his leg lift as he would to deliver a pitch. At the peak of the lift, right before he would normally start moving toward the plate, he shifts his weight to the outside of his back knee, and spins his body toward the glove-hand side until he faces second base. The pitcher should be able to plant his left foot (for a right-handed pitcher) or his right foot (for a left-handed pitcher, as shown) toward second base.

For the daylight spin move and the timing spin move, the pitcher uses a quick pivot in an attempt to pick off the runner and get an out. From the set position, the pitcher pivots his feet and turns his body toward first base (left-handed pitchers turn towards third base as shown). The pitcher then spins his head, torso, hips, and legs around 180 degrees, locates the target, points his non-throwing shoulder toward second base, and makes a quick throw. The difference between the two moves is in the middle infielders' actions. For the timing spin move, when the pick is called, the pitcher comes to the set position and looks at the runner. Once the pitcher turns back toward home plate, the infielder covering the base waits a certain amount of time and then breaks for second base. At the same time, the pitcher pivots and throws the pickoff. For the daylight spin move, the shortstop determines when to run the pickoff. The pitcher comes to the set position and looks at the runner. When the shortstop thinks they can pick off the runner, he breaks toward second base. Once the shortstop gets past the runner, and the pitcher can see "daylight" between the runner and the shortstop, the pitcher pivots and throws.

With each move, the middle infielder responsible for holding the runner has several duties. The first is to get to the bag on time, or early if necessary. The infielder's feet must be properly placed in front of the bag, putting the body in position to react to the throw. With a good throw, the infielder must catch and tag the runner.

To work on your team's choice of pickoff, have a pitcher, catcher, and base runner in place. Repeat the pickoff 10 times to ensure timing and execution.

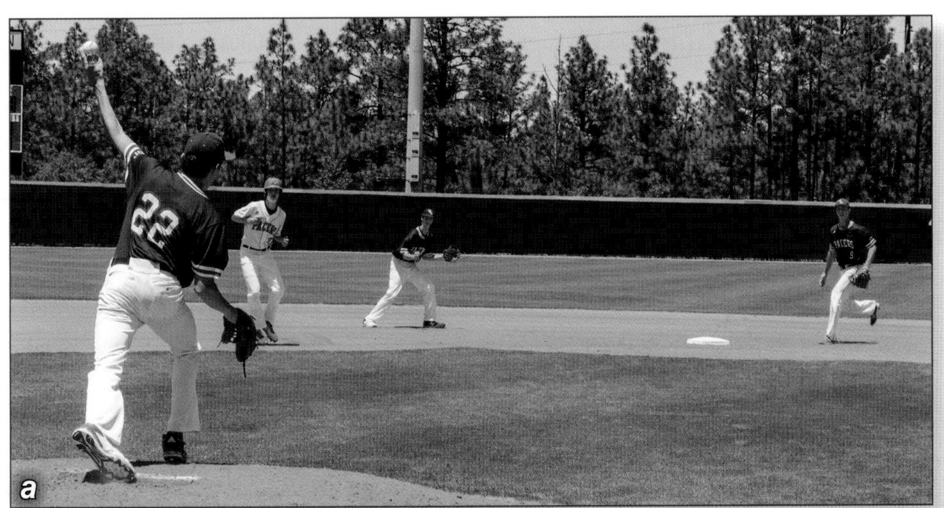

Figure 7.11 Picks with pitchers drill: *(a)* inside move.

(continued)

Middle Infield Drill 1 *(continued)*

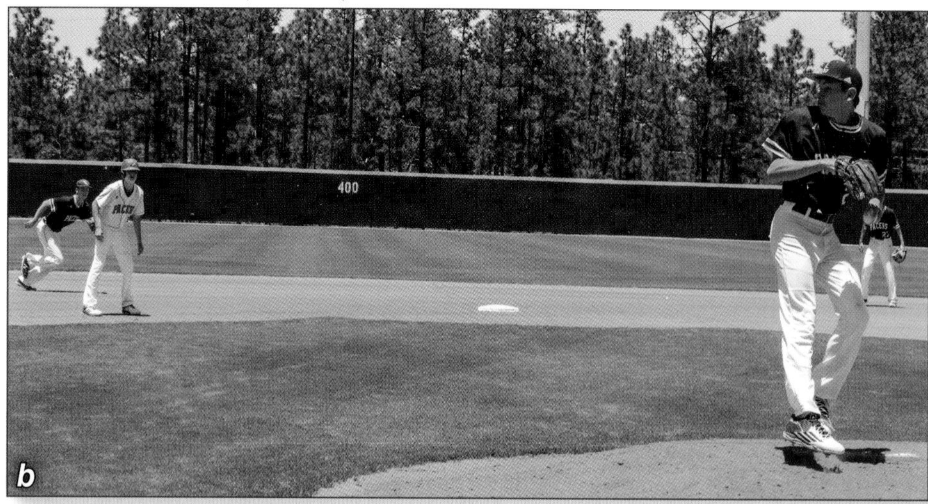

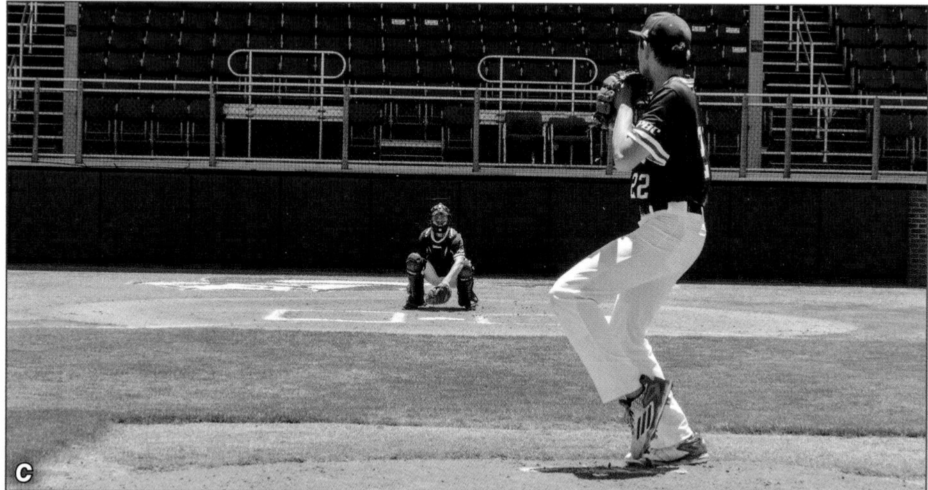

Figure 7.11 Picks with pitchers drill: *(b)* daylight spin move and *(c)* timing spin move.

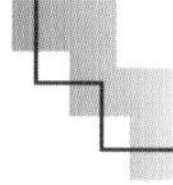

TO INCREASE DIFFICULTY

- Add a base runner.
- Work at game speed.

TO DECREASE DIFFICULTY

- Shorten the distance between the infielder and the base.
- Use oral timing cues.

Success Check

- Did you get in position at the base in time to receive the ball?
- How was your footwork around the base?
- Were you able to catch and tag, or move to keep the ball in front?

Score Your Success

You earn 1 point for every executed pickoff attempt.

You earn 0 points if the timing, footwork, or catch is flawed because of your faulty execution.

Your score ____ of 10

Figure 7.12 MIDDLE INFIELD DOUBLE-PLAY FEEDS

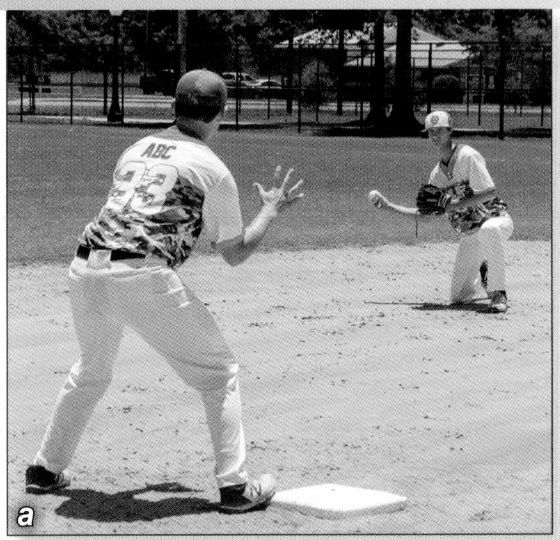

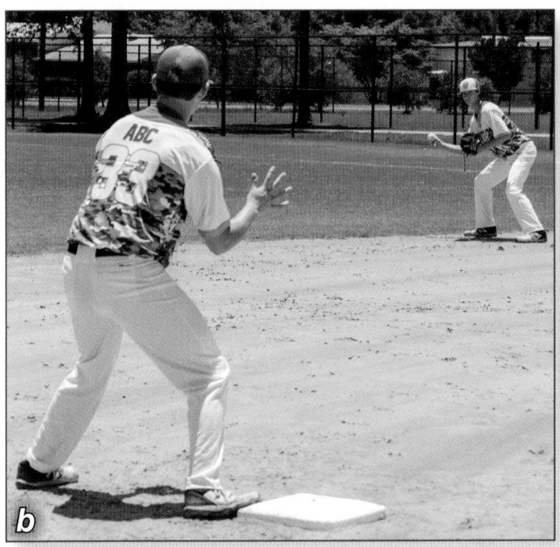

1. Say, "Flip" if the ball is hit near the base.
2. For a ball fielded slightly out of range for a flip, the infielder should go to a knee and angle the upper body to make the transfer (figure 7.12*a*). The fielder is then in good position to make a quick sidearm feed to second base.
3. For a ball to the forehand side of the second baseman (figure 7.12*b*) or the backhand side of the shortstop, the ball should be fielded cleanly, the feet should set quickly to open the body to the bag, and the transfer and feed should be made accurately. If the shortstop is covering the base, he places his right foot on the back corner of the base and faces the second baseman. If the shortstop fields and the second baseman covers, the second baseman will be at the back of the base with the left foot on the back corner.

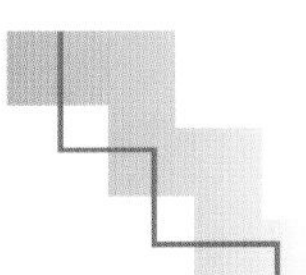

MISSTEP

Slow footwork and poor ball control will lead to inaccurate feeds and flawed timing of the turn at the second.

CORRECTION

Prepitch anticipation and taking good angles to the ball will speed up the feet and correct transfer flaws.

Figure 7.13 TURNING DOUBLE PLAYS FROM SECOND BASE

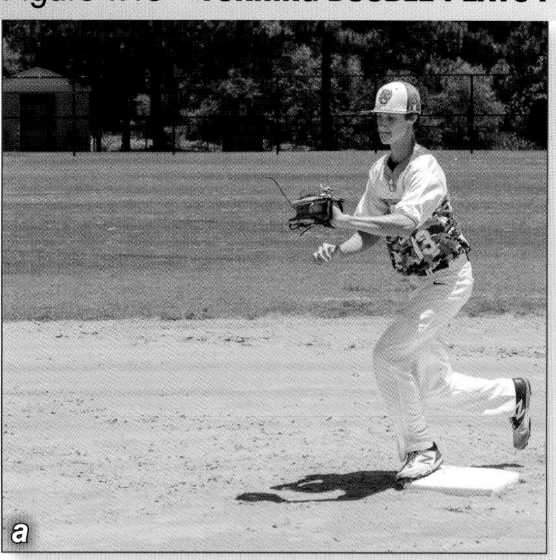

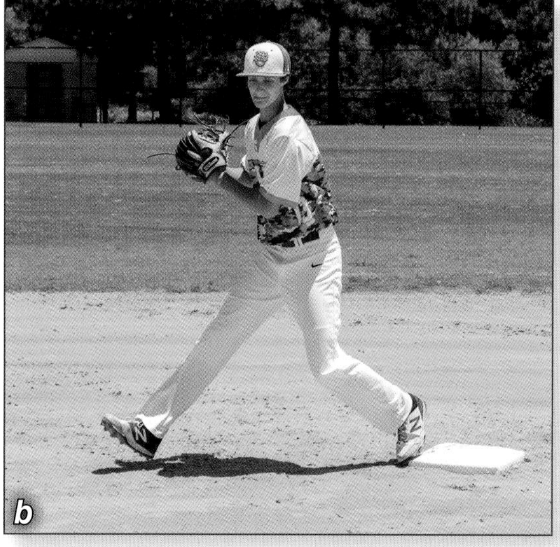

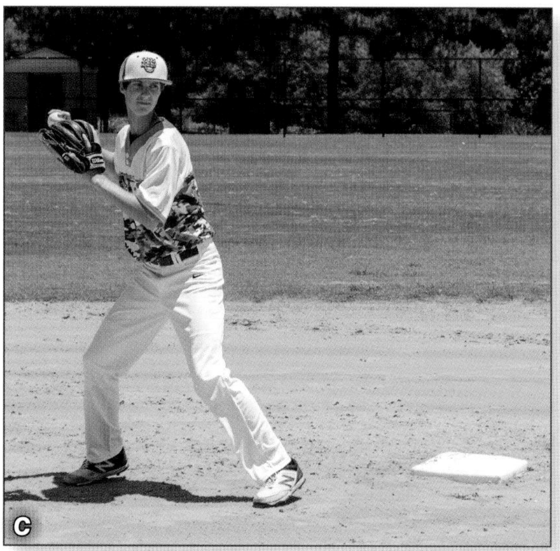

1. When the ball is hit to the third baseman or shortstop, the second baseman must get to the bag and give a target with the glove (figure 7.13*a*).
2. If the feed is being made from a distance, from third base, or from the backhand side of the shortstop, the second baseman should read the throw and step to the ball. An accurate throw will bring the second baseman across the bag with the left foot in contact with the base (figure 7.13*b*). As he receives the ball, the second baseman makes the transfer and throws as the right foot plants past the bag (figure 7.13*c*).

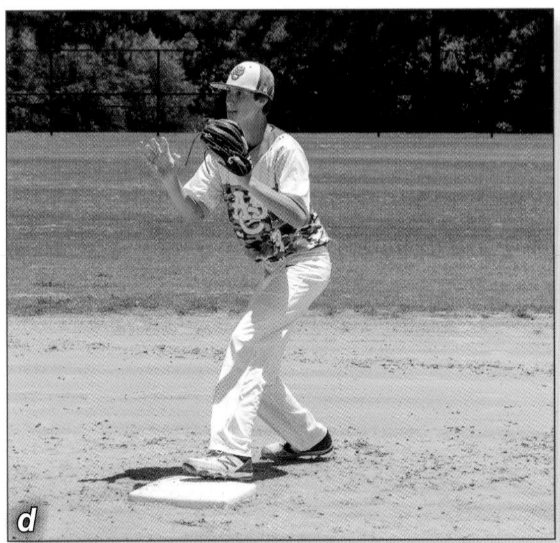

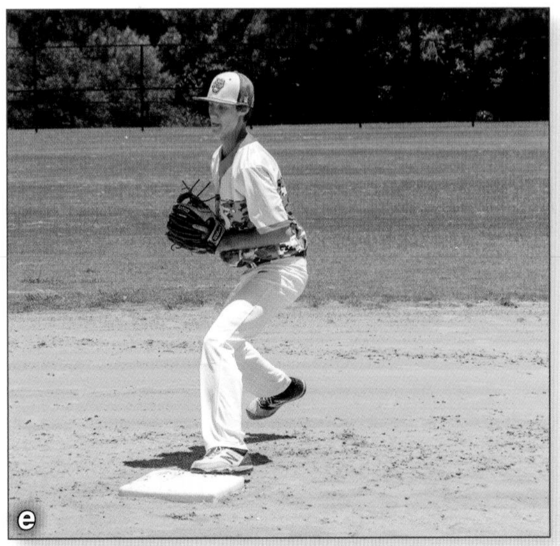

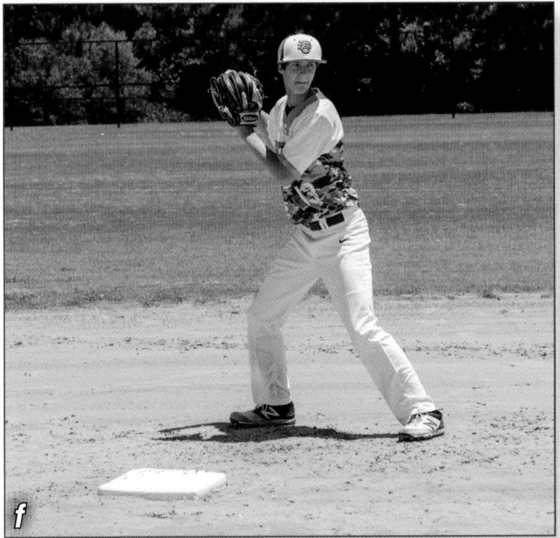

3. If the feed is coming from a shorter distance, the second baseman should push backward off the bag with the left foot (figure 7.13*d*), transfer (figure 7.13*e*), and throw as the right foot sets (figure 7.13*f*).

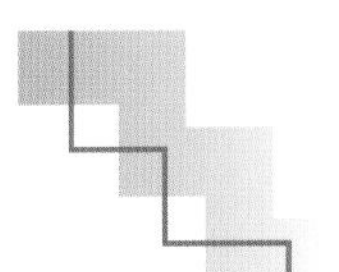

MISSTEP

Timing to the bag is vital. If you are late while playing second base, the feed may draw you away from the bag, preventing you from using the proper footwork. If you are on time but begin stepping through the bag before reading the throw, the entire play could be flawed.

CORRECTION

The correct prepitch positioning and anticipation should resolve timing issues before the feed, but you must also be able to read the throw and adjust your footwork accordingly. With repetition, you should develop a rhythm for your footwork that allows you to make the proper reads.

Figure 7.14 TURNING DOUBLE PLAYS FROM SHORTSTOP

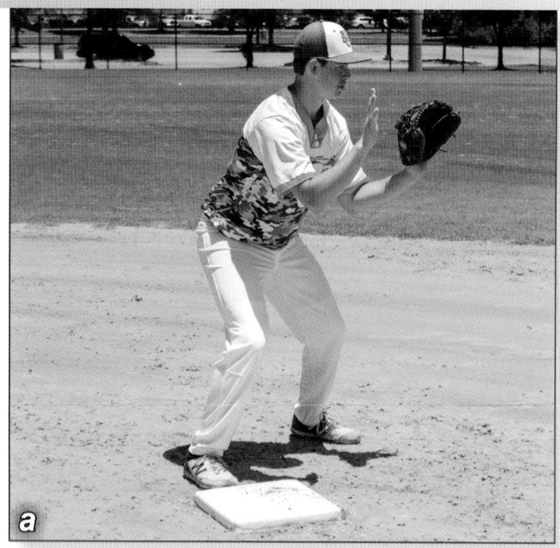

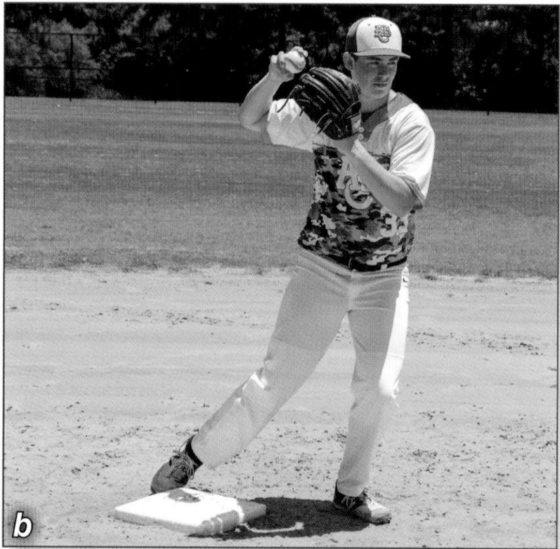

1. When the ball is hit to the right side of the infield, the shortstop should get to the bag and position himself behind the base while keeping his momentum moving forward (figure 7.14*a*).
2. As the feed is made, the shortstop should use his momentum to receive and transfer the ball to first while scraping the outfield side of the bag with his right foot (figure 7.14*b*), thus working around the outside of the baseline.

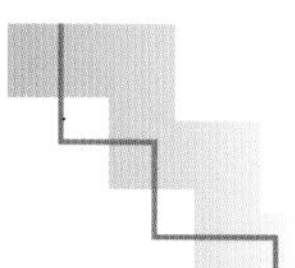

MISSTEP

If you lose your momentum, you will have difficulty adjusting your position to a flawed throw.

CORRECTION

You must use quick footwork with steady momentum to execute a variety of transfers depending on the feed you get.

Middle Infield Drill 2 **Rollers**

With the middle infielders at double-play depth, a coach kneels behind the pitcher's mound and rolls 10 balls to either the shortstop or second baseman (figure 7.15). The middle infielders work on fielding the ball with good body positioning, quality transfers and feeds, and fluidity throughout the turn as they throw to first base. After 10 rolls to one side, the coach switches to the other.

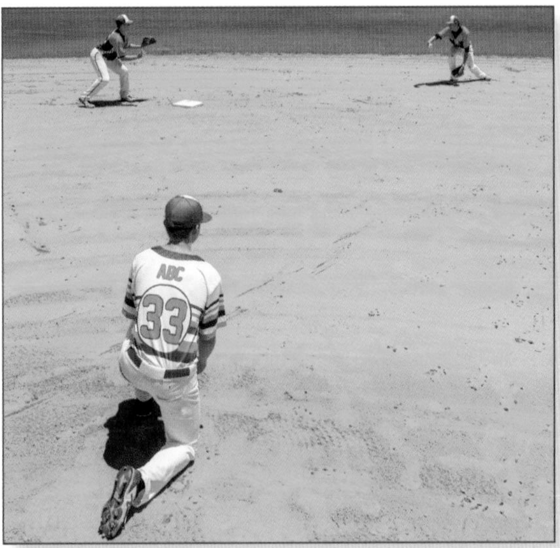

Figure 7.15 Rollers drill.

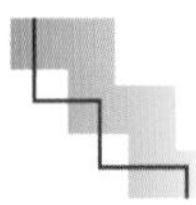

TO INCREASE DIFFICULTY

- Alter the spin on each ball.
- Challenge lateral range by delivering the ball to different areas.

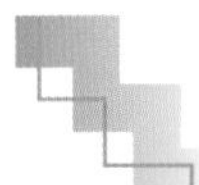

TO DECREASE DIFFICULTY

- Deliver all the balls to the same spot for the fielder to field.

Success Check

- Did you consistently make quality feeds?
- How was your positioning? Did it help or hurt your ability to make a clean transfer?
- How well did you execute your timing and footwork around the bag when turning the double play?

Score Your Success

Feeds _______ out of 10

Turns _______ out of 10

Total _______ out of 20

Middle Infield Drill 3 **Square Drill Focus**

For the middle infielders, the square drill is a time to focus on good rhythm and timing within their technique. This drill will enhance their overall consistency as they move into game speed. The goal is to develop fluidity with the functional movements, improve ball control, speed up transfers, improve accuracy, and strengthen the individual defender overall. As with the third baseman, the middle infielders typically field 10 balls straight ahead, throwing to first. Then they field 10 balls straight ahead, feeding double plays. The same routine is used for forehands and backhands. The middle infielders also make 10 turns at second and finish with 10 slow rollers, throwing to first.

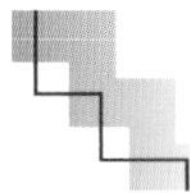

TO INCREASE DIFFICULTY

- Alter the spin on each ball.
- Challenge lateral range by delivering the ball to different areas.

TO DECREASE DIFFICULTY

- Deliver all the balls to the same spot for the fielder to field.
- Roll the ball.

Success Check

- Did you turn any routine plays into errors?
- How fluid was your timing and technique with your fielding, throwing, feeds, and turns?
- How accurate were your feeds and throws?

Score Your Success

You earn 1 point for every successfully executed play.

You earn 1/2 point for an executed play with flawed timing.

You earn 0 points for errors.

Straight up _______ out of 10

Double-play feeds ____ out of 10

Forehand _______ out of 10

Forehand double-play feeds ____ out of 10

Backhand _______ out of 10

Backhand double-play feeds ____ out of 10

Slow rollers _______ out of 10

Double-play turns _______ out of 10

Total _______ out of 80

STANDARD CUTOFF POSITIONING

As we move into situational defense, we need to address the standard cutoff positioning of the infielders for singles hit to the outfield. This standard positioning is the foundation for tandem relays later on. For details, see figure 7.16.

Figure 7.16 **CUTOFF POSITIONING FOR A SINGLE TO LEFT FIELD**

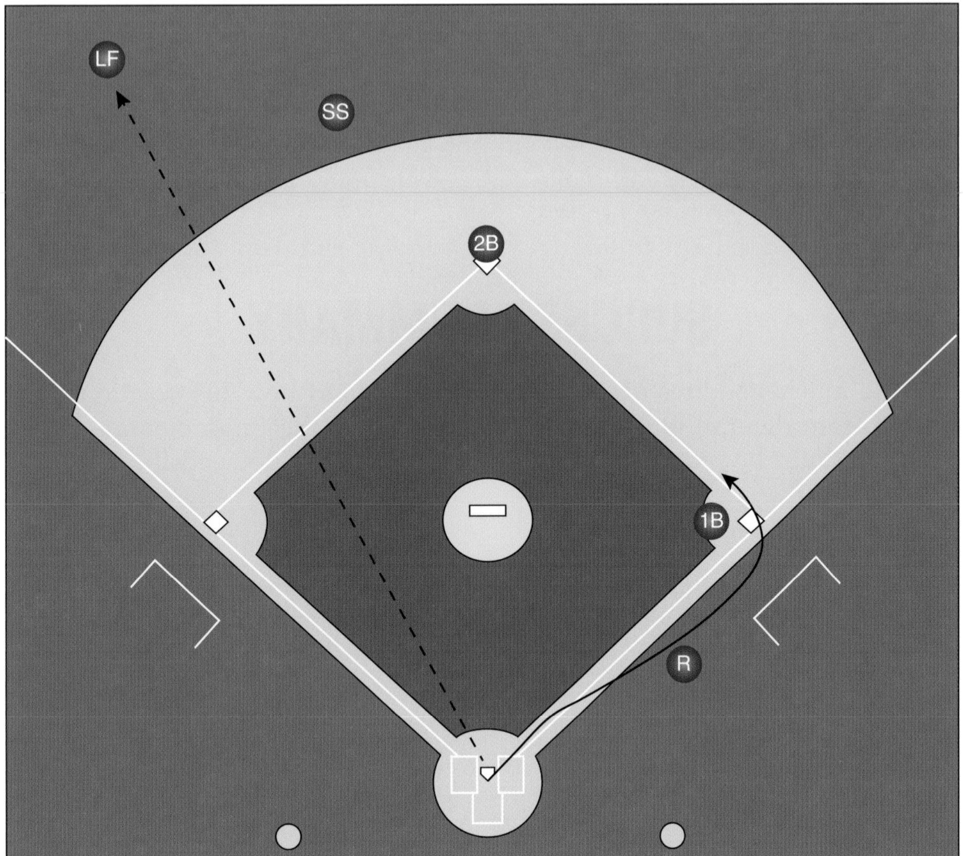

1. On any single hit to the left side of second base, the shortstop lines up between the base being thrown to and the outfielder fielding the ball, as shown in figure 7.16. The second baseman is the cutoff for any ball hit to the right side of second base.
2. The infielder covering the base that is being thrown to is in charge of lining up the cutoff man, the infielder who gets into position to line up a throw from the outfield. The cutoff man catches the throw from the outfield if the throw does not line up with the base to which it is intended to go.
3. The first baseman drifts inside the first-base bag as the runner rounds the base. The first baseman makes sure that the runner touches the base. If the runner does not attempt to advance, the first baseman should be prepared for a throw behind the runner from the cutoff man. If the runner attempts to advance to second, the first baseman trails the runner to the bag. While this is going on, the pitcher, catcher, and third baseman stay near their positions in case of overthrows.

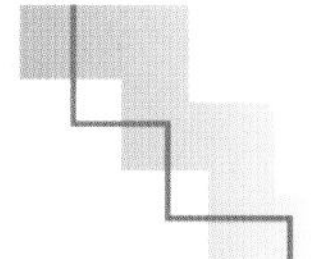

MISSTEP

If you are not lined up correctly, the relay will take longer to get to the base.

CORRECTION

Communication must be loud and crisp so that you are properly in line and so that you make the correct relay throw, given that your back is to the base runners.

SUCCESS SUMMARY

Playing the infield requires each player to understand how his position functions within the team defense. But to execute consistently, the fundamentals of playing each position must be practiced daily. How did you do at your position?

First-Base Drills

1. Angle throws and picks	____ out of 50
2. Square drill focus	____ out of 50
Total	____ **out of 100**

Third-Base Drill

1. Square drill focus	____ out of 70
Total	____ **out of 70**

Middle Infield Drills

1. Picks with pitchers	____ out of 10
2. Rollers	____ out of 20
3. Square drill focus	____ out of 80
Total	____ **out of 110**

Playing the infield requires a high level of concentration. As you take the next step to success, the knowledge that you must apply in your prepitch preparation will grow and the speed at which you must apply it will increase. If you scored 80 points as a first baseman, 50 points as a third baseman, or 90 points as a middle infielder, congratulations! You have taken the next step to success for playing the infield. As we move forward, you will be tested on all the skills you have developed and all the steps that you have taken as we begin to put together a situational team defense.

STEP

8

Playing the Outfield

As we move into step 8, you have seen how the individual skills you have developed are implemented within the position you play as part of an infield team defense. The next step you will take is learning to play the outfield. Playing the outfield involves specific skills beyond simply catching a fly ball. As you learned in step 7, each position on the infield has specific factors that determine prepitch and postpitch actions. This remains true for outfielders in step 8.

The goal of step 8 is to apply your individual skill set to the outfield position you will be playing. By understanding the individual responsibilities of the outfield positions, you will enhance your baseball IQ and be able to perform at a higher level than before. Your performance as an outfielder within a team defense is not graded by fielding percentage alone; it is also judged on your ability to fulfill your responsibilities concerning movement and positioning, communication, awareness, and decision making at the quickest rate possible.

As with the infield step to success, you need to keep in mind several outfield rules. The first rule is to know and understand the situation, including hitter tendencies, runner speed, score, outs, and so on. Each situation will alter the positioning and actions of each outfielder. The second rule is to keep the ball in front. As an outfielder, you should take pride in not letting anything past you. The last rule is to keep the double play in order. This rule entails hitting the cutoff man, keeping the ball in front, cutting down the distance on ground balls, not drifting on fly balls, and even backing up the infield. If you can play your outfield position with these rules in mind, you will be able to take the next step to success.

PREPITCH POSITIONING

Prepitch positioning at the higher levels is often based on scouting reports, but in this section our goal is to help you understand where you should stand in the outfield and the adjustments you should make based on certain factors. We discuss standard positioning (figure 8.1), shading left (figure 8.2*a*) and right (figure 8.2*b*), and no doubles positioning (figure 8.3) here.

Figure 8.1 STANDARD POSITIONING

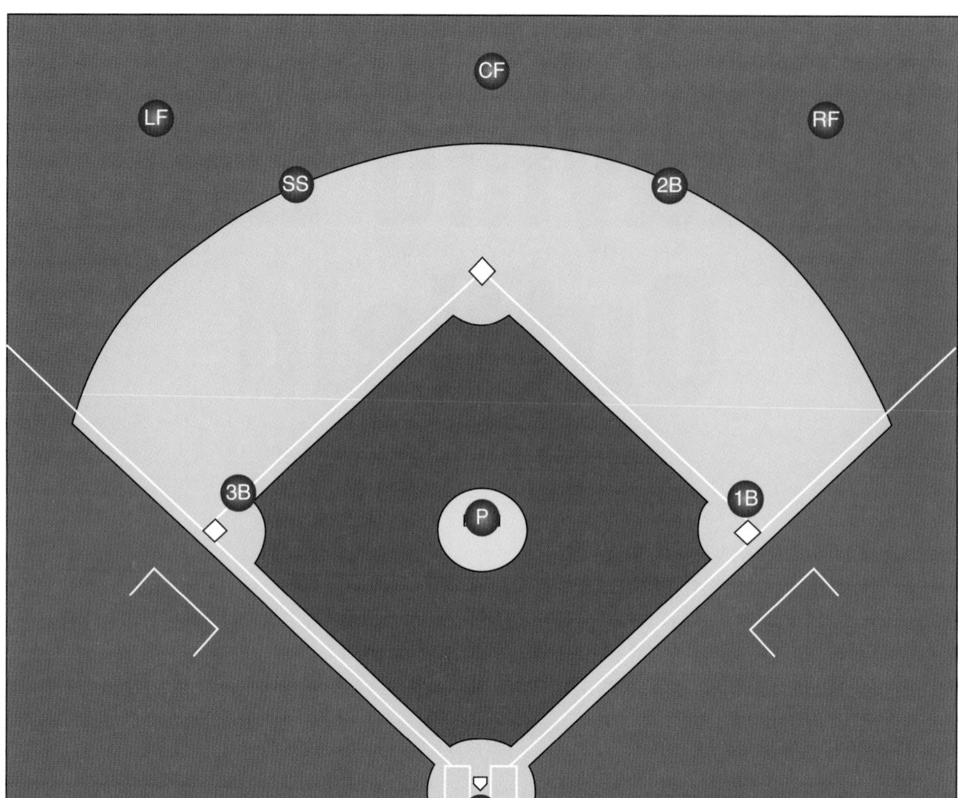

1. Against right-handed batters, the standard outfield positioning is commonly called "straight up" positioning. The outfielders play about mid-depth with the center fielder positioned directly behind second base, and the left and right fielders about 12 feet (3.5 m) off their respective foul lines. If you have access to scouting reports or know a particular hitter's tendencies, adjustments can be made based on the hitters. For a right-handed hitter known to be a pull hitter, a batter who usually hits the ball to the same side of the field that he bats from, the outfield will need to shift left. For an opposite-field hitter, the outfield should shift right.
2. Against left-handed batters, outfielders normally shift toward right field to better cover the pull-side, the side to where the batter will hit the ball. But the outfield can play in more standard positioning if a left-handed batter is known to be an opposite-field slap hitter.
3. The left fielder should be in line with first base and second base.
4. The right fielder should be in line with third base and second base.
5. Depth depends on each outfielder and the positioning where he is most comfortable.
6. If the outfielders have above average speed, the distance between them can be widened.

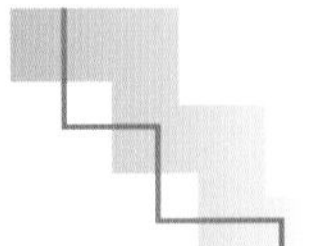

MISSTEP

Some outfielders may drift away from the correct alignment between pitches.

CORRECTION

Constant communication between outfielders can enhance focus.

Figure 8.2 **SHADING**

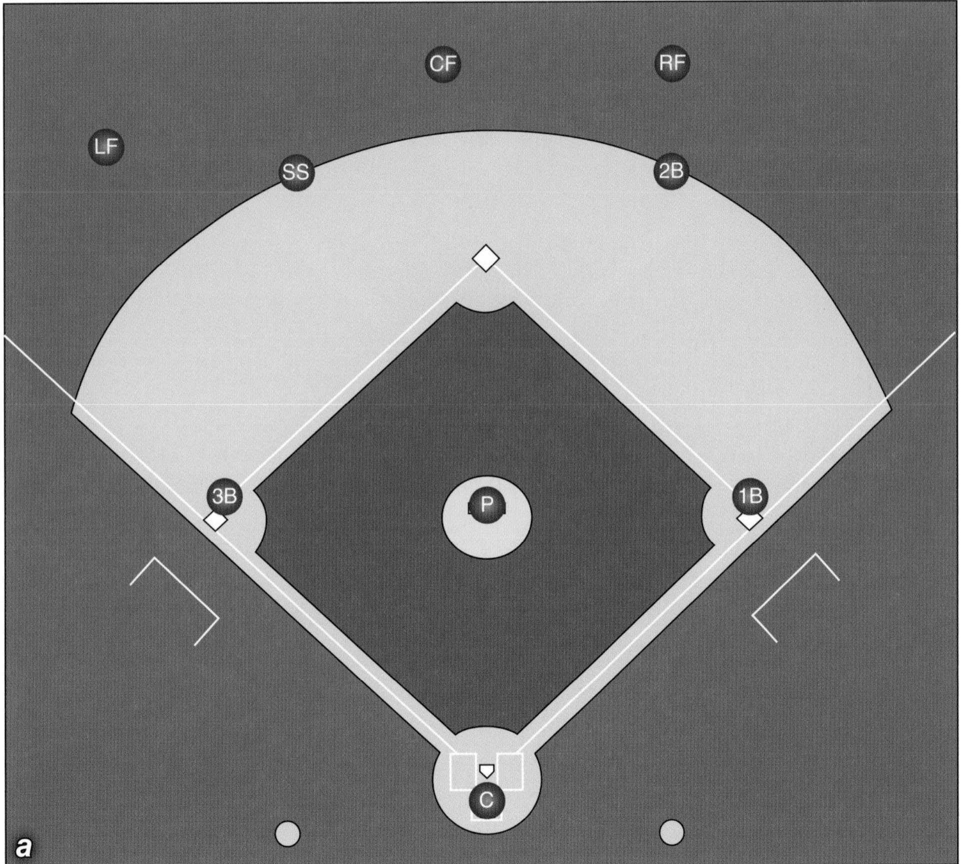

1. Hitter tendencies determine shading direction, whether to the left or right. Scouting reports or a coach's previous experience with a hitter will help inform where hitters are most likely to hit the ball.
2. As mentioned, for a right-handed pull hitter, the outfield should shade left (figure 8.2*a*). For an opposite-field slap hitter, who hits through the infielders to the opposite side of the field he bats from, the outfield should shade right.

(continued)

Figure 8.2 *(continued)*

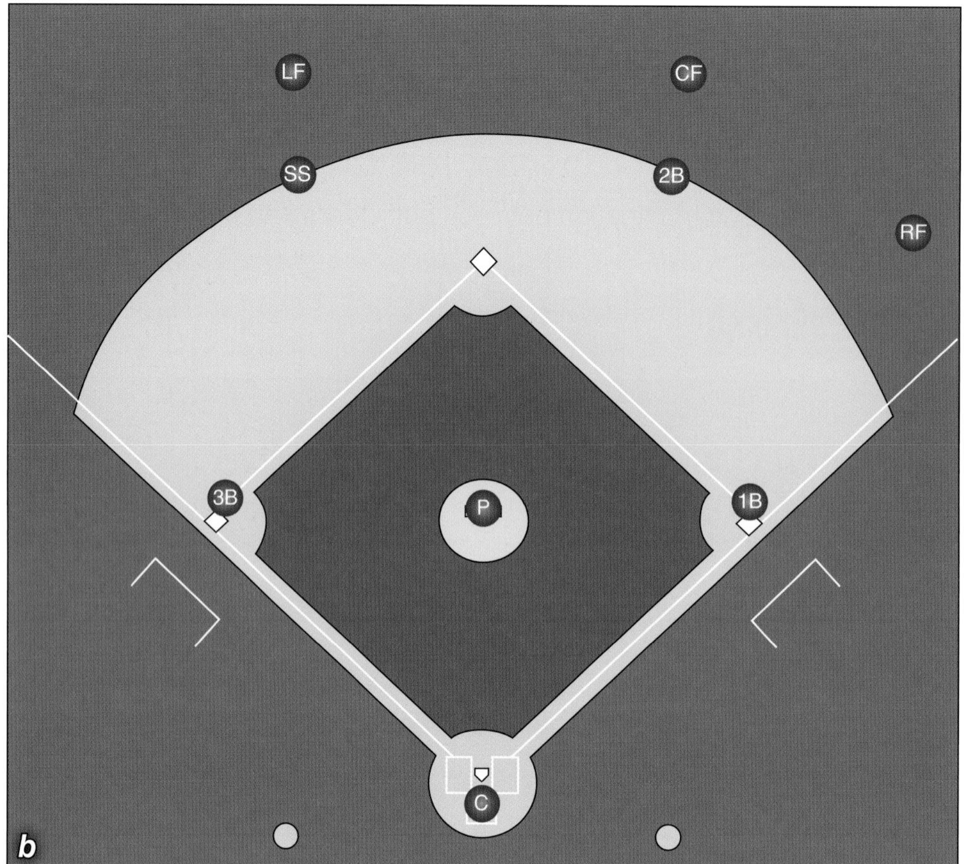

3. For left-handed batters, the shading is opposite: outfielders shade to right field (figure 8.2*b*) to better cover the pull-side unless the batter is known to be an opposite-field slap hitter.
4. The center fielder should communicate to the other outfielders on all shading.
5. Most of the time, all outfielders will shade together in the same direction.

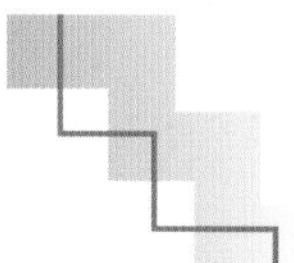

MISSTEP

Lack of communication can cause unwanted gaps between outfielders.

CORRECTION

The center fielder should always glance at the other outfielders to be sure they haven't realigned.

Figure 8.3 NO DOUBLES

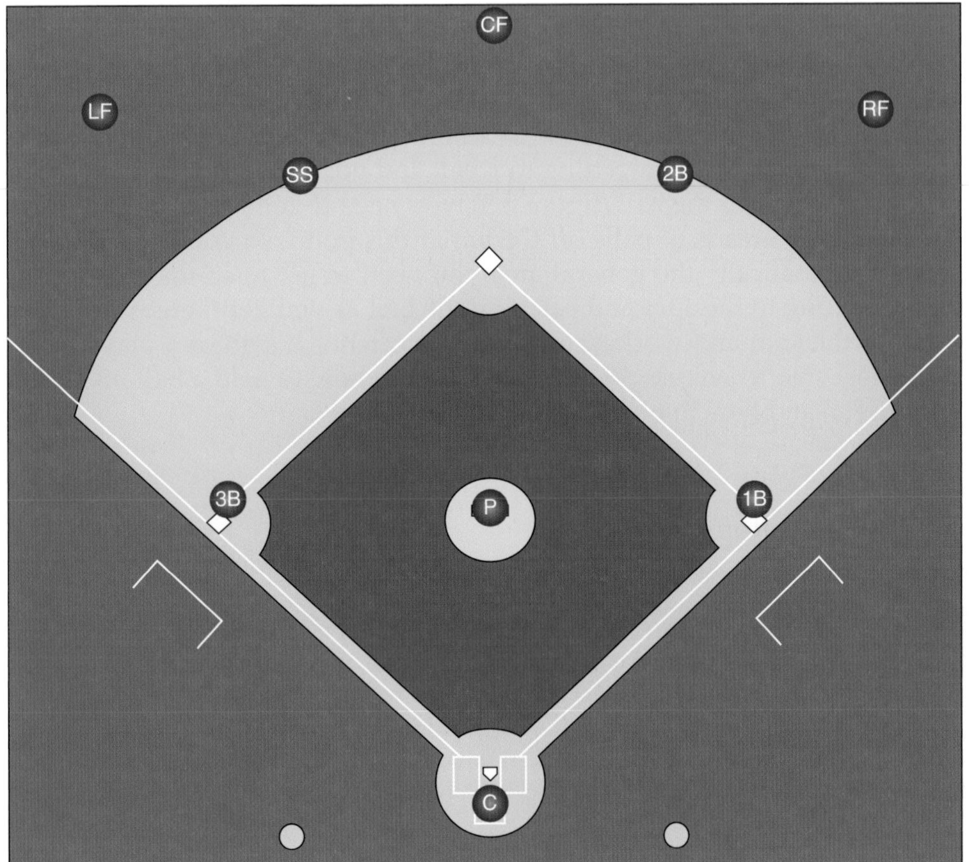

1. The "no doubles" defense is typically used late in games.
2. The outfielders play about 10 to 12 steps deeper than standard positioning at a distance from the wall that will not allow a ball to get over their heads, and they should shade the foul lines.
3. The purpose of "no doubles" positioning is for the outfielders to be able to close the gaps and create better angles in order to keep the batter from hitting a double, or to keep a base runner at first base from scoring on a deep hit.
4. When the outfielder is positioned at no doubles, he should be aware that all throws should go through the cutoff man.

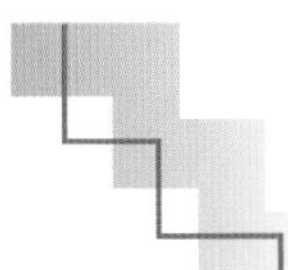

MISSTEP

If you are not deep enough or if you miss the cutoff man, you have defeated the purpose of the no doubles alignment.

CORRECTION

If you are not sure whether you're deep enough, then you probably are not. Keeping the double play in order and keeping the hitter out of scoring position is the first priority when in no doubles.

TRACKING FLY BALLS

Tracking fly balls is the most obvious of all the outfield skills. For this section you need to concentrate on a couple key elements. The main concentration point for a routine fly ball is the first step (figure 8.4). The first step you take needs to put you quickly in a direct line with the spot to where you are running. A good first step can be the difference between getting to a ball and not getting to the ball. After you are in line and tracking the ball (figure 8.5), you need to remember not to drift. You have taken enough reads of balls off the bat at this point, so you should be able to determine automatically the general area you need to get to so that you can make the catch. Drifting to the spot and catching the ball as you get there is bad practice. Sprinting to the spot and working through the catch is a sign of a player who has taken the next step to success. We will also discuss how to field a ball hit straight at you (figure 8.6) and how to play the wall (figure 8.7).

Figure 8.4 **ROUTINE FLY BALL**

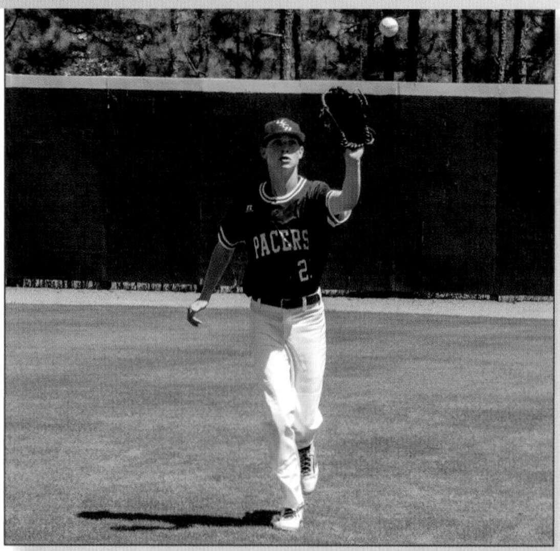

1. Take a good first step.
2. Get behind the ball.
3. Work through the catch.

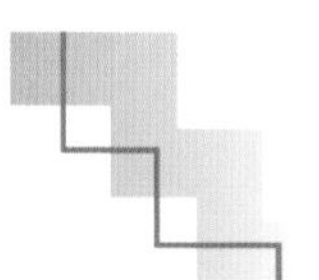

MISSTEP

Drifting to the ball is unacceptable.

CORRECTION

Get behind the ball and work through the catch. To do this, you need to sprint to a spot and then work back in.

Figure 8.5 ANGLES

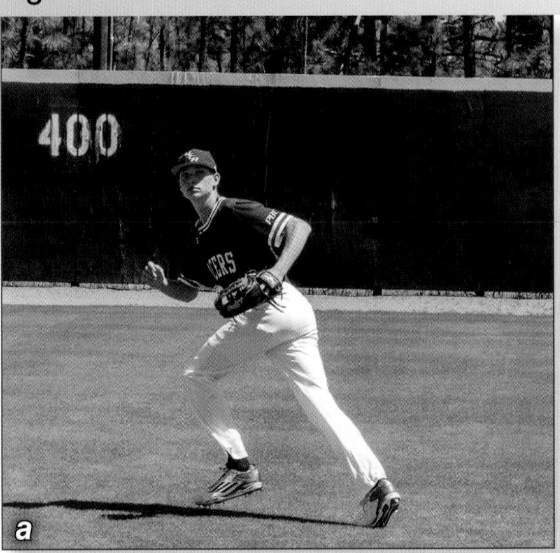

a

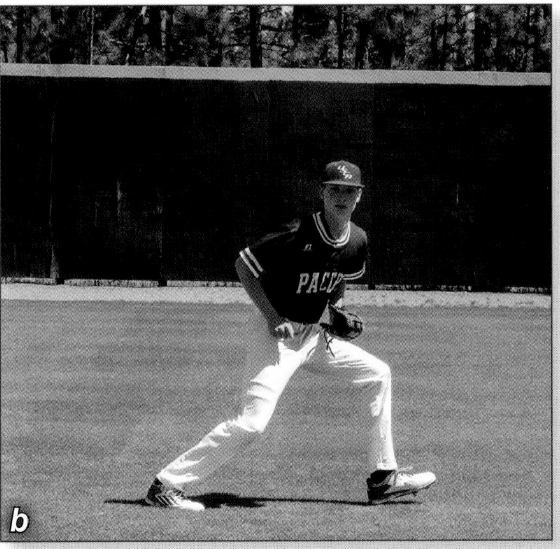

b

1. Judge the sound off the bat and read the flight of the ball.
2. Take a good first step and angle in the direction of the ball, either right (figure 8.5*a*) or left (figure 8.5*b*).
3. Some players may track the ball constantly as they run. For balls farther away, the best approach may be to drop your head, sprint to a spot, and then pick up the ball again.
4. After you make the catch, break down and get the ball back in quickly.

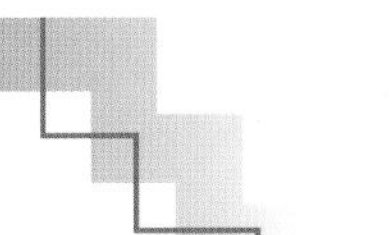

MISSTEP

A bad angle usually means that you did not track the ball to a point behind where it should land, thereby missing the ball completely.

CORRECTION

Everything starts from the first step. Be sure you put yourself in line with the point you are running to. If anything, you should set your angle deeper than necessary because you can adjust back in to the ball easier than you can adjust back.

Figure 8.6 **OVERHEAD, AT YOU, IN FRONT**

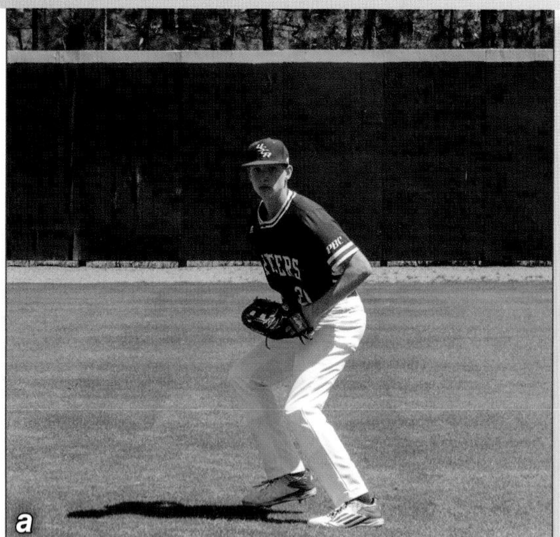

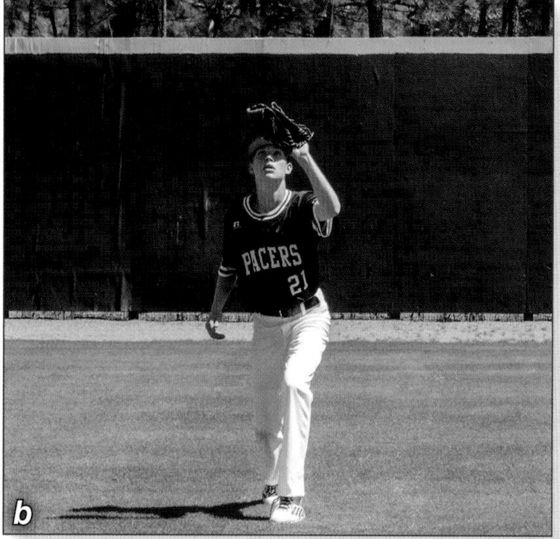

1. For a ball hit straight in line with your position, the sound off the bat and the initial angle of the ball should give you an idea of whether the ball is going over your head, at you, or in front of you.
2. If you are unsure initially, freeze or take a step back (figure 8.6*a*).
3. After you have the ball tracked, take a good first step and get to the ball (figure 8.6*b*).

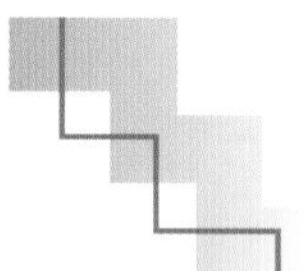

MISSTEP

The worst misread is taking the first step in and having the ball land behind you.

CORRECTION

By freezing on the initial contact, you have the opportunity to track in either direction and keep the ball in front of you.

Figure 8.7 PLAYING THE WALL

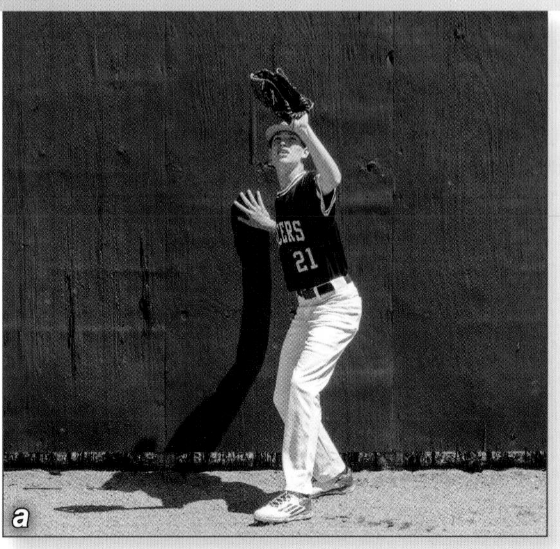

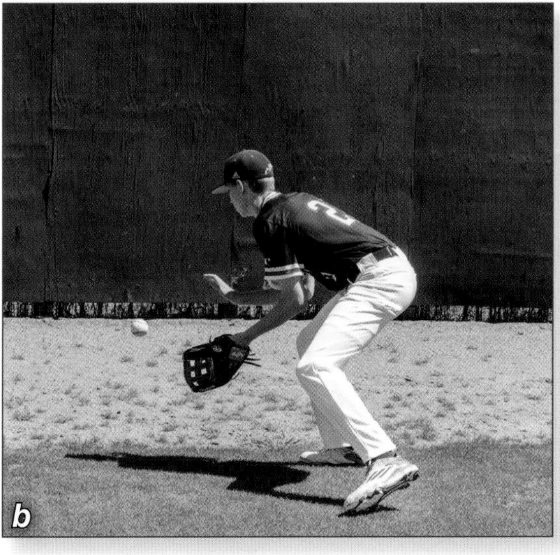

1. Take a good first step.
2. Get to the wall using your throwing hand as you track the catch (figure 8.7*a*).
3. If the ball is over your head and is going to beat you to the wall, break down and line yourself up to play the ball off the wall (figure 8.7*b*).

MISSTEP

Poor tracking can cause you to run to the wall on an uncatchable ball, thus allowing the ball to bounce away and giving the runners extra bases.

CORRECTION

Don't drift. You should have a read on the ball and a feel for where you are in relation to the wall. You should make the decision early enough to give you a chance to break down and play the ball off the wall.

Fly Ball Drill 1 **Bare-Handed Work**

The coach and the player stand 20 feet (6 m) apart facing each other. The coach has a ball in hand ready to flip or lob. The object is to concentrate on proper footwork. The player takes a good first step angled back and right (figure 8.8*a*). As he starts, the coach lobs the ball in the same direction. The player tracks the lobbed ball, gets behind it, and makes the catch with the bare glove hand (figure 8.8*b*) only as he works through the ball and transitions into a crow hop. After five repetitions to the right side, he does five more to the left side.

The next part of the drill focuses on footwork as well as tracking skills. Again, the player takes five repetitions breaking right, but the coach lobs the ball directly over the starting location. As the ball is released, the player switches directions by turning right, forcing him to take his eyes off the ball and relocate it after he has switched direction. After he relocates the ball, he must finish the catch by getting behind and working the ball through the glove. After the five repetitions of the right switch, he does five more in the opposite direction.

The last segment of the drill focuses on coming in and going back on balls in line with the player's position. In this drill, the coach releases the ball before the player breaks, forcing a simulated freeze and read. For balls in front of him, the player should work on getting to the spot, slowing down, and controlling the body through the catch and transition. For balls overhead, the player should work on a first step that sets the body in line to run straight back. He should still make the catch with one hand.

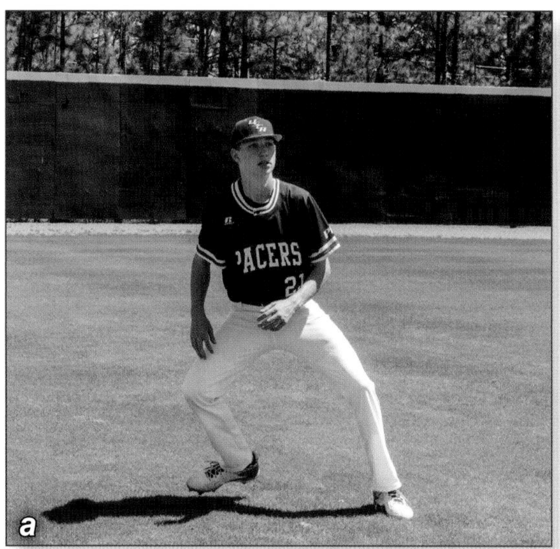

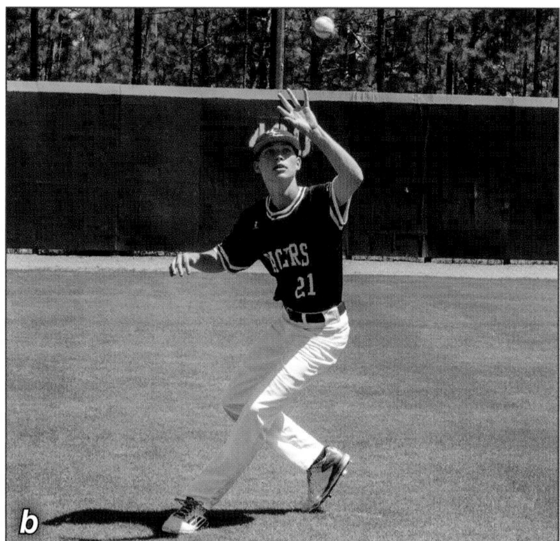

Figure 8.8 Bare-handed work drill.

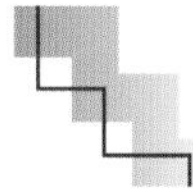

TO INCREASE DIFFICULTY

- Increase the distance and speed.

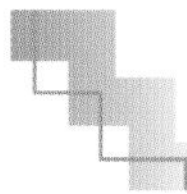

TO DECREASE DIFFICULTY

- Have the coach throw the ball from a shortened distance.
- Use a softer ball.

Success Check

- Did your first step put you in proper alignment with the spot you were going to?
- Did you get behind and work through the catch?
- Did you make the catch?

Score Your Success

You earn 1 point for every successful repetition.

You earn 1/2 point if your technique was good but you dropped the ball or used two hands.

You earn 0 points for being out of position because of slow or poor footwork.

First step right _____ of 5

First step left _____ of 5

First step right _____ of 5

First step left—switch _____ of 5

Coming in—basket _____ of 5

Going straight back _____ of 5

Your score _____ of 30

Fly Ball Drill 2 **Fungoes or Machine**

After the player completes the bare-handed drill, he is ready to put the glove on and transition straight into fly balls. The player stands 200 to 250 feet (61 to 76 m) away from a coach who is hitting fungoes. For this drill, the player goes through the same format used for the bare-handed drill, but every break starts after the ball is hit.

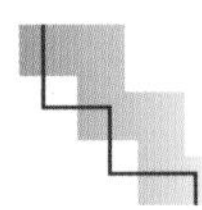

TO INCREASE DIFFICULTY

- Have the player start facing away from the coach and listening for contact. After he hears contact, he turns, finds the ball, and begins to track.

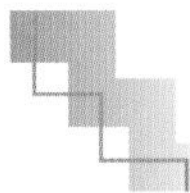

TO DECREASE DIFFICULTY

- The coach uses a machine to feed the fly balls.

Success Check

- Did your first step put you in proper alignment with the spot you were going to?
- Did you get behind and work through the catch, or did you drift to the ball?
- Did you make the catch?

Score Your Success

You earn 1 point for every successful repetition.

You earn 0 points if your technique was good but you dropped the ball.

You earn 0 points for being out of position because of slow or poor footwork.

First step right _____ of 5

First step left _____ of 5

First step right—switch _____ of 5

First step left—switch _____ of 5

Coming in—basket _____ of 5

Going straight back _____ of 5

Your score _____ of 30

Fly Ball Drill 3 **Two-Man Communication**

From the same distance, the outfielders split to 100 to 150 feet (30.5 to 46 m) apart. The coach hits fly balls between the two outfielders. Both outfielders break and track the ball. As the ball reaches the highest point, the two players must communicate who will catch it. The player catching the ball should work through the proper technique. The other player should peel behind where the catch is made to back up.

For this drill, the outfielder or group of outfielders who have authority on calling for the ball must be clarified. This understanding should reduce the possibility of the outfielders colliding or one of them failing to go for the ball.

Success Check

- Did you communicate correctly?
- Did you catch the ball using proper technique?
- Did the partner back up?

Score Your Success

You earn 1 point for a successful repetition.

You earn 1/2 point for a good catch but no back up.

You earn 0 points if the ball falls between you and the other outfielder or you come together.

You earn 0 points for using poor technique.

Your score ____ of 10

Fly Ball Drill 4 **Two-Man Wall Communication**

Using the same two-player setup, the distance apart should shrink to 100 feet (30.5 m) and the coach should be centered 100 feet in front. The coach throws or hits a fungo fly ball to the wall between the two outfielders. The outfielder who calls the ball should use the technique just discussed. The other outfielder should communicate the player's distance to the wall and, if possible, tell the player to stop on an uncatchable ball.

Success Check

- Were you under control as you approached the wall?
- Did the partner communicate well?
- Did you break down if the ball was uncatchable?

Score Your Success

You earn 1 point for every successful repetition.

You earn 0 points for a poor read.

Your score ____ of 5

APPROACHING GROUND BALLS

Ground balls are often overlooked when practicing with outfielders, but this aspect of outfield play may be the most important. For this section, the key point to concentrate on is cutting down the distance. Whenever the ball is hit on the ground through the infield, the outfielder must sprint to the ball. Drifting or coasting will create bad habits and allow a fast runner to take an extra base. Cutting down the distance by being at full speed at contact will eliminate the base runner's thought of taking the extra base. In addition, the outfielder will have time to slow down and get in rhythm with the ball without chopping his feet or having to rush a throw. Here we will discuss the three ways to approach an outfield ground ball: the one-knee approach (figure 8.9), infield style (figure 8.10), and do or die (figure 8.11). Depending on the hitter and offensive situation, an outfielder can determine which approach to use.

Figure 8.9 **ONE-KNEE**

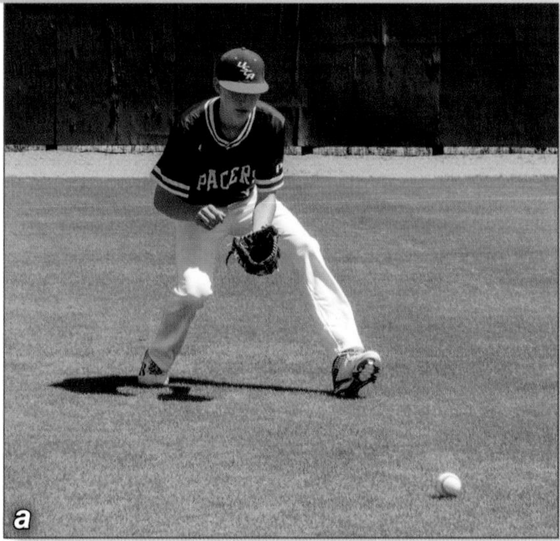

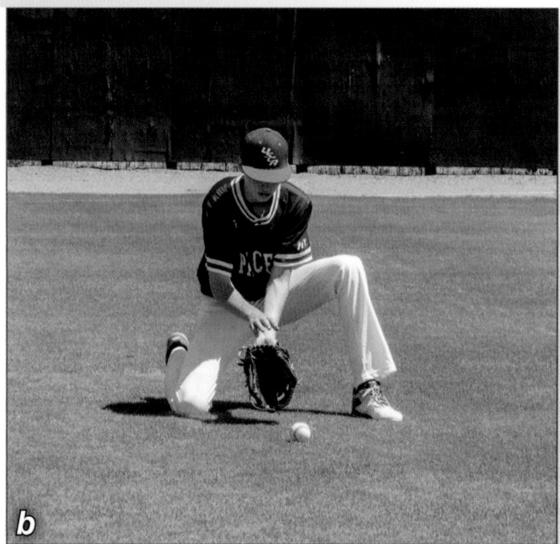

1. The situation for this technique is a slow runner hitting with no one on base.
2. When the ball is hit, cut down the distance (figure 8.9*a*).
3. Break down and center the ball with your body on one knee (figure 8.9*b*).

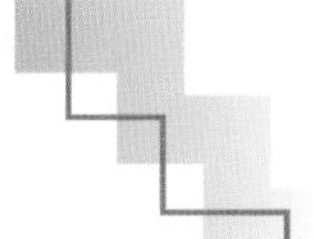

MISSTEP

Going to one knee too soon may allow the ball to kick away.

CORRECTION

Be sure your timing is correct so that if the ball does take an unusual bounce, it will hit your body.

Figure 8.10 INFIELD TRIANGLE STYLE

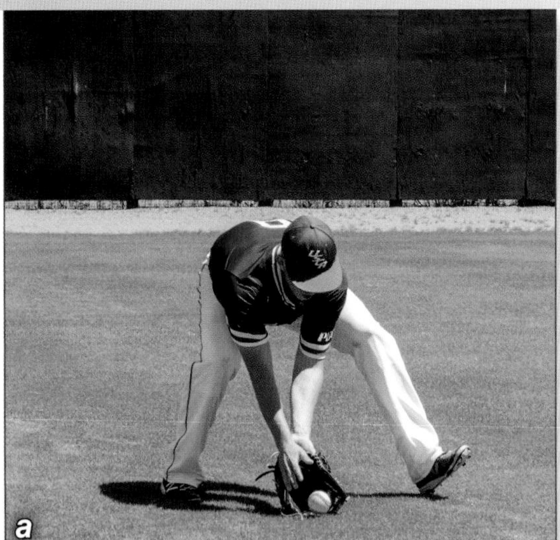

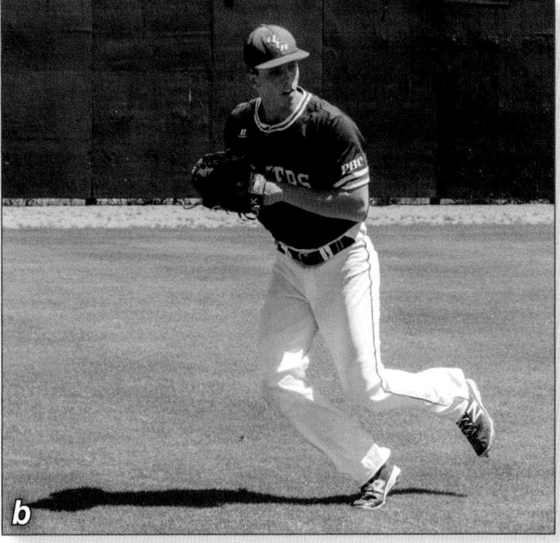

1. Use this technique when a good runner is hitting or when runners on base are not attempting to advance.
2. When the ball is hit, cut down the distance.
3. Using the footwork you learned as an infielder, work through the ball and get to the triangle position (figure 8.10*a*).
4. Transition and make the throw (figure 8.10*b*).

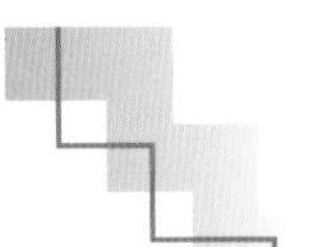

MISSTEP

Fielding the ball to the side of the body.

CORRECTION

Be sure that you can keep the ball in front.

Figure 8.11 **DO OR DIE**

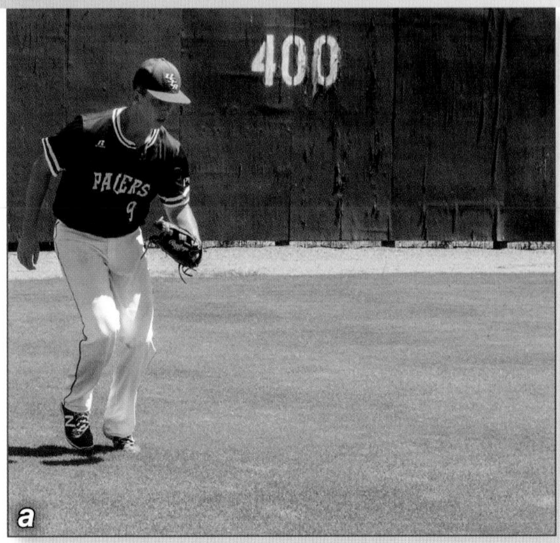

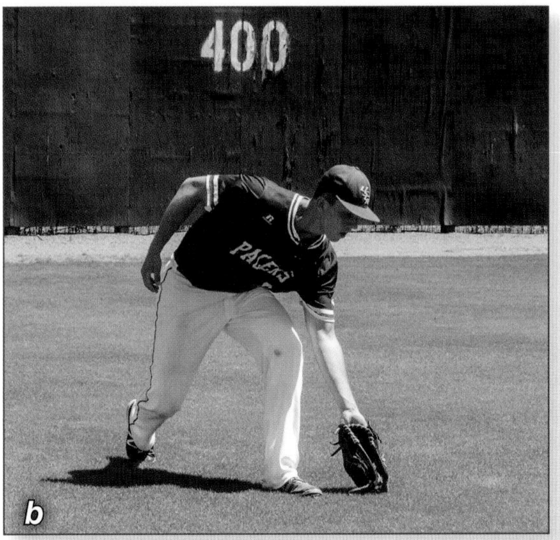

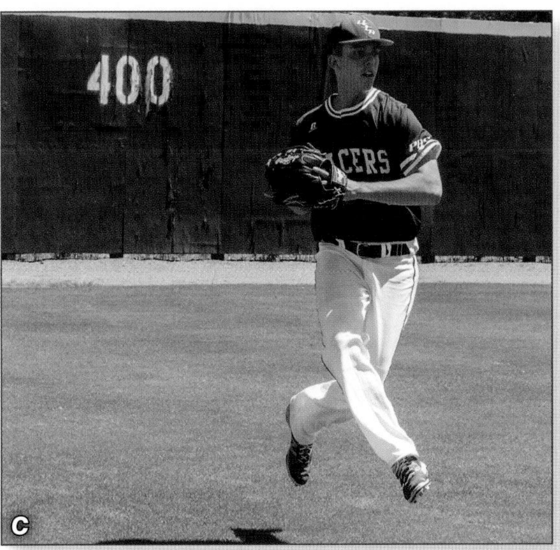

1. The do or die is only used in critical situations when the outfielder has no choice but to try and pick up the ball and attempt to throw out the potential winning runner or go ahead run late in the game. The risk is that it is a very difficult technique, and errors can result in a score, hence "do or die."
2. As you cut down the distance, set your angle to your target.
3. As you approach the ball, time your footwork with the catch (figure 8.11*a*). Your speed will slow a little, but your feet should not get choppy.
4. Field the ball in stride outside the glove-side foot (figure 8.11*b*).
5. As you field the ball, transfer into a crow hop and throw in one smooth motion (figure 8.11*c*).

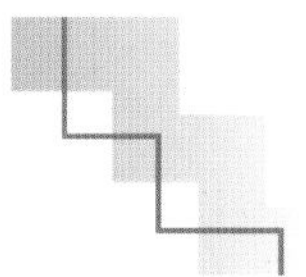

MISSTEP

Chopping your feet will cause your eyes to move, making the catch more difficult and slowing the entire process.

CORRECTION

If you have cut down the distance from contact, you will have extra time to slow down and time your feet without chopping. You can then have one fluid motion through the throw.

Ground Ball Drill 1 **Fungoes or Machine**

Using the same setup used for the fly ball drills, the coach this time hits ground balls to the outfielders. Each outfielder should go through five repetitions of one-knee and infield-style fielding.

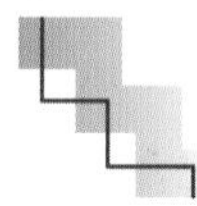

TO INCREASE DIFFICULTY

- Increase the distance and pace of the ball delivery.

TO DECREASE DIFFICULTY

- Have the coach deliver the ball from a shortened distance.

Success Check

- Did you cut down the distance with each repetition?
- Was your timing and footwork correct as you fielded the ball?
- Did you keep the ball in front on a bad hop?

Score Your Success

You earn 1 point for each successful repetition.

You earn 1 point for a bad hop that you keep in front.

You earn 0 points if the ball gets past you or you use poor technique.

One-knee _____ of 5

Infield style _____ of 5

Your score ____ of 10

Ground Ball Drill 2 **Reverse Steps Do or Die**

From 15 to 30 feet (4.5 to 9 m) apart, the player and coach face each other. The player starts in the do-or-die fielding position with the glove-side bare hand on the ground outside the glove-side foot. The coach rolls a ball to the player's hand (figure 8.12*a*). The player catches the ball and transitions into the crow hop without taking a step before the catch (figure 8.12*b*).

After five repetitions, the player adds one step to the process. This step puts him back into fielding position. For a right-handed thrower, the step is with the left foot. The player backs up slightly and stands up squared to the coach. As the coach rolls the ball, the player times the ball and steps with his glove-side foot, fields the ball, and continues through the process in one motion.

After five one-step reps, the player repeats the drill, adding two and then three steps to the process. After performing all 20 repetitions, the player starts the process over using his glove.

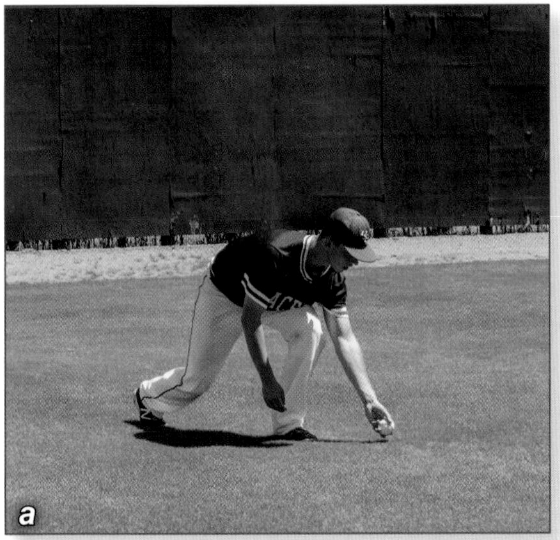

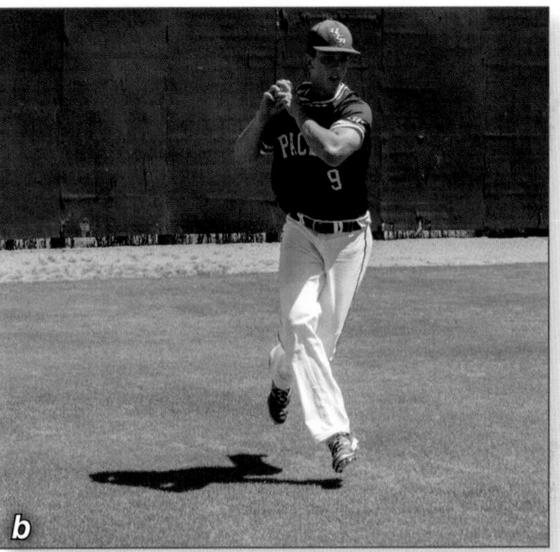

Figure 8.12 Reverse steps do-or-die drill.

Success Check

- Did you get into a good fielding position?
- Was your timing with the ball right?
- Were you able to field the ball cleanly and consistently and have a smooth transition?

Score Your Success

You earn 1 point for every successful rep with good timing.

You earn 1/2 point if you bobble the ball with the bare hand.

You earn 0 points if the ball gets by because of poor timing and footwork.

No steps—stationary bare-handed _____ of 5

One step—bare-handed _____ of 5

Two steps—bare-handed _____ of 5

Three steps—bare-handed _____ of 5

No steps—stationary with glove _____ of 5

One step with glove _____ of 5

Two steps with glove _____ of 5

Three steps with glove _____ of 5

Your score ____ of 40

Ground Ball Drill 3 **Angles With Cones**

Return to the 150-foot (46 m) distance between player and coach. Set up two cones, 20 to 30 feet (6 to 9 m) diagonally in front of the player, one on each side. The coach hits the ground balls at or outside either cone (five reps to each). The player should explode to the cone the ball is rolling to (figure 8.13*a*), cutting down the distance to the ball. He works around the outside of the cone as he changes direction so that his momentum is going back toward the coach. He should then field the ball with the proper technique (figure 8.13*b*) and transition.

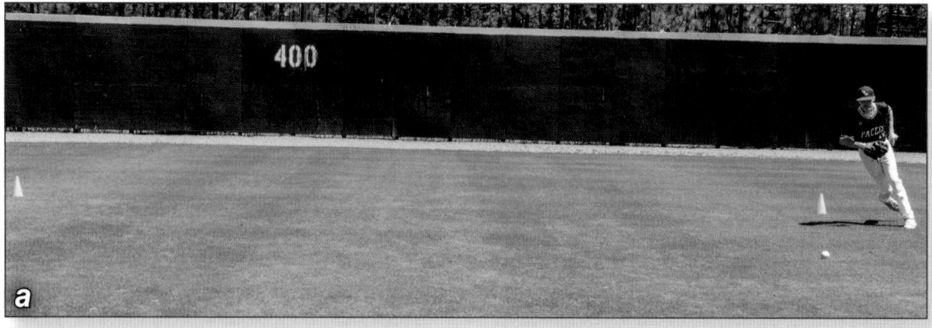

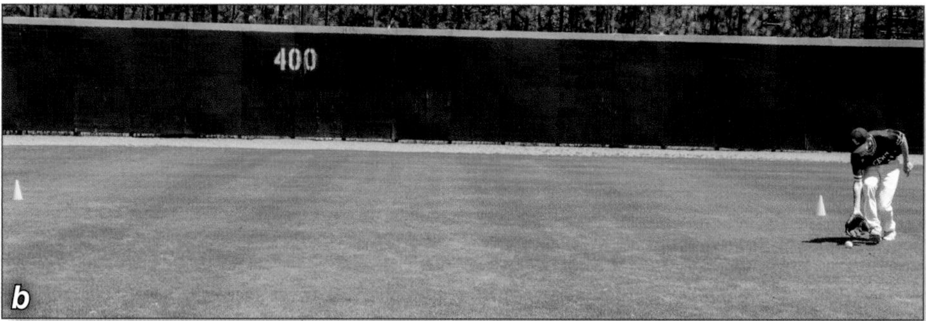

Figure 8.13 Angles with cones drill.

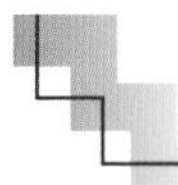

TO INCREASE DIFFICULTY

- Increase the distance to each cone.

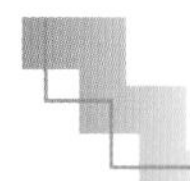

TO DECREASE DIFFICULTY

- Have the coach deliver the ball from a shortened distance.

Success Check

- Did you beat the ball to the cone?
- Did you have good footwork as you changed direction, allowing you to get into a good fielding position?

Score Your Success

You earn 1 point for every successful repetition.

You earn 1/2 point if you use choppy footwork around the cone.

You earn 0 points for not beating the ball to the cone or for letting the ball get by.

Angle right _____ of 5

Angle left _____ of 5

Your score ____ of 10

Ground Ball Drill 4 **Reverse Pivot**

The reverse pivot drill is used for a ball hit to the player's glove side that he can get to but cannot create an angle around. For this drill, the setup remains the same as that for the previous drill. The coach hit ground balls (five reps) harder and farther outside the cone to the glove side of the player. The player breaks to the ball at full speed. Taking a steeper angle to the ball is often better to ensure that it doesn't get by. When the player is within fielding range, he catches the ball in front of his glove-side foot (figure 8.14*a*). After he catches the ball, the player quickly plants his back foot as he turns his glove-side foot toward the target (figure 8.14*b*). If he does the reverse pivot perfectly, the player releases the ball as the front foot lands (figure 8.14*c*). Most of the time, the player takes a shuffle toward the target to build momentum on the throw. This is fine.

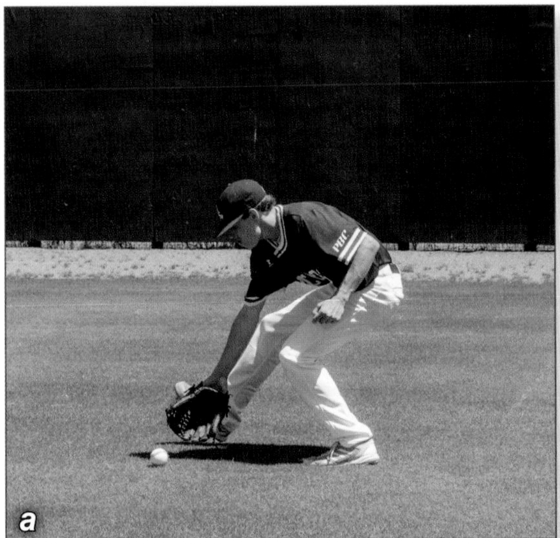

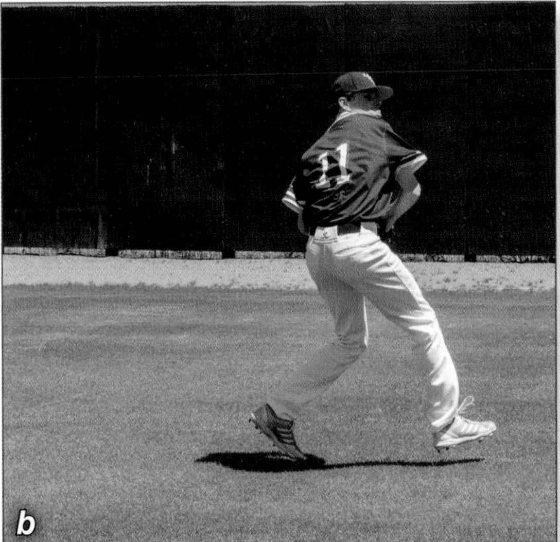

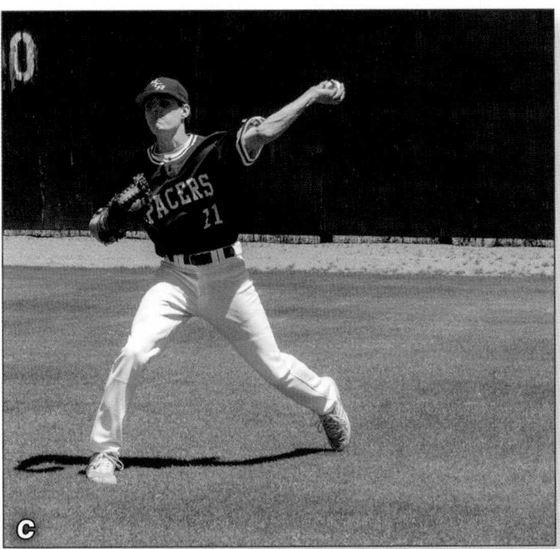

Figure 8.14 Reverse pivot drill.

(continued)

Ground Ball Drill 4 *(continued)*

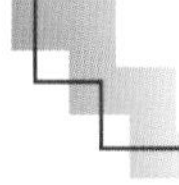

TO INCREASE DIFFICULTY

- Increase the distance and challenge the fielder's range.

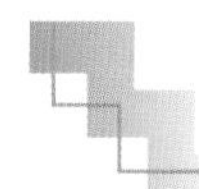

TO DECREASE DIFFICULTY

- Have the outfielder start with the ball in the glove.

Success Check

- Were you able to cut off the ball and prevent it from getting by?
- How quickly were you able to reverse pivot after cutting off the ball?
- Did you get turned enough to line up with the target?

Score Your Success

You earn 1 point for every quick and successful repetition.

You earn 1/2 point if you had to take more than one shuffle before you threw the ball.

You earn 0 points for taking too long to break down and make the transition.

Your score ____ of 5

POSTPITCH POSITIONING

Positioning yourself as an outfielder after the ball is in play is important to team defense, whether the ball is hit to you or not. A miscue or error can occur on every play on a baseball field, so each outfielder must anticipate and move into a position that will back up a misplay by a teammate. Here we discuss backing up between outfielders (figure 8.15) and backing up the infield (figure 8.16).

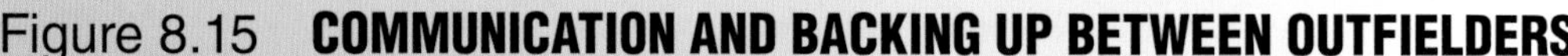

Figure 8.15 **COMMUNICATION AND BACKING UP BETWEEN OUTFIELDERS**

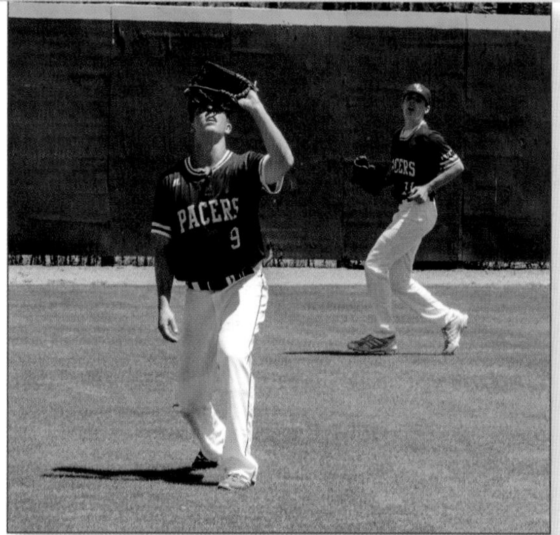

1. As a reminder, balls that are hit between two outfielders should be handled by one and backed up by the other.
2. The ball should be called for as soon as possible, while the other outfielder moves into position to back up.
3. The center fielder is the authority on these calls and should direct traffic accordingly.

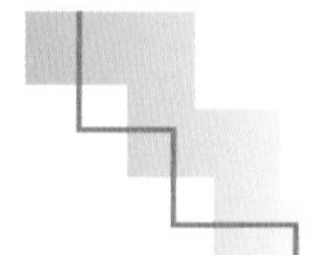

MISSTEP

Having two players collide or having neither player go for the ball is unacceptable. Both are a direct result of poor communication.

CORRECTION

Each player must want the ball yet understand who has priority. With that in mind, the sooner the call is made, the better.

Figure 8.16 BACKING UP THE INFIELD

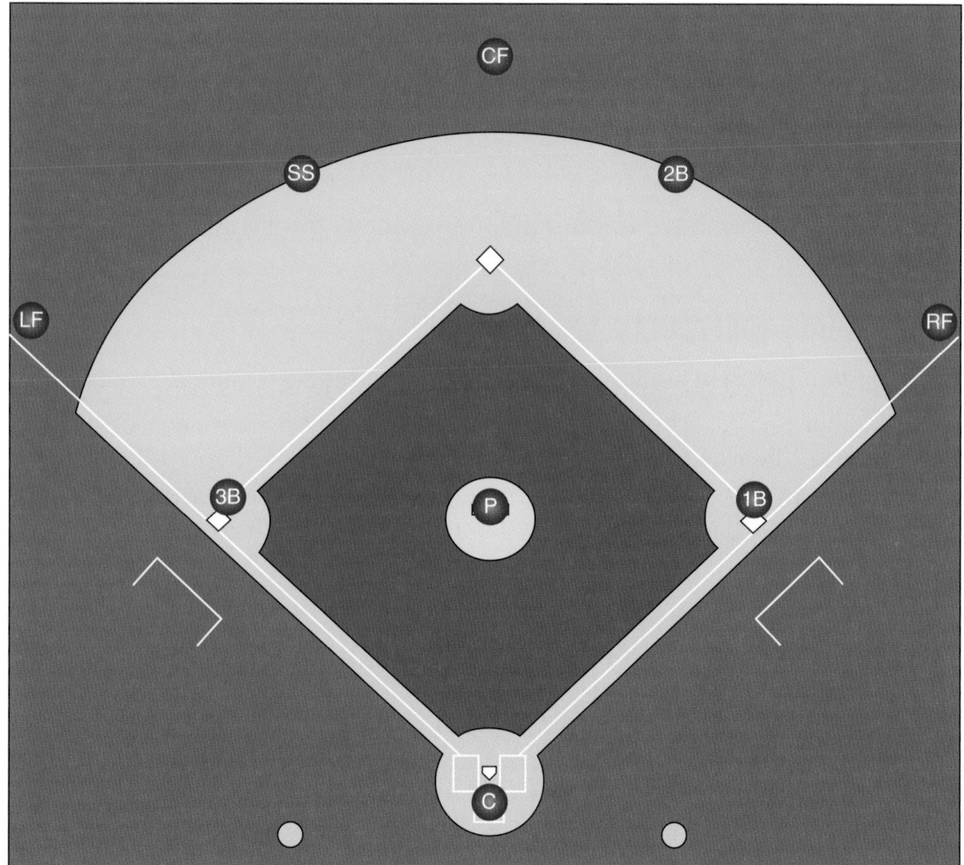

1. When the ball is in play on the infield or elsewhere in the outfield, the other outfielders should always be moving to back up whatever may happen on the infield.
2. The right fielder has the most important responsibilities of the outfielders because most throws on the infield are to first base.
3. The right fielder must always get into position for an errant throw by the first baseman. The center fielder should back up the area between the shortstop and the second baseman.
4. The left fielder, therefore, should back up the area from the shortstop to the third-base line.

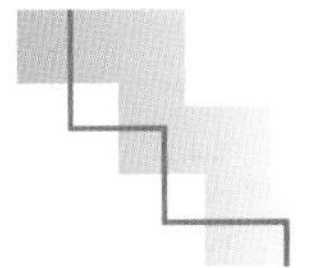

MISSTEP

A common misstep is getting caught watching the play and forgetting to move to back up. Most of the time, this inattention will go unnoticed, but the one time that you are caught out of position on a bad throw is the one time that it hurts the most.

CORRECTION

Backing up the infield is a major responsibility for each outfield position. This job should be made a habit.

Postpitch Positioning Drill **Team Defense or Intrasquad**

The positioning drill can be done during a team defense or intrasquad setting. The idea is to check on each outfielder's position as a play concludes.

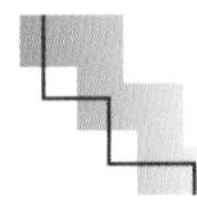

TO INCREASE DIFFICULTY

- In a live setting, have each outfielder react to the situation at game speed.

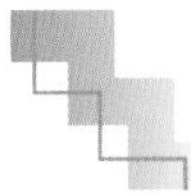

TO DECREASE DIFFICULTY

- In a team defense setting, walk through where each outfielder should move to.

Success Check

- Did the outfielder move to back up?
- Was he in the correct spot just in case?

Score Your Success

You earn 1 point for getting to the right spot.

You earn 0 points for being late or not moving.

Your score ____ of 10

SUCCESS SUMMARY

As you can see, playing the outfield can be a lot more detailed than it may look on TV. These drills are designed to help you develop the skills you need to play at a higher level and make the game look as easy as it does on TV.

Fly Ball Drills

1. Bare-handed work ____ out of 30
2. Fungoes or machine ____ out of 30
3. Two-man communication ____ out of 10
4. Two-man wall communication ____ out of 5

Ground Ball Drills

1. Fungoes or machine ____ out of 10
2. Reverse steps do or die ____ out of 40
3. Angles with cones ____ out of 10
4. Reverse pivot ____ out of 5

Postpitch Positioning Drill

1. Team defense or intrasquad ____ out of 10

Total ____ **out of 150**

Playing the outfield is more than just standing around waiting for a pop-up. If you scored higher than 120, you are not that guy and have successfully taken the next step to success. Congratulations! As we continue, you will need the skills you have learned in these first eight steps to put together your complete skill package as a team player.

STEP

9

Situational Defense

As we move into the final two parts of your steps to success, you have the skills you need to fulfill your responsibilities as part of a team defense. These next two steps show how defenders work together to get outs. As you will notice, communication is a big part of a successful team defense. Good communication requires each player to have good knowledge of the game, sufficient understanding of the situation, and enough baseball savvy to get into proper position and make good decisions in an instant.

In this step, we look at how to defend the bunt, the first-and-third defense, rundowns, fly ball communication, and tandem relays. Communicating, controlling the baseball, and getting an out go a long way as part of a team defense.

BUNT DEFENSE

Defending the bunt can make or break a team defensively. Teams that can control the baseball and get an out will have much more success than those that are constantly out of position and do not control the baseball. Bunting is usually used in sacrifice situations when an offense is willing to give up an out to advance the base runner or base runners. These situations typically occur late in a game with a runner on first or second, or runners on first and second with zero outs. By sacrificing a runner into scoring position, the offense assumes that a base hit will then score that runner. By sacrificing a runner from second to third, the offense can then score in various ways other than a base hit, such as a sacrifice fly. In addition, some hitters might use a bunt as a way to get on base outside of these typical sacrifice situations.

Here we discuss defending the bunt with runners on first (figure 9.1), defending the bunt with runners on first and second (figure 9.2) and defending against a bunt for a hit (figure 9.3).

Figure 9.1 **RUNNER ON FIRST**

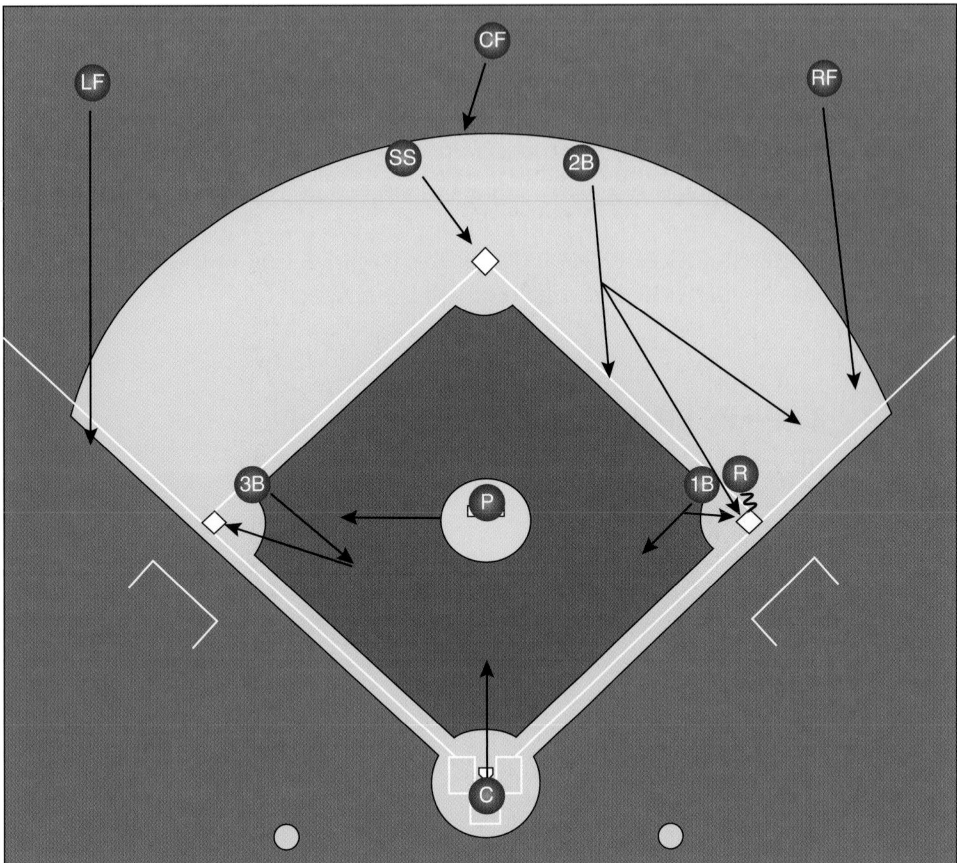

1. The first baseman holds the runner. As the pitch is delivered and the bunt is laid down, the first baseman reads the ball. Anything past the range of the pitcher and within a small vicinity to the right, he fields the ball; otherwise, he returns to the bag.
2. In this bunt situation, the second baseman should move away from double-play depth and toward first base. He is responsible for the triangle communication, attacking anything past the pitcher and directing the first baseman.
3. The shortstop stays in double-play depth and covers second base when the bunt is put in play.
4. The third baseman starts in on the grass. He is responsible for the entire third-base side.
5. The pitcher is responsible for the middle of the field and the first-base side.
6. The catcher is responsible for anything that stops close to home plate.
7. If the third baseman fields the ball, the pitcher should sprint to cover third. The catcher should stay to cover home plate in this situation, and if he can't tell for sure if the lead runner can be tagged out at second he calls out for a throw to first. If anyone else fields the ball, the third baseman should get back to cover the bag.
8. The outfielders back up their assigned bases, as was discussed in figure 8.16 in step 8.

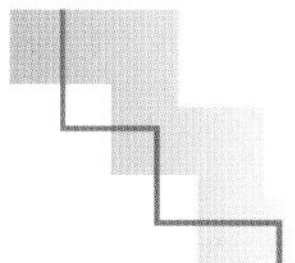

MISSTEP

If the ball is bunted in the triangle between the pitcher, first baseman, and second baseman, communication is often the misstep that leads to issues.

CORRECTION

The second baseman can solve the communication issue if his first priority is to get the ball bunted past the pitcher. If the first baseman understands this and does not break to get a ball in the triangle but instead covers first, most issues will be solved.

Figure 9.2 **RUNNERS ON FIRST AND SECOND**

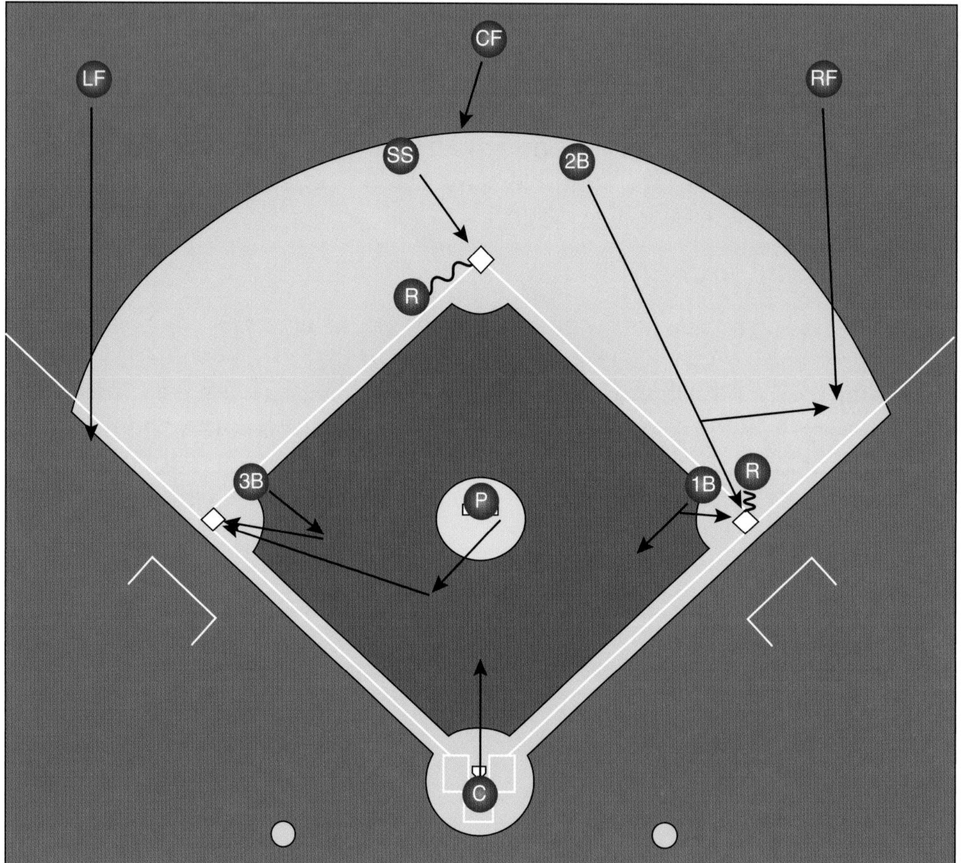

1. In a bunt situation with runners on first and second and no outs, the first baseman plays in front of the runner and charges the bunt. If the ball is bunted on the third-base side, the first baseman gets back to cover the base.
2. The second baseman moves toward first base and covers first if the first baseman does not get back to the bag.
3. The shortstop covers second base.
4. The third baseman starts in front of the third-base bag. He reads the bunt and fields anything toward the line or past the pitcher. If the pitcher can field the ball, the third baseman covers the third-base bag.
5. The pitcher is responsible for whatever he can get on the third-base side.
6. The catcher gets anything he can in front of the plate. He is also responsible for making the call on where the ball should be thrown.

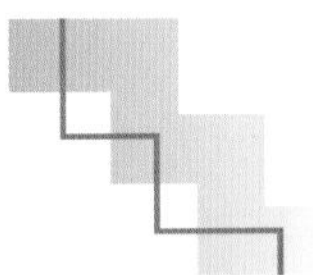

MISSTEP

A common misstep is a bad read by the third baseman on a ball that the pitcher cannot field. He may also charge too soon with a left-handed pitcher on the mound.

CORRECTION

If the third baseman has any doubt about whether the pitcher can field the ball, he should charge. Remember the importance of getting an out. A left-handed pitcher typically finishes the pitch by falling toward the third-base side, so he can cover more area and does not have to spin to throw to third.

Figure 9.3 BUNT FOR A HIT

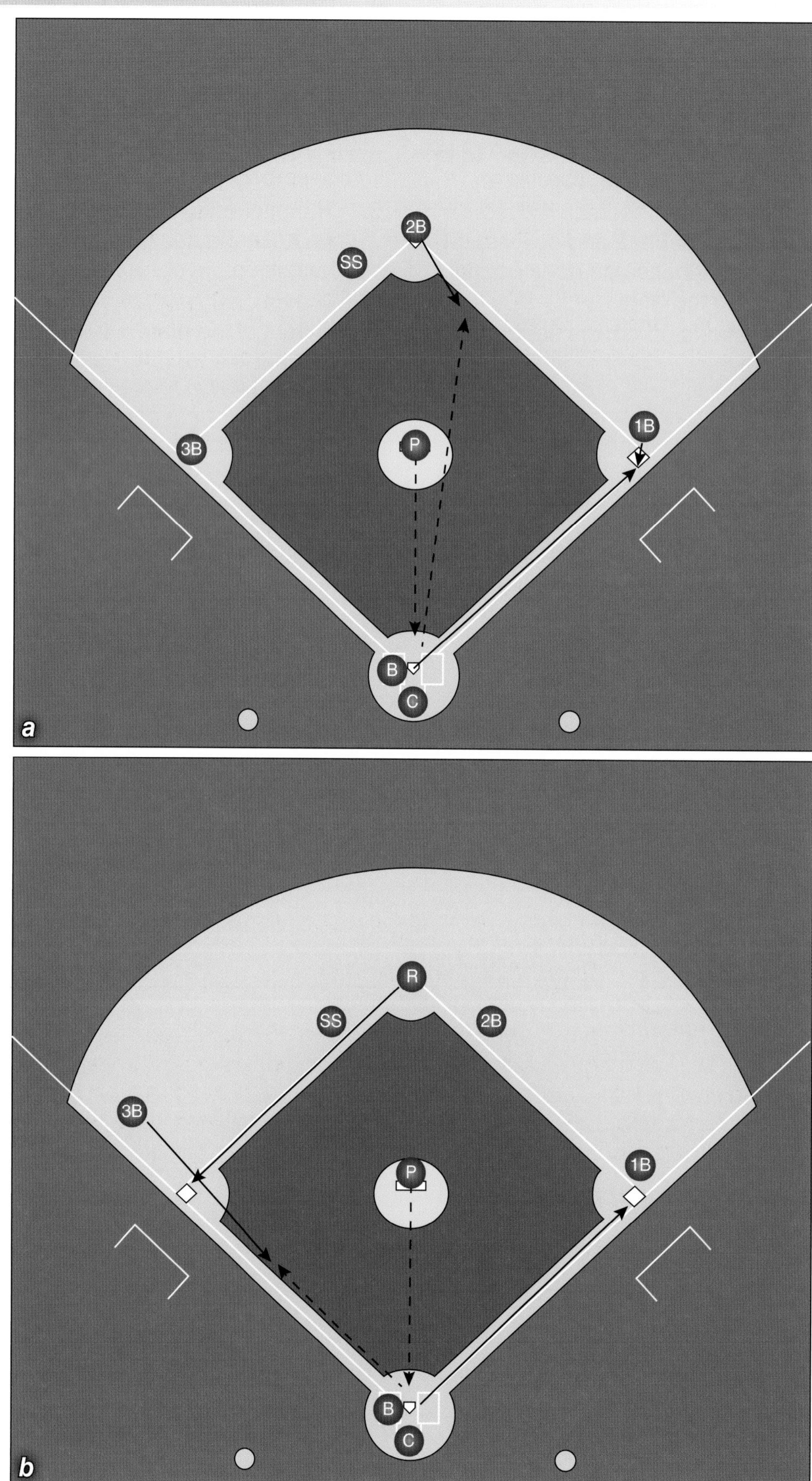

1. Each defensive player should be aware of hitters who may attempt to bunt for a hit. Bunting for a hit is often used by players with speed or those who are not accomplished hitters.
2. A push bunt is intended to be placed in the triangle area on the first-base side (figure 9.3*a*). It is commonly tried with a fast hitter when the second baseman is pulled up to the middle and you have a left-handed pitcher on the mound.
3. The second baseman should charge toward home as soon as he sees the hitter move his hands to bunt.
4. After the ball is bunted, the same triangle communication should take place; the second baseman directs traffic.
5. The first baseman moves to cover first base and waits to take the throw to get the runner out.
6. For a drag bunt on the third-base side (figure 9.3*b*), the third baseman is usually in a do-or-die situation with his field and throw to first. This is because the drag bunt is usually employed when the third baseman is playing deep. So, if you know a hitter is an excellent bunter and is very fast, it may be a good idea to have the third baseman move closer to his standard position.
7. The first baseman moves to cover first and waits for the throw to get the runner out.

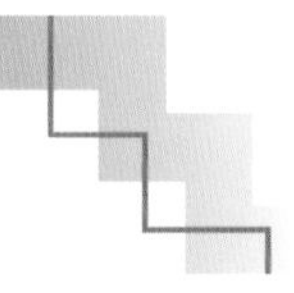

MISSTEP

In do-or-die situations for the third baseman, overthrows are common.

CORRECTION

The second baseman and right fielder should move behind the first baseman to back up on a potential overthrow.

Bunt Drill 1 **Team Pitcher's Fielding Practice (PFP) for Bunt Defense—Coach Rolling Bunts**

This team drill begins with the defense in position and the pitcher on the mound. This drill can be done with outfielders in position working on backing up bases or with just the infielders. A coach is in the batter's box with a ball in hand. The situation is given, and the bunt defense play is called. The pitcher simulates throwing the pitch, and the coach rolls the ball to different areas, simulating a bunt.

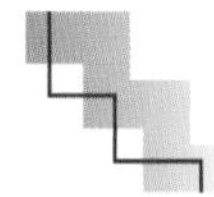

TO INCREASE DIFFICULTY

- Have base runners play the bunts live.

TO DECREASE DIFFICULTY

- Use no base runners and no ball. Have each player move accordingly based on specifics given by the coach.

(continued)

Bunt Drill 1 *(continued)*

Success Check

- Was there good communication between infielders?
- Did players read the bunt and move to the appropriate positions quickly?
- Were no overthrows, particularly by the third baseman covering a drag bunt, made?

Score Your Success

The defense earns 1 point for executing and getting an out.

The defense earns 0 points for not getting an out.

Your score ____ of 15

Bunt Drill 2 **Defensive Bunt Intrasquad**

The bunt intrasquad is designed to focus on defending every possible bunt. The team can be divided up for this drill. Preferably, this drill is done with just the infielders and the pitcher on the field and with the rest of the team on offense. The pitcher throws live, and the game is played out with the offense only being able to bunt.

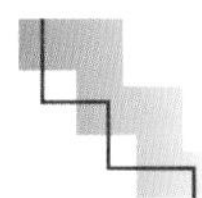

TO INCREASE DIFFICULTY

- Go at game speed, including signs and a live offense.

TO DECREASE DIFFICULTY

- Have the coach roll the bunt.

Success Check

- How many runs were scored? This will determine if the defense is reading and executing well.
- How many errors were made? Overthrows are common from the third baseman on the drag bunt. Players need to move into position to back up their man.

Score Your Success

The defense earns 1 point for executing and getting an out.

The defense earns 0 points for not getting an out.

Your score ____ of 25

FIRST-AND-THIRD DEFENSE

Defending a first-and-third offense (when there are runners on first base and third base) requires each player to understand the situation and the goal of the defense at that moment. Each defender has a responsibility and should be aware of the common goal for the defense; each situation may change what that goal is. To break it down, let's look at these responsibilities based on what an offense might do. We'll discuss the throw through (figure 9.4), which is the standard first-and-third defense, as well as the middle infielders' cut (figure 9.5), covering a hit back to the pitcher (figure 9.6), and a throw to third (figure 9.7).

Figure 9.4 **THROW THROUGH**

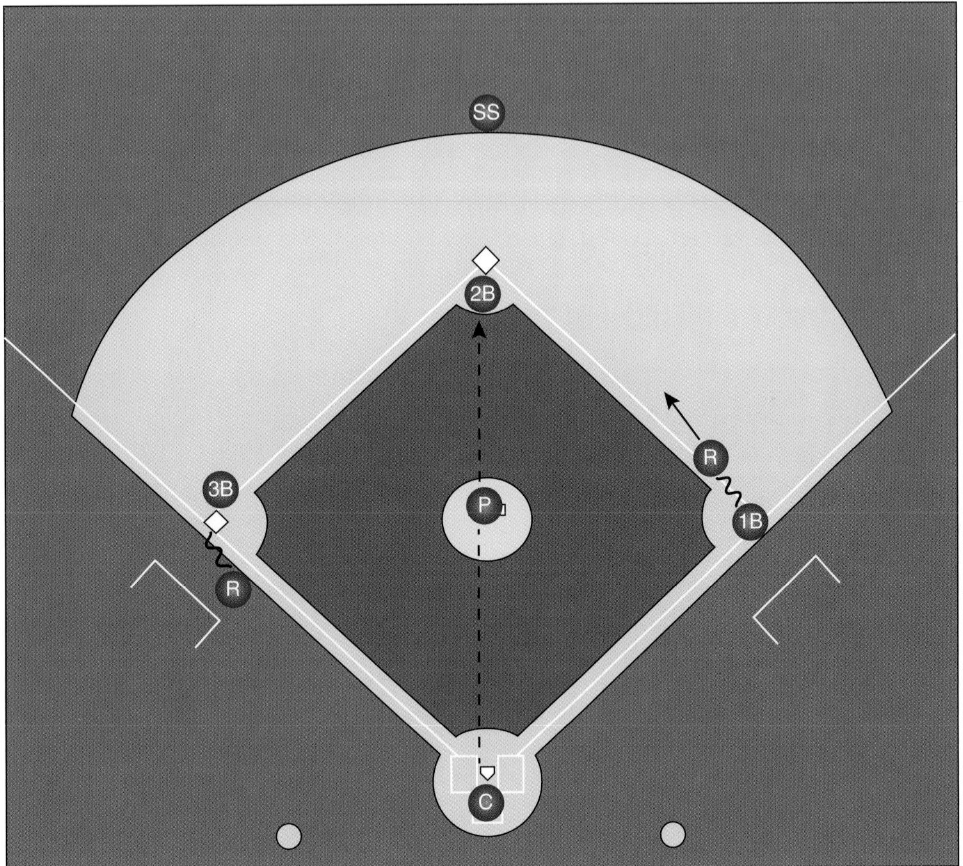

1. The standard first-and-third defense is set up with the infield at double-play depth, the first baseman holding the runner, and the third baseman even with the bag.
2. As the runner steals, the catcher peeks at the runner at third base (if he is coming home, the catcher doesn't make the throw to second). If the runner is stationary, the throw goes straight to second.
3. A middle infielder should take the throw at the bag, and the other middle infielder should be backing up.
4. Depending on the situation, the runner at third base may attempt to run home as the catcher makes the throw. The third baseman should yell, "Runner" if this happens.
5. At this point, the middle infielder can catch and tag the runner at second, or come to the throw, catch it, and attempt to throw out the runner at home.
6. The pitcher just needs to get out of the way of the throw from home to second.

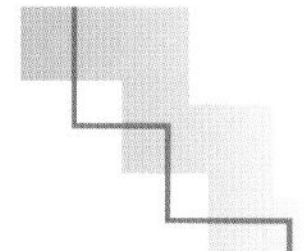

MISSTEP

The situation, especially the number of outs, determines what read the middle infielder should make. With two outs, the common misstep that the middle infielder will make is attempting to throw out the runner at home when he could have made the third out at second.

CORRECTION

The play call should remind the middle infielder of what read to make.

Figure 9.5 **MIDDLE INFIELDERS' CUT**

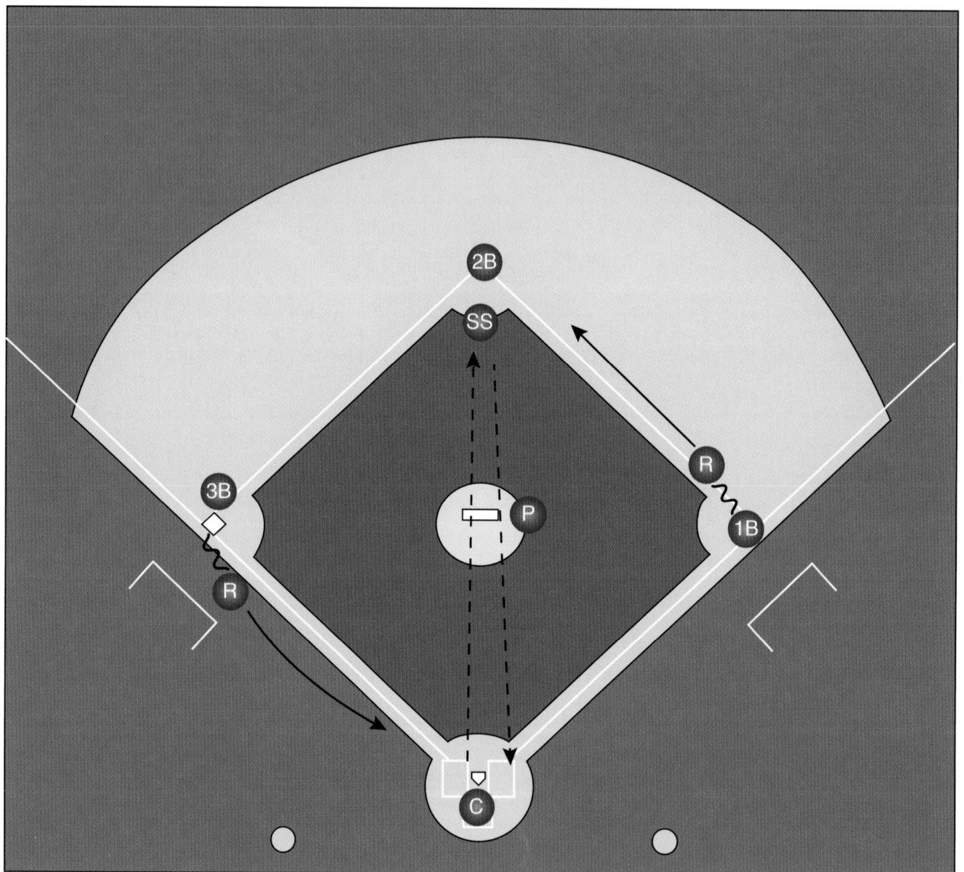

1. With the first baseman holding the runner and the third baseman even with the bag, the middle infielder in coverage takes the throw from the catcher in front of the second-base bag. Typically, this is where the cut of the grass is. The other middle infielder should be at the bag, which is also a position of backing up the throw.
2. The cutoff man is reading the runner at third base. If the runner breaks for home or is far enough away from third base, the infielder should cut the throw and look to get the runner out at third.
3. If the runner at third base is stationary near the bag, the throw should not be cut; therefore, the other middle infielder receives the ball at the bag and attempts to tag out the base stealer. In this case, the pitcher just needs to get out of the way of the throw by the catcher from home plate to second base.

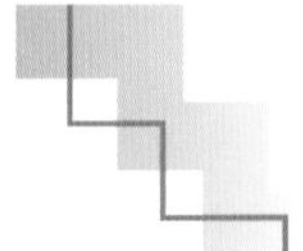

MISSTEP

The throw from the catcher is vital. If the throw is off target, the middle infielder will have no chance of handling the ball and getting an out.

CORRECTION

The catcher must throw the ball as he would if throwing straight through. The positioning of the cutoff man should not change anything about the throw.

Figure 9.6 **BACK TO PITCHER**

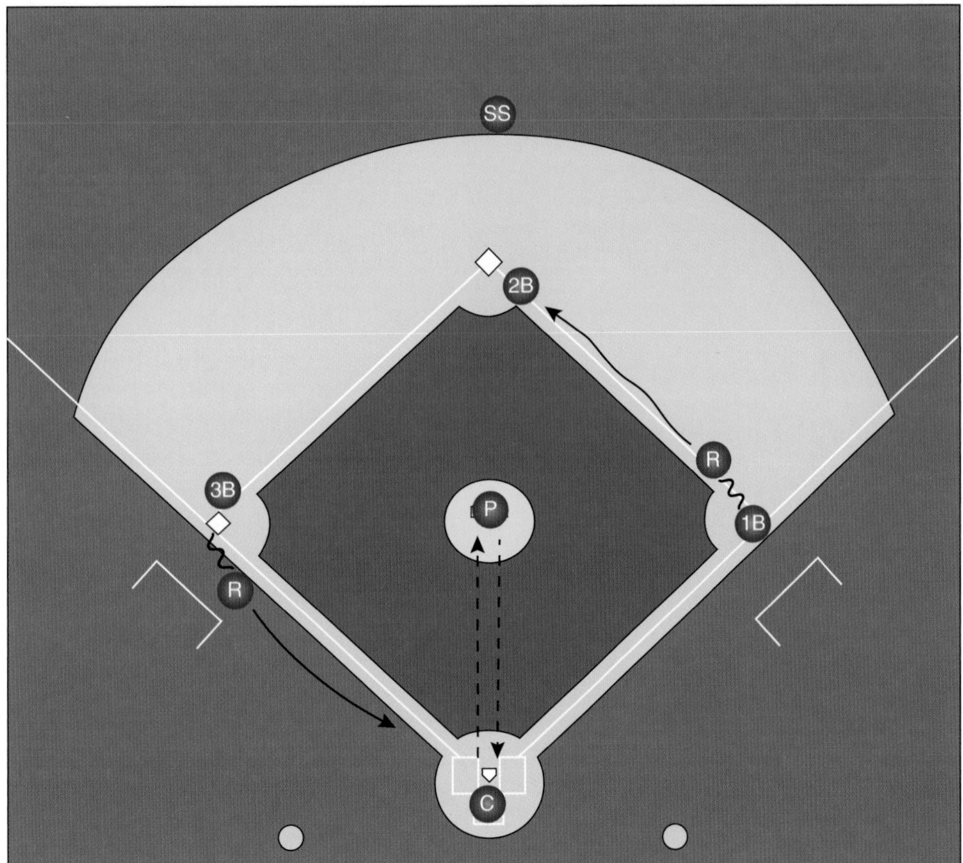

1. In this play call, the catcher does the same actions he would if throwing straight through.
2. The first baseman is holding the runner, and the third baseman is even with the bag. The second baseman covers the base and the shortstop backs him.
3. The pitcher is the cutoff man. He catches the throw from the catcher and looks to catch the runner at third breaking toward home.

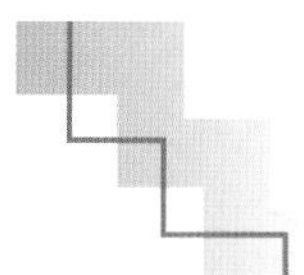

MISSTEP

If the pitcher does not get the call that the throw is coming to him, he may be in danger of having the catcher hit him with the throw.

CORRECTION

The catcher should make the throw chest to head high and straight through toward second base. If the pitcher does forget, he should be out of the way, allowing the middle infielders to catch the ball.

Figure 9.7 THROW TO THIRD

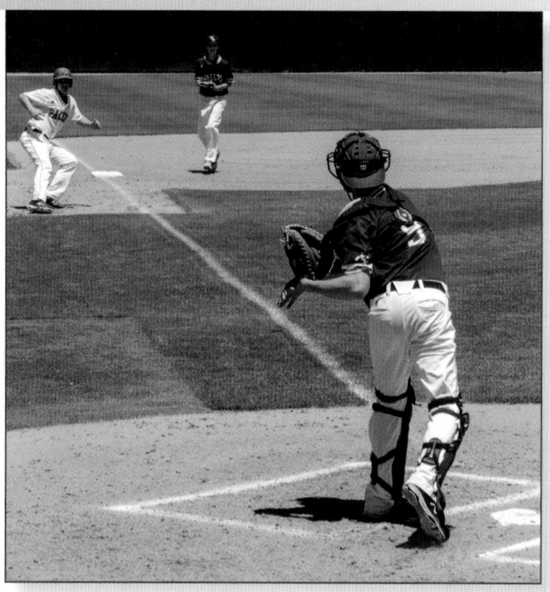

1. This call is often made with an exceptionally fast runner at first or perhaps a runner at third who is getting a big lead. The infielders are in standard first-and-third defense double-play depth and the first baseman is holding the runner.
2. The catcher should make the throw straight through the runner at third, chest high. If the runner has squared his shoulders to home, the throw at his chest will freeze him. If he does move, the third baseman will still be able to handle the throw.
3. The left fielder should back up the third baseman in case of an overthrow.

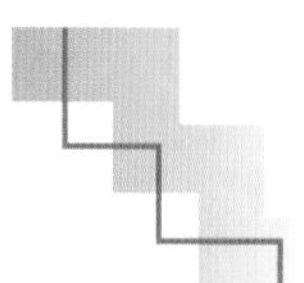

MISSTEP

The catcher may try to throw around the runner at third base, which increases the chance of throwing the ball away.

CORRECTION

Throwing through the runner gives the catcher a bigger target and keeps the ball in an area where the third baseman can handle it.

First-and-Third Drill 1 **Team Defense—No Hitter**

With the defense in position, the play is called out. The pitcher has a ball in his hand, and the coach stands in as a hitter. Base runners play live at first base and third base.

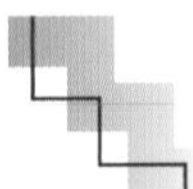

TO INCREASE DIFFICULTY

- Have an offense play live against the defense.

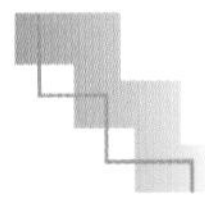

TO DECREASE DIFFICULTY

- Have a coach pitch.
- Slow each play down and explain what needs to happen in advance.

Success Check

- Did the defense control the baseball? Overthrows will allow for a score, so ball control is essential. Players must also back up their man.
- Did the defense get an out?
- Was the right decision made? Players need to be able to read the situation correctly.

Score Your Success

The defense earns 1 point for getting an out or making the correct decision with the ball.

The defense earns 0 points if a poor decision is made or the ball is not controlled.

Your score ___ of 15

First-and-Third Drill 2 **Controlled Intrasquad**

The controlled intrasquad is a live game setting with pitchers and hitters. For this drill, runners are placed at first and third to begin an inning. The defensive situation is played out in a live game setting.

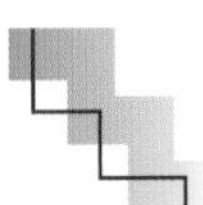

TO INCREASE DIFFICULTY

- Call out different inning, out, and score situations so that each defender must figure out the defensive goal and adjust accordingly.

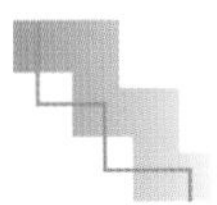

TO DECREASE DIFFICULTY

- Have the offense run only certain plays.
- Let the defense know what is coming.

(continued)

First-and-Third Drill 2 *(continued)*

Success Check

- Did the defense control the baseball? Overthrows will allow for a score, so ball control is essential. Players must also back up their man.
- Did the defense get an out?
- Was the right decision made? Players need to be able to read the situation correctly.

Score Your Success

The defense earns 1 point for getting an out or making the correct decision with the ball.

The defense earns 0 points if a poor decision is made or the ball is not controlled.

Your score ___ of 10

RUNDOWNS

Rundowns should be a simple part of a team defense, but they are often overlooked. Rundowns require players not only to control the baseball precisely but also to understand and anticipate the actions of their teammates so that they move together. Here is how it's done (figure 9.8).

Figure 9.8 **RUNDOWN TECHNIQUES**

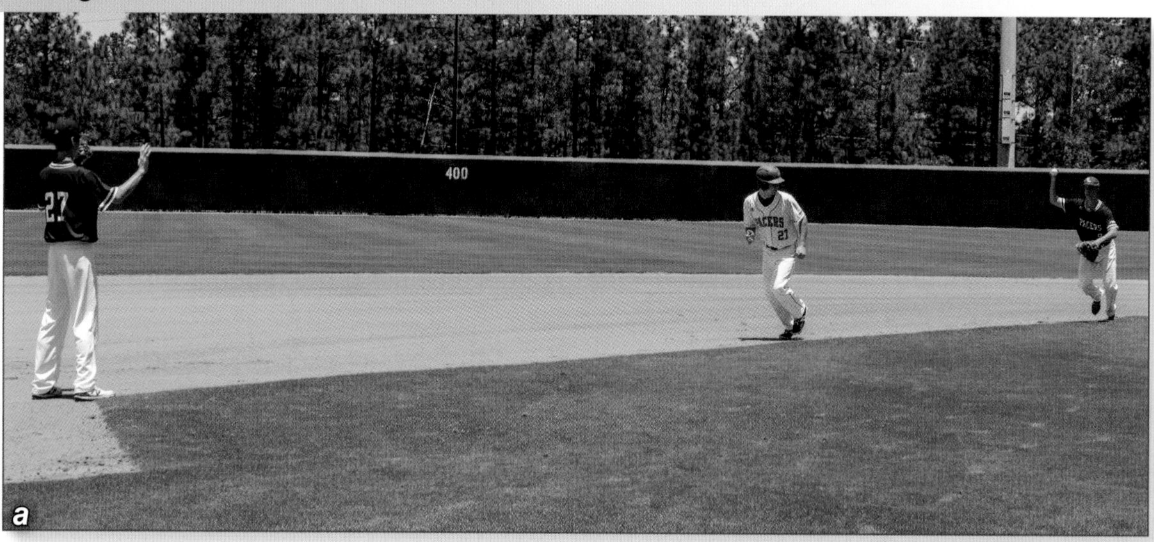

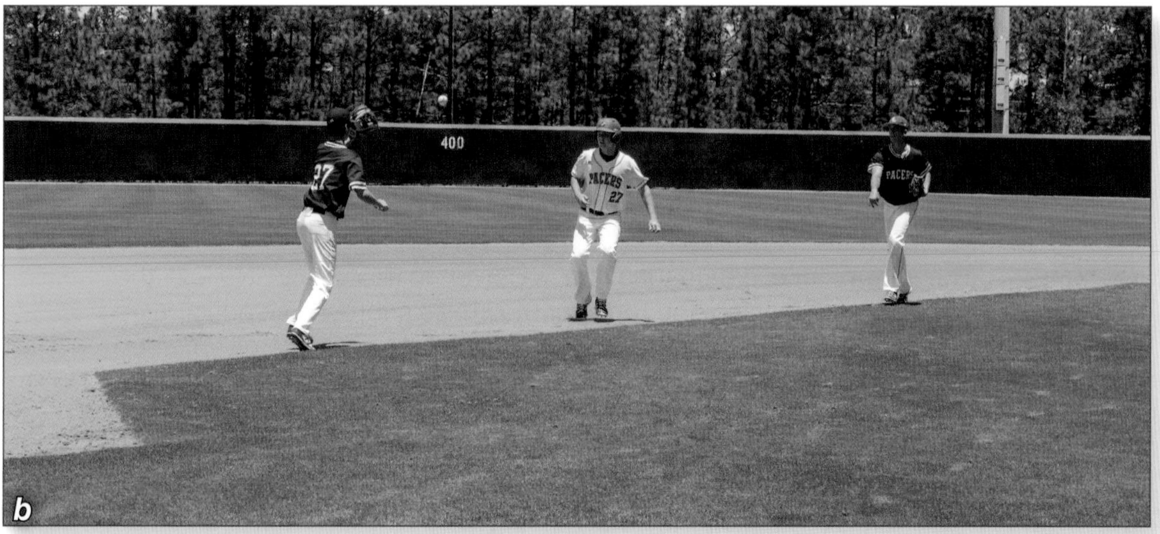

b

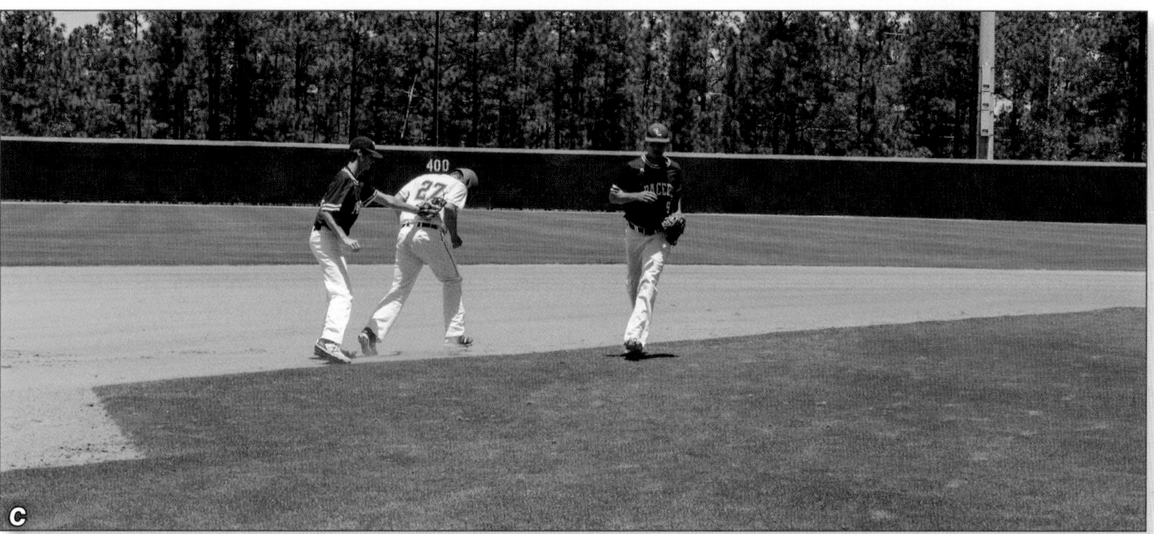

c

1. When the rundown begins, the thrower and receiver should line up with each other inside the base line.
2. The receiver should slowly shrink the gap while holding both hands up to give the thrower a chest-high target.
3. The thrower should move toward the runner with the ball up and in throwing position (figure 9.8*a*).
4. As the runner gets near the receiver, the receiver should call, "Ball," signaling the thrower to give up the ball (figure 9.8*b*).
5. After the thrower releases the ball, he should peel inside the throwing and running lanes and rotate around to the base that he was moving toward (figure 9.8*c*).
6. The receiver should be able to catch and tag the runner immediately.
7. If the offense has a trail runner who advances to the base behind the rundown, the defense should run the runner back to that base and tag both runners.

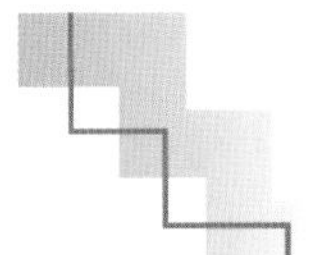

MISSTEP

A couple common mistakes are made in rundowns. The first is the pump fake by the thrower, where the thrower has the ball in hand and moves his arm in a throwing motion without releasing the ball. The second is making contact with the runner without the ball.

CORRECTION

The pump fake can cause the receiver to freeze as well. If the runner keeps moving, the receiver may miss a throw if he anticipates another pump fake. The pump should be done immediately or when the thrower is not going to throw the ball at all and is going to attempt to make a tag.

To eliminate making contact with the runner if you do not have the ball, keep inside the running lane and peel off after making a throw. If you stop moving or drift into the lane, base runners will look for an opportunity to make contact. This circumstance will create a dead ball and give the runner the next base.

Rundowns Drill 1 **Three-Man Rundowns**

The three-man rundown drill is done with two defenders standing 80 feet (24 m) apart and a runner in the middle. One defender has the ball. The defender with the ball works on closing the distance and the timing of the throw for an immediate catch and tag (figure 9.9).

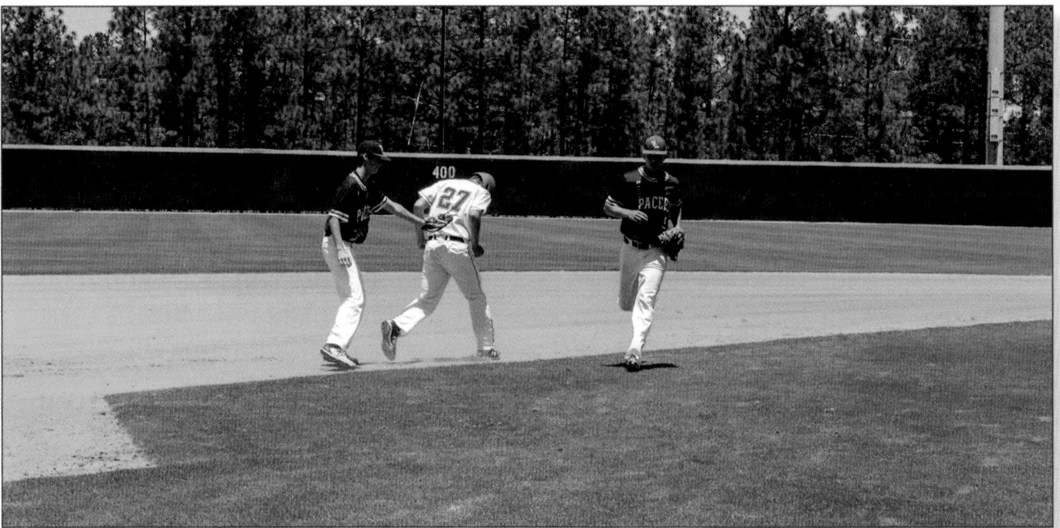

Figure 9.9 Three-man rundowns drill.

Success Check

- Feeds should be executed correctly.
- Receivers need good timing and should shrink the gap in a controlled manner.
- Good communication between the receivers is necessary.

Score Your Success

The defense earns 1 point if they execute the rundown correctly.

The defense earns 1/2 point if the throw is made too soon but the ball is controlled.

The defense earns 0 points for throwing late, not controlling the ball, or making contact with the runner without the ball.

Your score ____ of 10

Rundowns Drill 2
Team Pitcher's Fielding Practice (PFP)—Picks to Rundowns

In a team defensive setting with the infield in place and the pitchers on the mound, base runners are placed at first, second, and third. The first pitcher picks to first base, and the base runner simulates getting picked off and getting into a rundown (figure 9.10*a*). When the rundown between first and second ends, the next pitcher picks to second base, creating a rundown between second and third (figure 9.10*b*). The final rundown has the pitcher throw home and the catcher back pick to third base, creating a rundown between third and home.

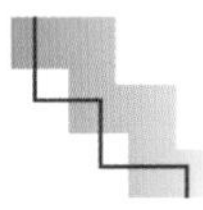

TO INCREASE DIFFICULTY

- Have all sections going simultaneously.
- Have base runners go at game speed.

TO DECREASE DIFFICULTY

- Work on only one section at a time.
- Have the base runners go only at 50 percent of game speed.

(continued)

Rundowns Drill 2 *(continued)*

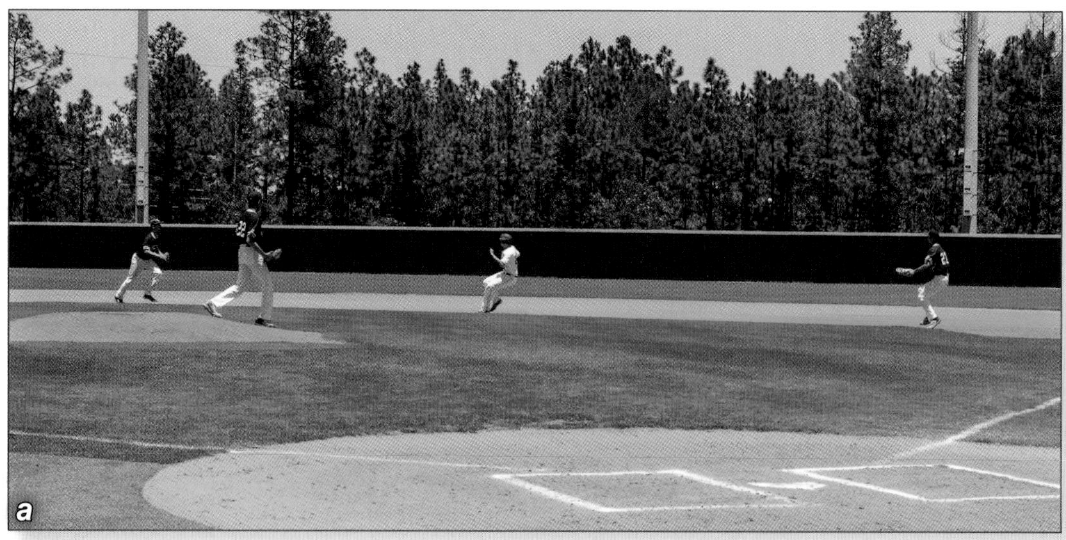

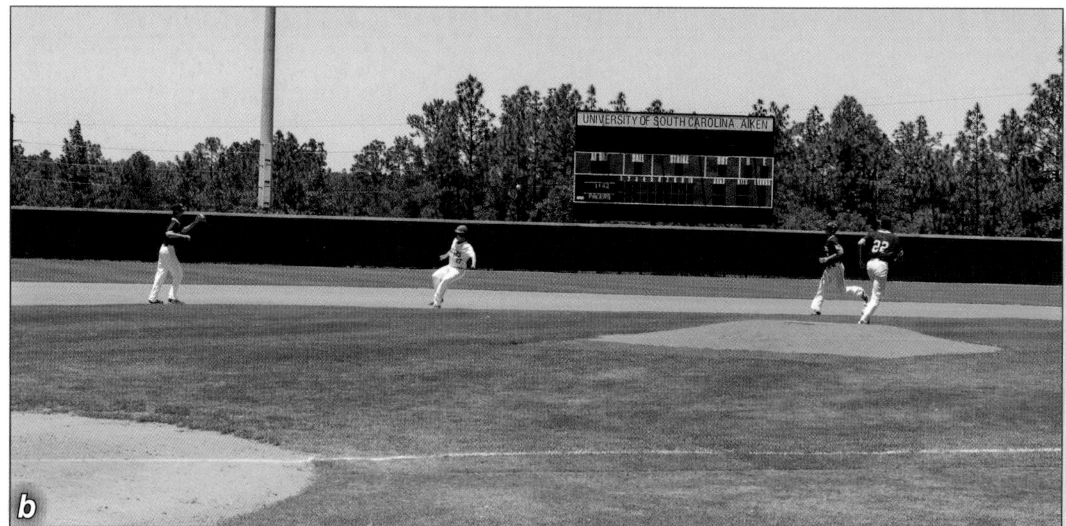

Figure 9.10 Team PFP—picks to rundowns drill: picks to first base *(a)* and picks to second base *(b)*.

Success Check

- Feeds should be executed correctly.
- Receivers need good timing and should shrink the gap in a controlled manner.
- Good communication between the receivers is necessary.

Score Your Success

The defense earns 1 point for an executed rundown.

The defense earns 1/2 point if the rundown required more than two throws but still produced an out.

The defense earns 0 points if they do not get an out.

Your score ____ of 15

FLY BALL COMMUNICATION

Communicating about fly balls in both the infield and the outfield (figure 9.11) is imperative because the lack of it can create dangerous situations that can result in collisions and injuries. Lack of communication can also cause the embarrassing moment of a ball falling between two players. Regardless, communication between fielders must be practiced regularly so that none of the previous events happen.

Figure 9.11 **COMMUNICATION**

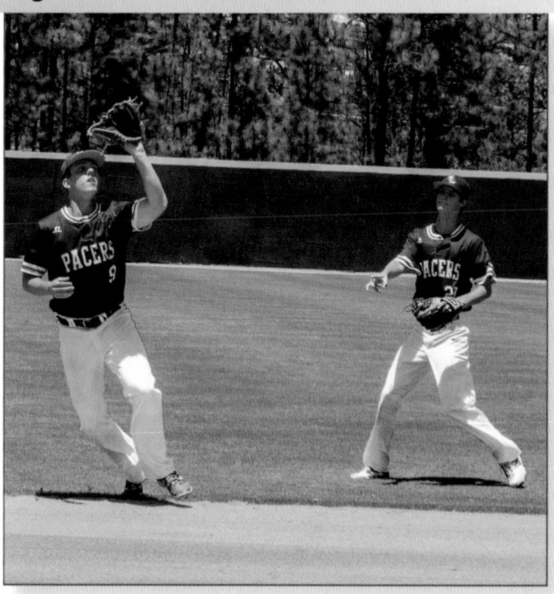

1. The center fielder is top authority on all fly balls.
2. The outfielders have priority over the infielders.
3. The middle infielders have priority over the corner infielders.
4. The corner infielders have priority over the pitcher and catcher.
5. On fly balls, the ball should be called at its highest point.

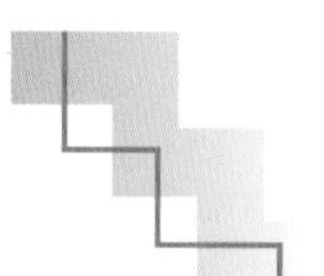

MISSTEP

One misstep occurs when you have priority and call a ball you cannot catch. Another happens when two players converge on each other without one peeling off.

CORRECTION

If you are called off by a teammate with priority, get out of the way immediately. If you have priority, but your teammate is camped under the ball, let him have it.

Fly Ball Communication Drill
Team Defense—Machine or Coach Fungoes

Fly ball communication is practiced with the defense in place and a coach hitting fungoes or feeding a machine from home plate. As the fly balls are fed all over the field, the defense works on good communication and technique for calling and catching fly balls.

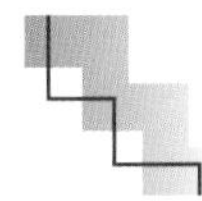

TO INCREASE DIFFICULTY

- Have the outfielders start with their backs turned to the ball.

TO DECREASE DIFFICULTY

- Have the coach throw the ball from a shorter distance.

Success Check

- Good communication—the ball should be called at the highest point.
- Getting out of the way—players need to let the person who called the ball field it.

Score Your Success

The defense earns 1 point for proper communication and a catch.

The defense earns 1/2 point if the wrong person makes the catch.

The defense earns 0 points if the ball is not caught.

Your score ____ of 20

TANDEM RELAYS

The tandem is a way that the defense can control a ball thrown from the outfield and relay it quickly to the infield. This play requires proper alignment and a good read of the flight of the ball so that the right decision is made and the quickest relay is executed. Take a look at figure 9.12 and the tandem relay drill following it, which demonstrate the way to learn this defensive skill.

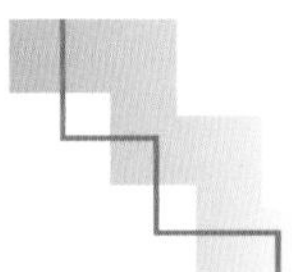

MISSTEP

If the cutoff men are late getting into position, the result could be poor ball control and loss of a chance to throw out a base runner.

CORRECTION

The tandem should be called for as soon as the need for it is recognized.

Figure 9.12 **TANDEM SETUP**

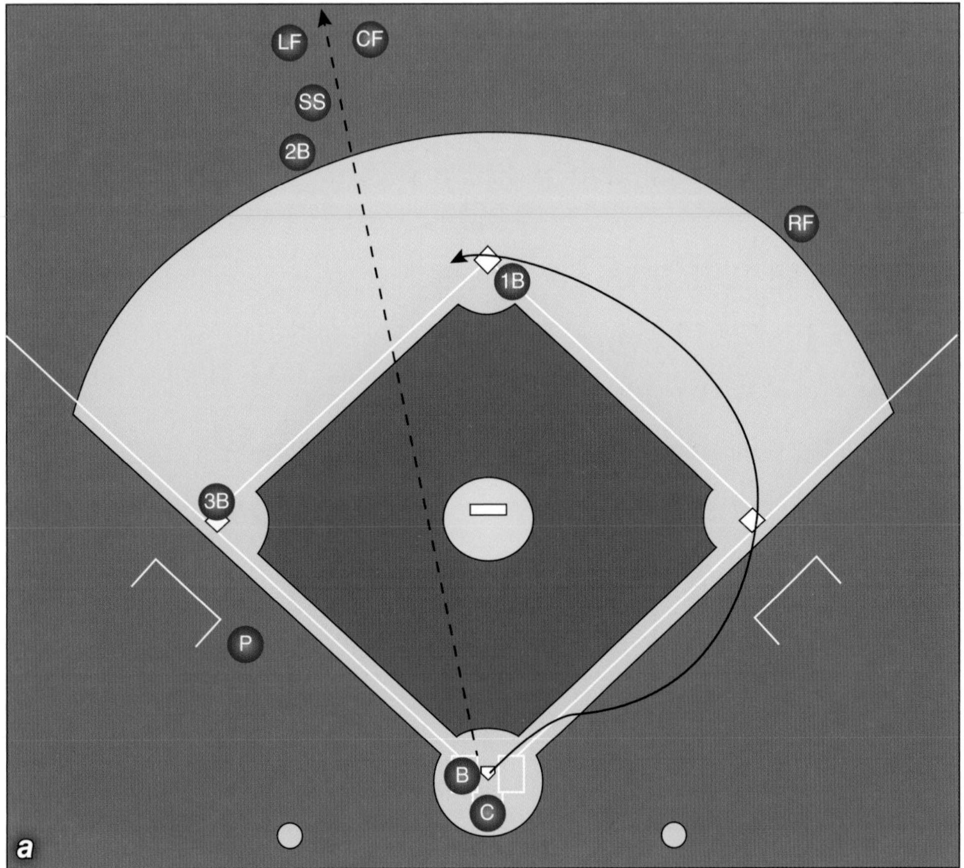

1. For a true double hit down the left-field line or to left-center field, the shortstop and second baseman rotate into a cutoff position.
2. With no runners on base, the tandem lines up to third base. With a runner on first base, the tandem lines up with the catcher at home plate.
3. For doubles down the left-field line and to left-center field, the shortstop is the initial cutoff and the second baseman is approximately 10 to 20 feet (3 to 6 m) behind him (figure 9.12*a*).
4. For balls in right-center field, the initial cutoff switches to the second baseman, and the shortstop is the trail.

(continued)

Figure 9.12 *(continued)*

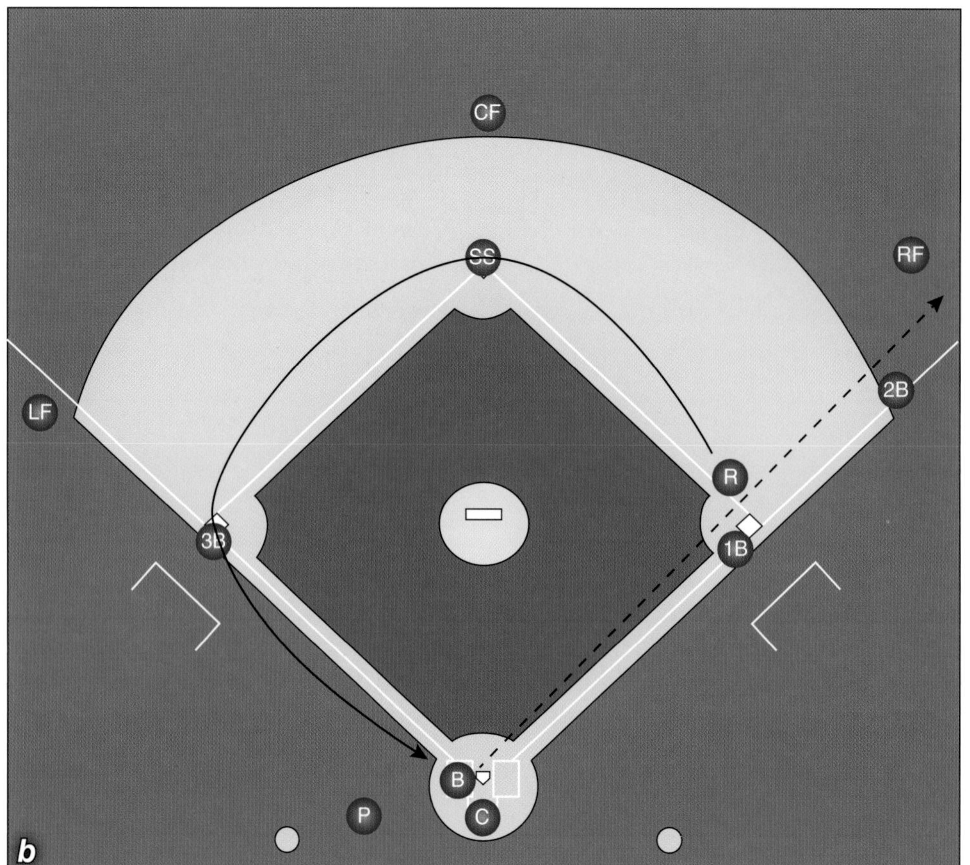

5. For balls down the right-field line with no runners on base, the tandem to third is the same as the one used on a ball hit to right-center field. With a runner on first, the second baseman is the initial cutoff man, and the first baseman is the trail for the tandem relay to home plate (9.12*b*).
6. The catcher makes all calls on where the ball is relayed.
7. The third baseman or the catcher, depending on the situation, aligns the tandem relay with the outfielder's position as he fields the ball.
8. The first baseman watches the hitter touch the bag at first base and trails him into second base, unless he is the cutoff man with a runner on first and a ball down the right-field line.

Tandem Relay Drill **Team Defense—Coach Fungoes**

The tandem relay drill has a coach in the center of the infield hitting fungoes to the defense. Balls are hit down both lines and in both gaps, simulating true doubles. The defense shifts into tandem positions and makes the throws or cuts called by the catcher.

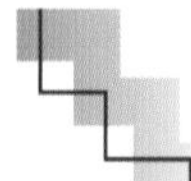

TO INCREASE DIFFICULTY

- Have base runners run live.

TO DECREASE DIFFICULTY

- Let the outfielders start with the ball and have the infielders already in proper alignment.

Success Check

- Proper communication should be used.
- The alignment should be correct.
- The correct person should make the relay.

Score Your Success

The defense earns 1 point for controlling the baseball and making good throws.

The defense earns 0 points if the ball gets tangled between the tandem.

The defense earns 0 points for poor throws.

Your score ____ of 15

SUCCESS SUMMARY

Situational defense demands that the individual players understand the game. Whatever the situation, the goal should always be to get an out, and to do that the defense must control the baseball. As you increase the difficulty within each drill, you will see the success rate fall. Therefore, each team defensive situation must be covered constantly throughout the year, so that the pressure and speed of a live game is not a factor.

Bunt Drills

1. Team PFP—coach rolling bunts _____ out of 15
2. Defensive bunt intrasquad _____ out of 25

First-and-Third Drills

1. Team defense—no hitter _____ out of 15
2. Controlled intrasquad _____ out of 10

Rundown Drills

1. Three-man rundowns _____ out of 10
2. Team PFP—picks to rundowns _____ out of 15

Fly Ball Communication Drill

1. Team defense—machine or coach fungoes _____ out of 20

Tandem Relay Drill

1. Team defense—coach fungoes _____ out of 15

Total _____ **out of 125**

If you scored more than 100 points, congratulations! You have successfully taken the next step to success. The goal for your team defense should be 125 of 125, but if you were perfect then you would have nothing to learn. A reasonable goal for this section is 90 points. Any score less than 90 should not be considered failure. Rather, it should give you a better understanding of the holes in your team defense which opponents can expose.

STEP

10

Situational Offense

The final step we will look at is team offense and the way in which you implement the skills that you have developed. The situations we will discuss are bunting, hit and run and run and hit, first-and-third offense, and moving runners and scoring. As part of a team offense, you will use your individual skills as a hitter and base runner in coordination with your teammates to help the team succeed.

A big factor in team offense is the approach of its hitters. Being asked to sacrifice, to hit the ball on the ground, or to do a specific job is often tough for hitters to comprehend. Most hitters just want to hit. But certain situations call for the team player to do what is best for the team. As we move through these steps, understand that this aspect of the game makes both you and the team more successful.

SACRIFICE BUNTING

Bunting is a part of the offensive game that is often referred to as small ball. For some players, bunting for a hit can be a part of their individual skill set that forces a defense to adjust positioning, and we'll cover this skill later in the chapter. For others, bunting is used in sacrifice situations when an offense is willing to give up an out to advance the base runner or base runners. These situations typically occur late in a game with a runner on first (figure 10.1), a runner on second, or runners on first and second (figure 10.2), with zero outs. It can also occur with a runner on third (figure 10.3). By sacrificing a runner into scoring position, that is, from first to second, the offense assumes that a base hit will then score that runner. By sacrificing a runner from second to third, the offense can then score in various ways other than a base hit, such as a sacrifice fly, a ground ball out with the infield back, a passed ball (a ball that should have been caught by the catcher, but was not, leading to a runner or runners advancing to the next base or scoring), or a wild pitch (a pitched ball thrown in a manner that the catcher had no chance of catching, leading to a runner or runners advancing to the next base), and so on. An offense that can bunt typically puts pressure on a defense. In late-inning situations, this pressure can determine the outcome of a game.

Figure 10.1 **RUNNER ON FIRST—SACRIFICE TO FIRST-BASE SIDE**

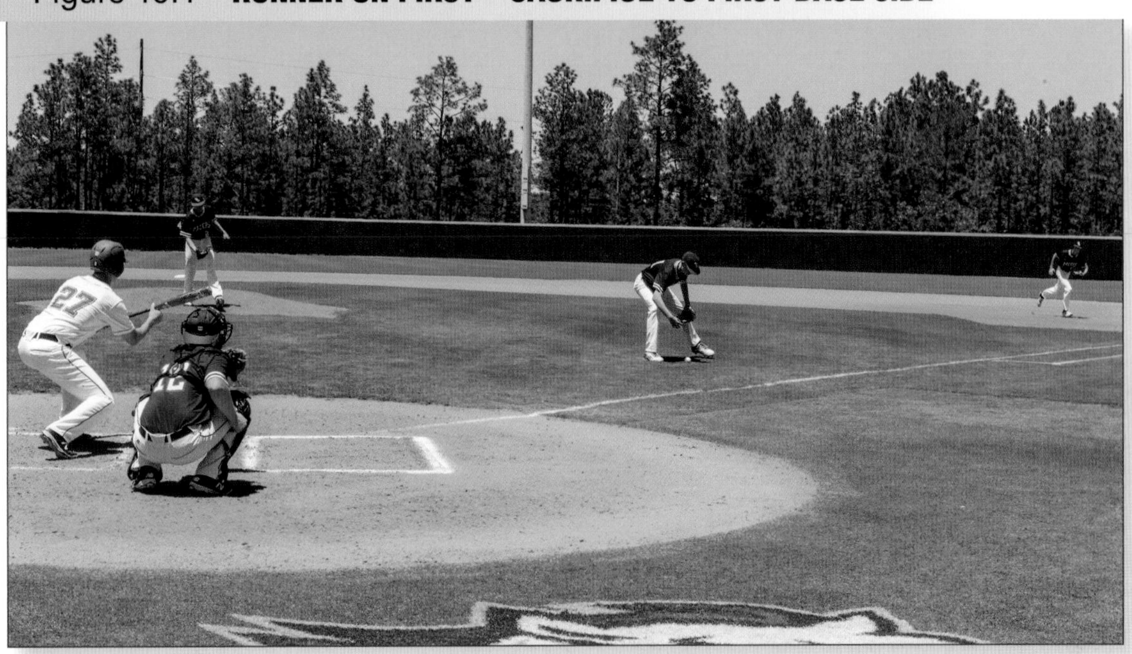

1. As the pitcher becomes set, the batter squares to bunt.
2. The batter should place the bunt on the first-base side between the pitcher and the first-base line.
3. The runner should get a normal secondary lead and read the angle of the bunt.

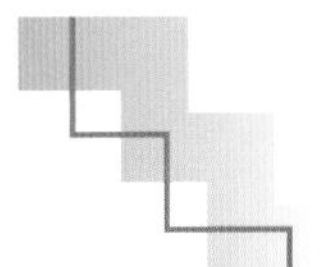

MISSTEP

If the runner drifts too far off first base in the secondary lead, expecting that the bunt will be executed, but the hitter takes the pitch, then the runner is in danger of getting thrown out by the catcher.

CORRECTION

The runner must be aware that the hitter is taught to bunt only strikes in a sacrifice situation. Therefore, he must see contact and a downward angle before he breaks to second.

Figure 10.2 **RUNNERS ON FIRST AND SECOND—SACRIFICE TO THIRD-BASE SIDE**

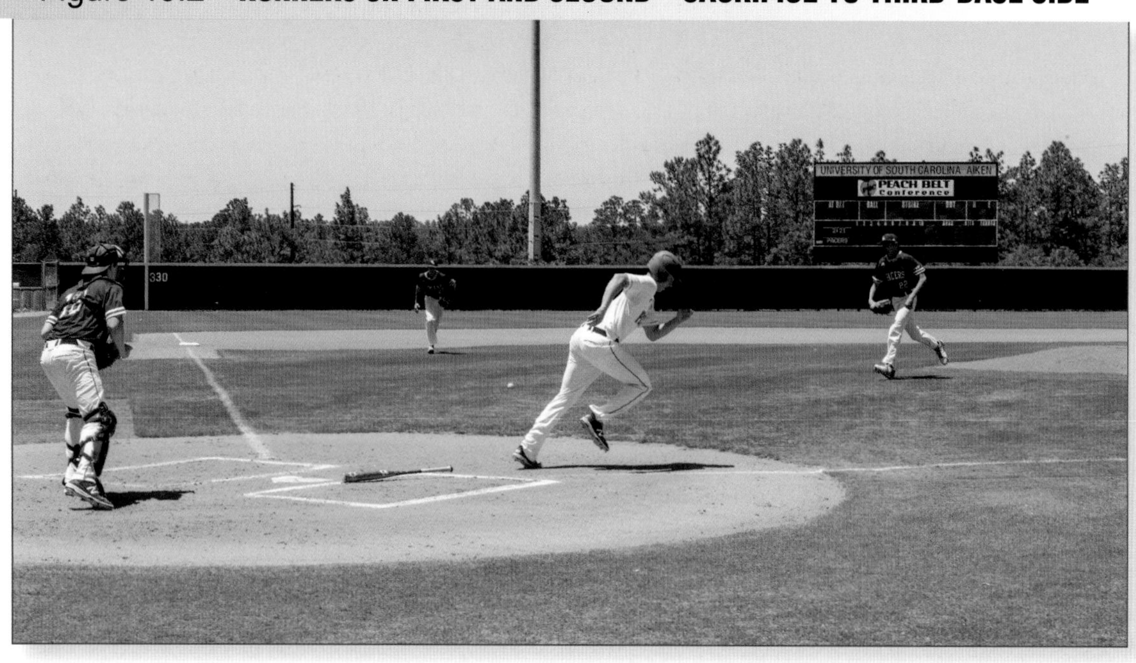

1. As the pitcher becomes set, the batter squares to bunt.
2. The hitter should place the bunt on the third-base side of the infield, preferably hard enough to force the third baseman to field it.
3. Both runners should get a normal secondary lead and read the angle of the bunt.

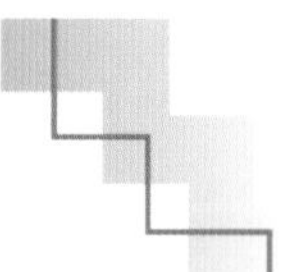

MISSTEP

Bunting the ball back to the pitcher is a big misstep, especially with a left-hander on the mound.

CORRECTION

You should be sure to get the bunt toward the line, far enough away from the mound so that the third baseman has to field the ball.

SQUEEZE BUNTING

A squeeze bunt is a sacrifice bunt with a runner on third base. The batter bunts the ball, expecting to be thrown out, but his bunt gives the runner at third base an opportunity to score. Since the bunt is a sacrifice, a squeeze bunt would not be performed with two outs. You would also not attempt a squeeze bunt with two strikes because a foul ball would mean a third strike and an out.

There are two types of squeeze bunts: the suicide squeeze (figure 10.3) and the safety squeeze. It is called a suicide squeeze because the runner at third base goes without knowing if the bunt is successfully placed. If the bunt is misplaced, it is likely that the runner will be out at home. But, if the bunt is good, it is a very hard play for the defense to cover and almost always results in a score.

The safety squeeze is performed like the suicide squeeze, but the runner at third base waits to make sure the bunt is placed correctly before going. It is easier to defend than the suicide squeeze, since the runner waits, and it is not quite as easy to score on.

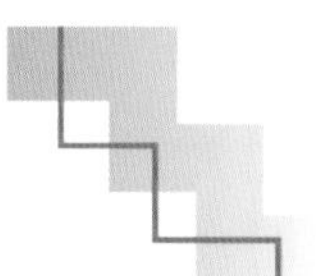

MISSTEP

Your failure to make contact with the ball gives the runner zero protection from being tagged out at home by the catcher.

CORRECTION

Get into a good position to put the bat on the ball.

Figure 10.3 **SQUEEZE BUNT**

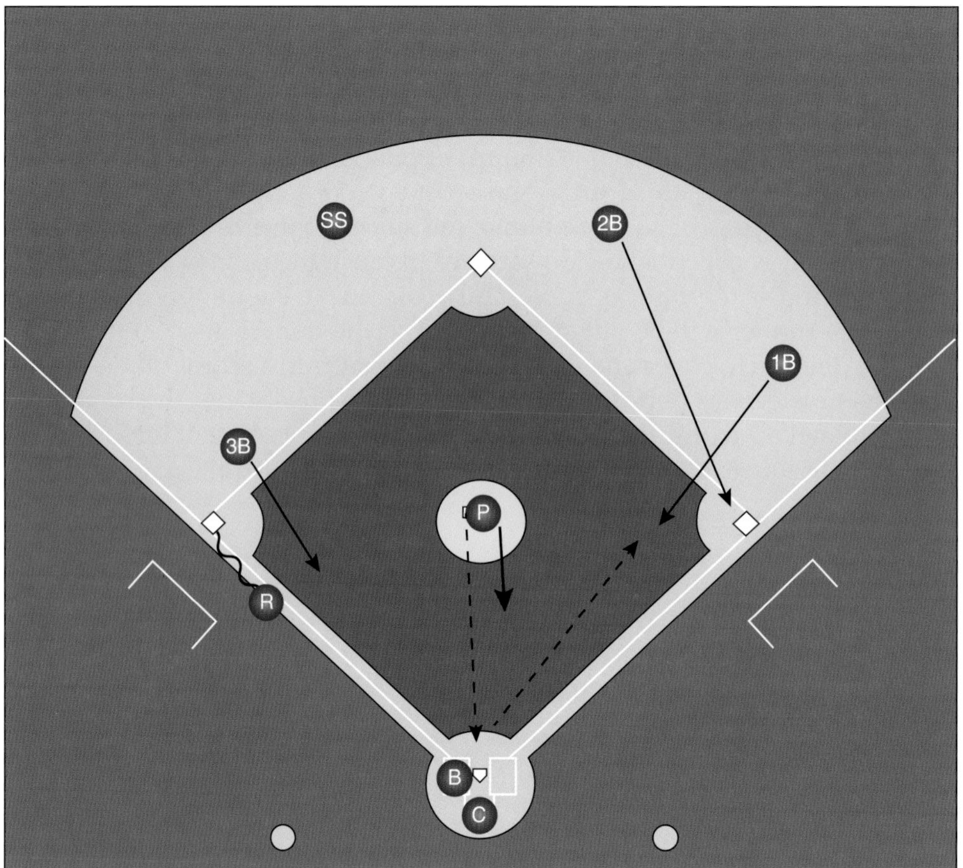

1. The technique for this bunt is the same as the standard bunt. The only difference is that the batter does not reveal he is bunting until the pitcher is mid-delivery.
2. As the pitcher delivers the ball to the plate, the hitter squares to bunt. Either pivot or take a small jab step in order to quickly get into position.
3. The hitter must make contact with the ball, regardless of where the pitch is located. The bunt just needs to be on the ground.
4. The runner at third should wait until the pitcher's arm is at its highest point in the arm swing as he delivers to the plate. The runner must be sure that the pitcher is not picking over to third before he breaks at full speed toward home plate.

BUNTING FOR A HIT

Bunting for a hit is a skill often used by players with speed or those who are not accomplished hitters. The push bunt (figure 10.4) and drag bunt (figure 10.5) are ways that a hitter can place the ball in various positions on the infield so that the defense cannot make a play to get him out. A player who can consistently use the push or drag bunts often sees a defense shift to protect against it, thus creating holes in the infield that give him a better chance to get a hit by swinging the bat. The push bunt and drag bunt are very similar, and are performed in much the same way. Both the push bunt and the drag bunt are difficult to perform correctly, and as a result, they are not performed very often by youth players.

Figure 10.4 **PUSH BUNT**

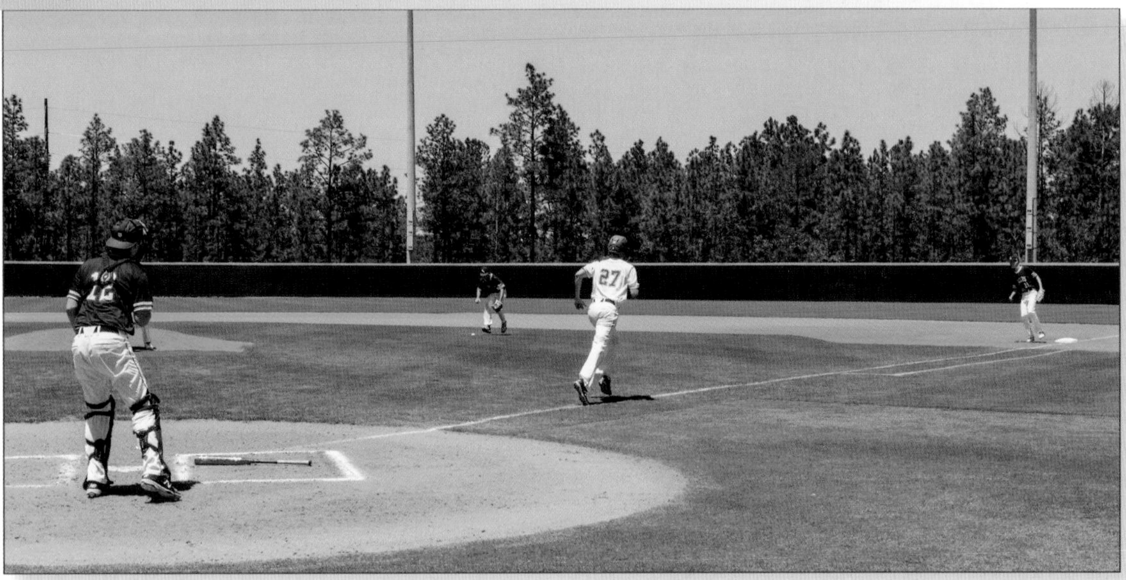

1. As the pitcher begins the delivery, the hitter gets into position to bunt, disguising his intention as long as possible yet setting up to bunt early enough to feel comfortable. The push bunt technique is basically the same as the basic bunt technique covered in step 5, figure 5.6. The main difference is that for a push bunt, the hitter disguises the intention to bunt for as long as possible so the infielders don't adjust their standard positioning.
2. The batter angles the bat with the tip slightly behind the handle and "pushes" the bat out at contact, keeping the angle consistent so that the ball is placed toward the right side of infield.
3. The hitter should place the push bunt in the triangle area between the first baseman, second baseman, and past pitcher (figure 10.4).
4. As soon as contact is made, the runner needs to go. A right-handed batter steps first with his right foot. A left-handed batter will lead with his left foot, crossing it over the right foot.

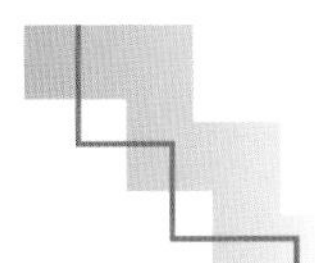

MISSTEP

Showing bunt too early gives the defense a chance to gain a step.

CORRECTION

Be sure to practice your timing, working on being able to wait longer while remaining in rhythm.

Figure 10.5 **DRAG BUNT**

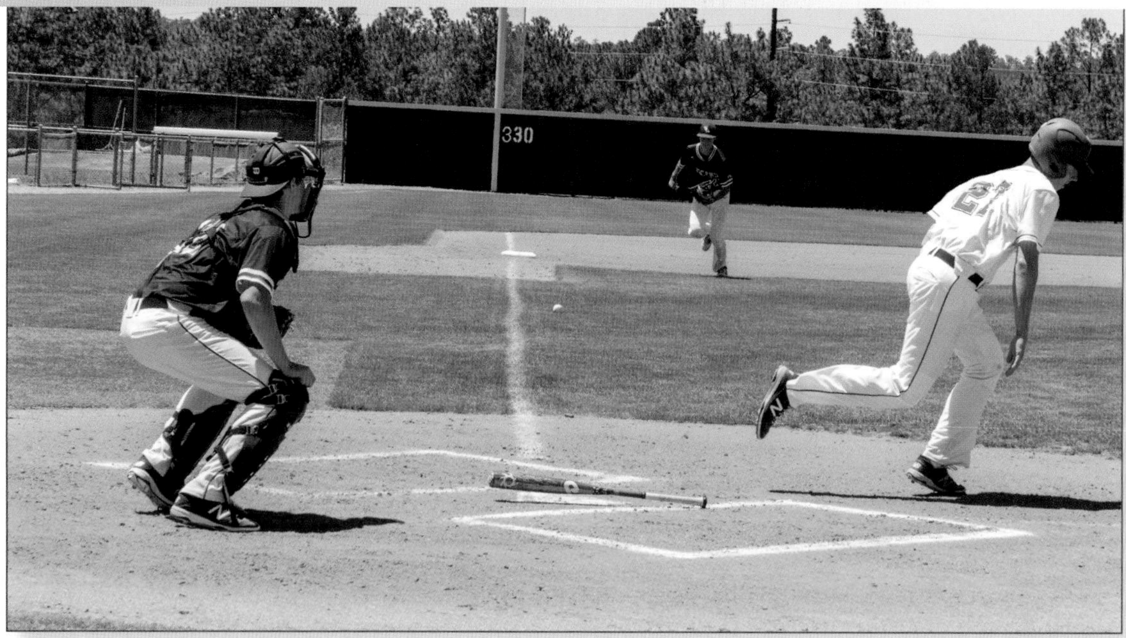

1. The drag bunt is typically used by left-handed batters and, as such, is performed like the push bunt, but with opposite ball placement. However, it can be used by a right-handed batter as well.
2. The hitter's timing of getting into position is the same that he uses for the push bunt, and the technique is the same as for the basic bunt.
3. With a left-handed batter, the batter angles the bat with the tip slightly behind the handle and "pushes" the bat out at contact, keeping the angle consistent so the ball is placed toward the third-base line. For a right-handed batter, the bat should be angled with the barrel end toward first base.
4. The hitter should place the drag bunt close to, or on, the third-base line and have it stop about halfway to third base or little farther (figure 10.5).
5. As soon as contact is made, the runner needs to go. A right-handed batter steps first with his right foot. A left-handed batter will lead with his left foot, crossing it over the right foot.

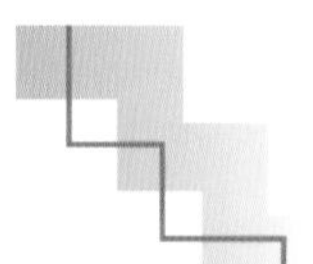

MISSTEP

If the ball is not close enough to the line, the third baseman will have an easier time making the play.

CORRECTION

The thought behind the drag bunt is to place it on the line; if you are going to miss, be sure to miss in foul territory.

Bunting Drill 1 **Breakdown**

The bunting breakdown focuses on each player's ability to lay down specific bunts. Each round has the hitter lay down two bunts of each kind—sacrifices, bunts for hits, and squeezes. Moving runners without swinging the bat shows the focus that the team is putting on this aspect of the game. The drill can be run with a defense and runners to work on both offensive and defensive bunt techniques. Alternatively, it can be run with only hitters to work on bunt technique and placement if you don't have a lot of time or just want to focus on the offensive aspect.

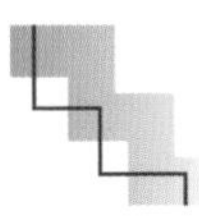

TO INCREASE DIFFICULTY

- Use a pitching machine.
- Increase or decrease the pitch speed without the hitter's knowledge.
- Throw pitches other than a fastball.

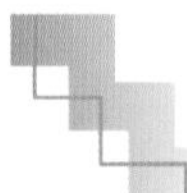

TO DECREASE DIFFICULTY

- Slow down the speed that the pitcher is delivering the ball.

Success Check

- The batter should consistently get into the correct bunt position.
- The batter must place the ball correctly for each type of bunt.
- For the push and drag bunts, the batter should get a good break toward first base after making contact.

Score Your Success

You earn 1 point for every successful bunt.

You earn 1/2 point if the technique was correct but the bunt was off target.

You earn 0 points for poor technique, popping up the ball, missing the ball, or bunting back to the pitcher.

Sacrifice to first _____ of 2

Sacrifice to third _____ of 2

Push bunt _____ of 2

Drag bunt _____ of 2

Squeeze _____ of 2

Your score ____ of 10

Bunting Drill 2 **Batting Practice Rounds With Bunts**

When bunts are inserted into a batting practice round, hitters must focus on getting the bunt down properly either before or after taking their swings. For this drill, have hitters execute a different bunt at the beginning or end of every round.

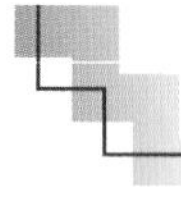

TO INCREASE DIFFICULTY

- Mix pitches and locations.
- Pressure the hitter by allowing him more swings after a successful round and by reducing the number of swings after an unsuccessful round.

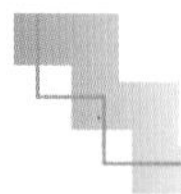

TO DECREASE DIFFICULTY

- Slow down the pitch speed during the bunting segment.

Success Check

- The batter should consistently get into the correct bunt position.
- The batter must place the ball correctly for each type of bunt.
- For the push and drag bunts, the batter should get a good break toward first after making contact.

Score Your Success

You earn 1 point for every successful bunt.

You earn 1/2 point if the technique was correct but the bunt was off target.

You earn 0 points for using poor technique, popping up the ball, missing the ball, or bunting back to the pitcher.

Round 1: Sacrifice to first _____ of 2

Round 2: Sacrifice to third _____ of 2

Round 3: Push bunt _____ of 2

Round 4: Drag bunt _____ of 2

Round 5: Squeeze _____ of 2

Your score _____ of 10

Bunting Drill 3 **Bunt Only Intrasquad**

As we talked about with the defensive bunt intrasquad, the focus now shifts to the offensive side. In a live intrasquad game setting, the offense can only bunt. The offensive players will be graded on both bunting and reading the bunts as a base runner.

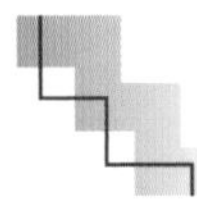

TO INCREASE DIFFICULTY

- Have pitchers throw live to the bunters.

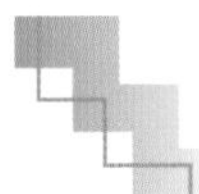

TO DECREASE DIFFICULTY

- Slow down the pitch speed.

Success Check

- The bunter should utilize the correct bunt for situation.
- For the push and drag bunts, the batter should get a good break toward first base after making contact.
- The runner should read the bunt correctly.
- The runner should advance bases.

Score Your Success

You earn 1 point for a successful bunt and a good baserunning read.

You earn 1/2 point if the push or drag bunt was good but the defense made a great play.

You earn 0 points for poor reads and poor execution of the bunts.

Bunting _____ of 5

Reads at first base _____ of 5

Reads at second base _____ of 5

Reads at third base _____ of 5

Your score _____ of 20

HIT AND RUN AND RUN AND HIT

The hit and run and run and hit portion of an offense is a way to put pressure on a defense. The theory is that a base runner in motion will cause one or more defensive players to shift as the pitch is being delivered, creating gaps in the defense for the hitter. Depending on the team, the personnel, and the situation, these two aspects of situational offense, if used consistently, can be a dynamic factor that puts pressure on opposing defenses.

Hit and Run

The runner or runners are put in motion as the pitcher delivers to the plate. The hitter's job is to hit a ground ball on or through the infield but away from the middle of the field. As the runner or runners get halfway to the next base, they should look to see where the ball has been hit.

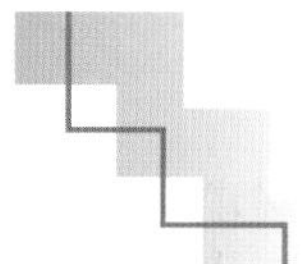

MISSTEP

A common misstep is the runner getting picked off while trying to get a good jump. For the hitter, the common belief is that hitting the ball behind the runner, to right field, is the proper technique for the hit and run.

CORRECTION

The hit and run is not a straight steal for the runner. It simply gets the runner in motion to stay out of a double play or to get the defense out of position. As for the hitter, although hitting the ball to the right side is good, doing so is not always possible. As long as the ball is put on the ground and away from the middle of the field, the hit will be considered a success.

Run and Hit

The run and hit is used when a base stealer is on first. The base runner's job is to get a jump and steal the base. The hitter should be aware of the runner's jump, taking the pitch if the runner has the bag stolen or protecting the runner with a swing if his jump is bad.

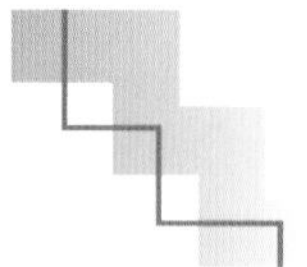

MISSTEP

The batter fouls off a pitch when the bag is stolen.

CORRECTION

If the bag is stolen, taking the pitch would be best, but if you are going to swing, be sure to put the ball on the ground and in play.

Hit and Run, Run and Hit Drill 1 **Batting Practice Rounds**

Use one or two rounds during batting practice to focus on the hit and run or run and hit. Have the players run the bases as well to work on getting good jumps and picking up the baseball.

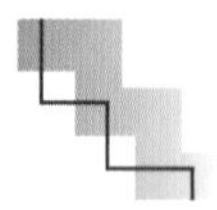

TO INCREASE DIFFICULTY

- Increase pitch speed.
- Mix in different pitches and locations.
- Pick off to keep the base runner honest.

TO DECREASE DIFFICULTY

- Slow the pitch speed.
- Throw the ball only in the area where the hitter will be most successful.

Success Check

- As a hitter, did you hit a ground ball on or through the infield, away from the middle of the field?
- Did you make the right decisions as a runner?

Score Your Success

You earn 1 point for a hit and run on the ground away from the middle.

You earn 1/2 point for a hit and run line drive.

You earn 0 points for hitting a pop-up or not swinging.

You earn 1 point for good baserunning.

Hitting _____ of 10

Running _____ of 10

Your score _____ of 20

Hit and Run, Run and Hit Drill 2 **Intrasquad**

Another time to practice the hit and run and run and hit is during a live setting, such as intrasquad. This gives the defense a chance to work on defending against the hit and run and the run and hit. It also gives the offensive players an opportunity to work on practicing their technique. The batters should work on placing the hit correctly for the hit and run and reading the pitch and runner correctly on the run and hit, taking the pitch if the runner has the bag stolen, or protecting the runner with a swing if his jump is bad.

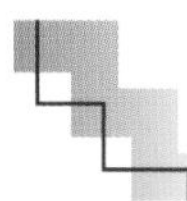

TO INCREASE DIFFICULTY

- Give signs as in a game situation.

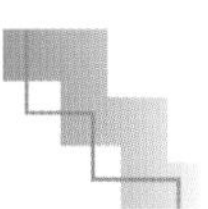

TO DECREASE DIFFICULTY

- Announce the situation to the team.
- Allow the pitchers to throw fastballs only.

Success Check

- For the hit and run, the batter should place the hit correctly.
- For the run and hit, the runner needs to get a good jump. The batter needs to read the runner's jump, taking the pitch if the runner has the bag stolen or protecting the runner with a swing if his jump is bad.

Score Your Success

Hitting _____ of 5

Running _____of 5

Your score _____ of 10

FIRST-AND-THIRD OFFENSE

Having runners on first and third creates a unique situation for an offense. The offense has several ways to add pressure, force decisions and throws, and create uncomfortable situations that challenge a defense. Each play can be used at any time. However, the situation, including the speed of the runners on the bases, the inning, the score, the pitcher-hitter matchup, and the number of outs, determines which play is best suited for that time. Some offensive options for a first-and-third situation are the straight steal (figure 10.6), the steal stop (figure 10.7), the delay steal (figure 10.8), and the get picked—early break (figure 10.9).

Figure 10.6 **STRAIGHT STEAL**

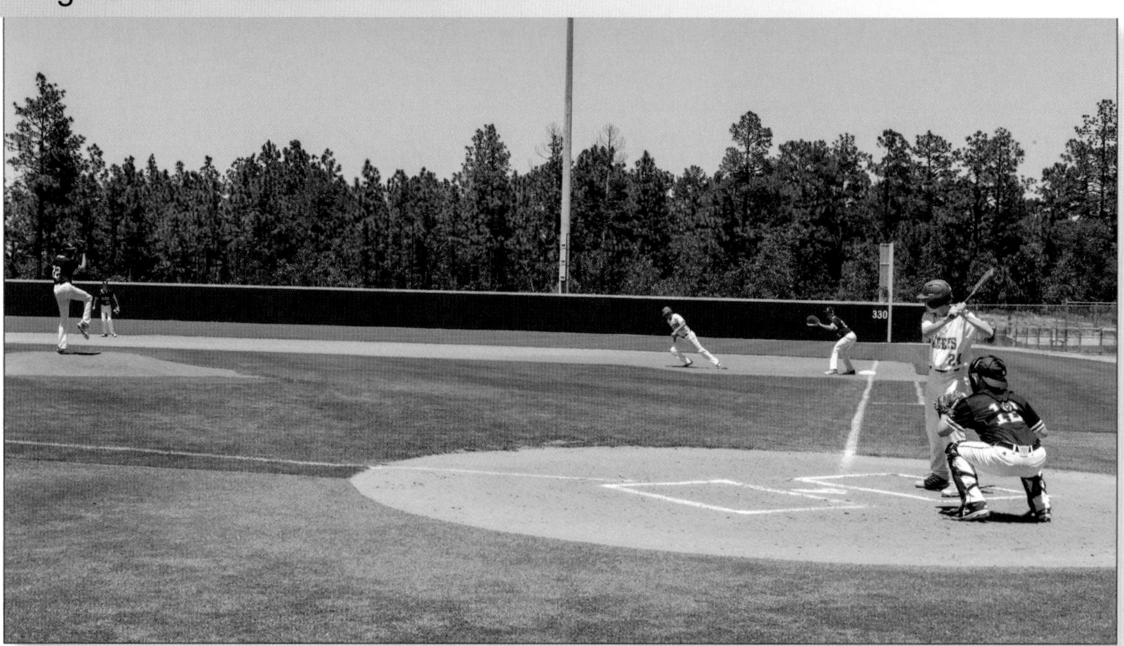

1. The runner at first is on a steal break.
2. The runner at third reads the throw from the catcher; he remains at third base unless the ball is thrown away. The goal is to advance the runner at first base to second base.

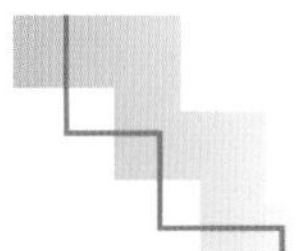

MISSTEP

The runner at third makes an out.

CORRECTION

The runner at third must be aware of both the defense and where the ball is thrown. He should always anticipate having to get back to the bag.

Figure 10.7 **STEAL STOP**

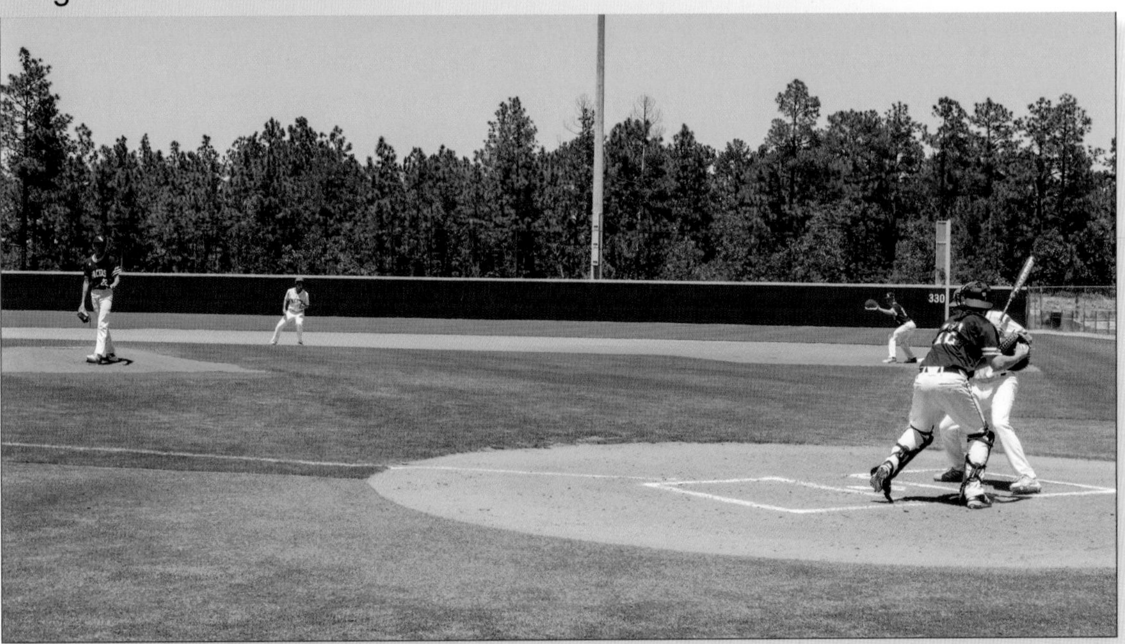

1. The runner at first is on a steal break.
2. At the halfway point, as the catcher throws the ball to second, the runner stops.
3. The runner at third breaks toward home as the catcher releases the ball.
4. The goal is to score the runner at third by having the catcher throw toward second. There will likely not be enough time for the defenseman covering second to throw the ball back home.

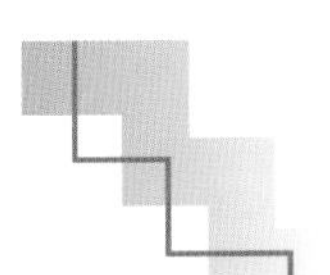

MISSTEP

The runner at first gets picked off.

CORRECTION

Treat the steal stop as a hit and run.

Figure 10.8 **DELAY STEAL**

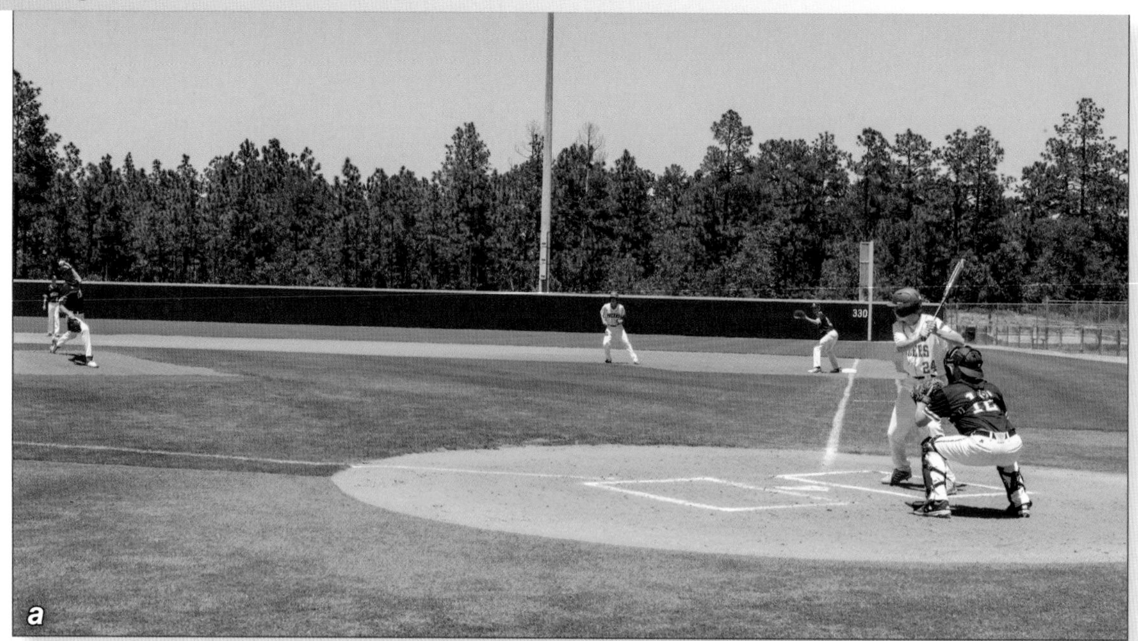

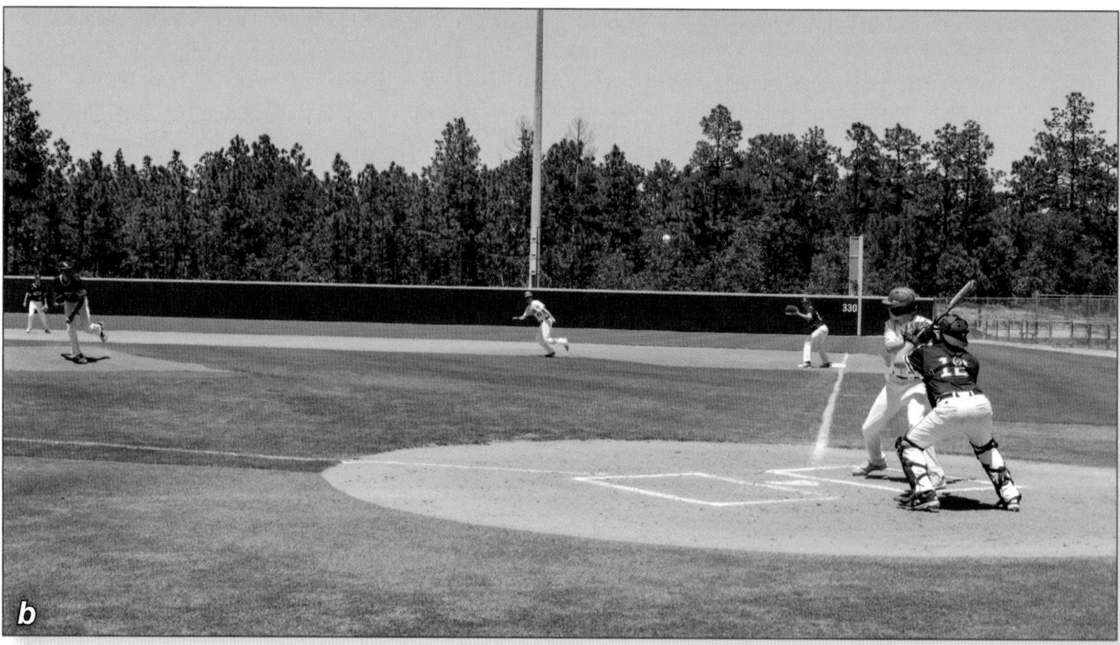

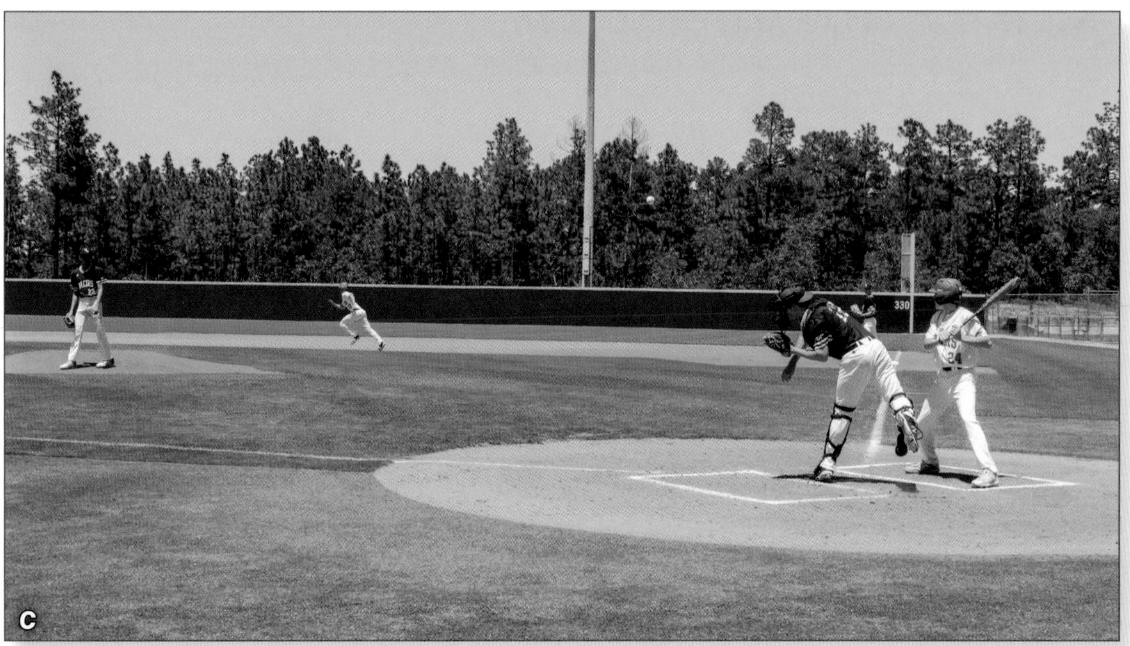

1. The runner at first takes a normal secondary lead (figure 10.8*a*) and breaks for second base as the catcher catches the ball (figure 10.8*b*).
2. The runner at third base reads the throw to second from the catcher (figure 10.8*c*).
3. If the runner delay steals, he can also stop halfway and create a rundown situation.
4. The runner must stay in the rundown as long as possible, trying to get the first baseman to throw the ball.
5. The runner at third breaks home only as the first baseman releases the ball in the rundown.
6. The goal is to score the third base runner.

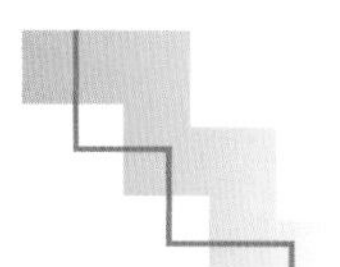

MISSTEP

The runner at first runs into an out.

CORRECTION

The runner at first must find the ball when the catcher throws it. If he runs into an out, the play was pointless. He needs to stay in the rundown situation.

Figure 10.9 **GET PICKED—EARLY BREAK**

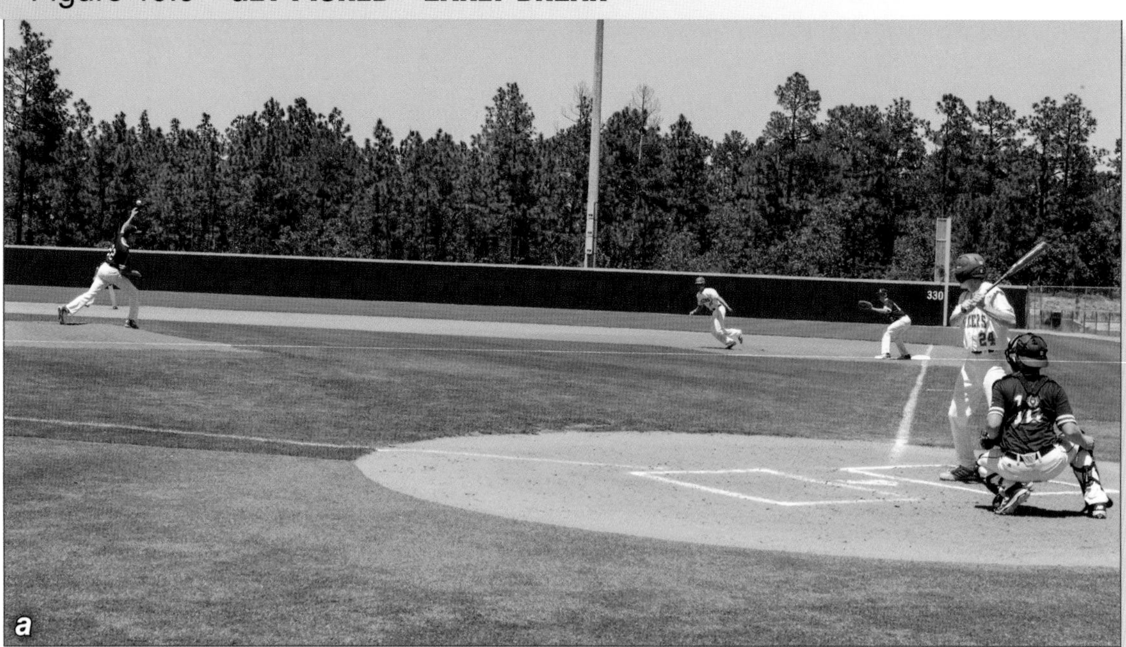

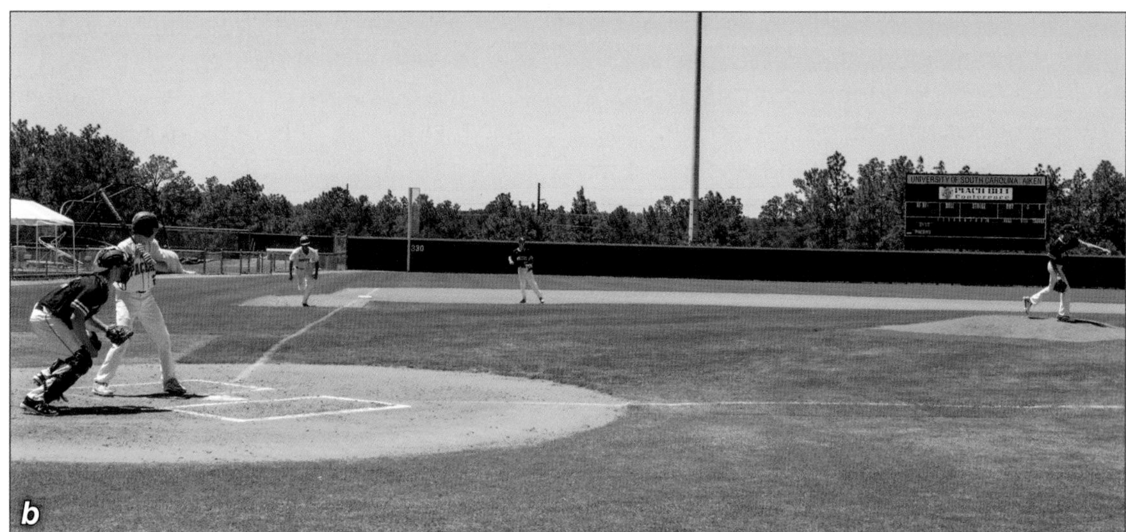

1. As the pitcher becomes set, the runner at first expands the lead to draw a pickoff from the pitcher (figure 10.09*a*).
2. At this point, the runner at first should remain in the rundown.
3. The runner at third breaks toward home as the pitcher releases the ball (figure 10.09*b*).
4. The goal is to score the runner at third.
5. Against a left-handed pitcher, the runner at third can break at the moment the pitcher begins to become set.
6. The runner at first breaks as soon as the runner at third breaks. This forces the pitcher either to balk or step off, giving the runner at third enough of a window to score.

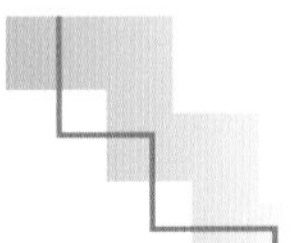

MISSTEP

Poor timing leads to easy outs.

CORRECTION

The runner at third cannot break too soon, and the runner at first cannot break too late.

First-and-Third Offense Drill 1
Team Offense—Baserunning Without a Hitter

This drill is done with a coach or pitcher on the mound. A defense can be put into place, or the drill can be run dry. The object is for the base runners to work on the proper timing and techniques of each offensive play call. There is not hitter, but the pitcher pitches to the catcher if the drill is run with a defense in place so that runners can work on reading and proper timing. The runners will be looking for signs from the base coaches to see what they should do.

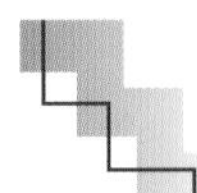

TO INCREASE DIFFICULTY

- Perform the drill live, at game speed, with a defense in place.

TO DECREASE DIFFICULTY

- A coach can act as the pitcher, slowing the tempo so that the players can understand the concept.

Success Check

- The runners need to respond correctly to the coaches' signs. This mean both looking for the signs and knowing what they mean.
- Runners should get the right lead and a good break.
- Good timing between the two runners is essential.

Score Your Success

You earn 1 point for executing the play.

You earn 0 points for poor timing or missing signs.

Running at first base _____ of 5

Running at third base _____ of 5

Your score _____ of 10

First-and-Third Offense Drill 2 Simulated Team Intrasquad

Another time to practice first-and-third offense is during a live setting such as intrasquad. This drill is run similar to the baserunning without a hitter drill, but now includes a batter and always includes the defense. The base runners should work on the proper timing and technique for each offensive play call. The runners will be looking for signs from the base coaches to see what they should do, but should now also be reading the pitches and watching the hitter.

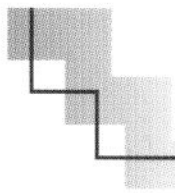

TO INCREASE DIFFICULTY

- Give signs and play at game speed.

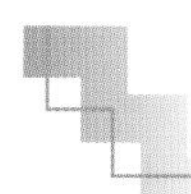

TO DECREASE DIFFICULTY

- Announce the situation and slow down the game.

Success Check

- The base runners read the hitter and the pitcher, and watch the coaches' signs.
- Runners lead correctly based on their read of the situation and break when appropriate.

Score Your Success

Running at first base _____ of 5

Running at third base _____ of 5

Your score _____ of 10

MOVING RUNNERS AND SCORING

Situational hitting is a significant aspect that often determines the overall success of an offense. Moving runners as a hitter is similar to moving runners in the sacrifice situations discussed earlier in this chapter. The idea is to let the hitter swing, but to hit the ball to certain areas of the field so that the runner can advance successfully to the next base. The same applies to driving in a runner from third. The hitter should focus on making contact to specific areas according to the defensive positioning. Here are a few common offensive situations.

Runner On Second Base and No Outs—Move Him

The hitter's job is to get the runner to third base with less than two outs. To do this, the approach must be to hit the ball to the right side of the field. The runner must read the ball. On a hard-hit ground ball at the runner or a ground ball to the third baseman, the runner stays at second. Any ground ball hit behind the runner will advance him. Fly balls are a judgment read by the third-base coach, but with no outs, the runner should be tagging up and listening for the call.

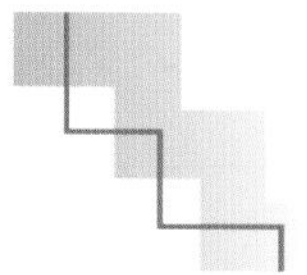

MISSTEP

The runner gets thrown out at third base on a ball hit to the left side of the infield.

CORRECTION

If there is any doubt, just stay at your base.

Infield In—Score Him

With the infield in, the hitter's job is to hit a fly ball to the outfield deep enough so that the runner can tag and score. Alternatively, the hitter can hit a hard line drive through the middle of the field. The runner must be sure that a ground ball gets through the infield or he must be ready to tag up on a fly ball.

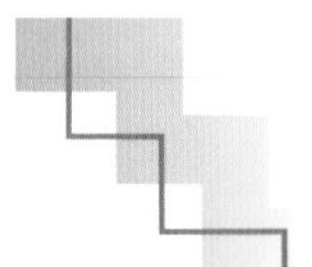

MISSTEP

The runner at third breaks on contact.

CORRECTION

The runner must see the ball through the infield. Shortening up the lead is a good reminder not to break on contact.

Infield Back—Score Him

The runner may break on contact, holding only if the ball is hit back to the pitcher. The hitter's job is to hit a ground ball in the middle of the field. If he does that, he gets an easy RBI.

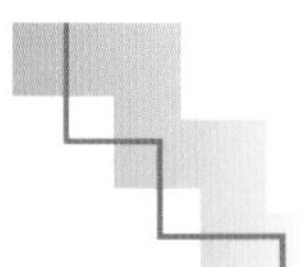

MISSTEP

The batter strikes out.

CORRECTION

This situation is the easiest run in baseball. The hitter just has to make contact and hit a ground ball to the shortstop for an RBI.

Moving Runners and Scoring Drill 1
Batting Practice With Base Runners

Use one or two rounds during batting practice to focus on moving runners. Have the players run the bases as well to work on getting good jumps and picking up the baseball. The base runners should work on proper timing and technique. They should be looking for signs from the base coaches to see what they should do. They should also be reading the pitches and watching the hitter.

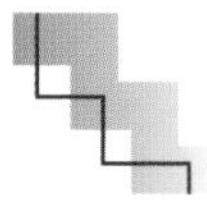

TO INCREASE DIFFICULTY

- Have runners split between bases.
- Each runner and hitter is given his own situation and reads the ball at contact.

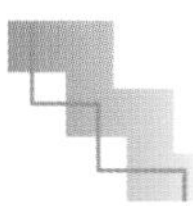

TO DECREASE DIFFICULTY

- Allow base runners to run from only one base at a time.
- Use only one specific situation at a time.

(continued)

Moving Runners and Scoring Drill 1 *(continued)*

Success Check

- The runner should make the right decision based on his read of the situation, and also be keeping an eye on the base coaches for guidance.
- The hitter should hit the ball properly and place it correctly to advance the runner.

Score Your Success

Runner on second base and no outs—move him _____ of 5

Infield in—score him _____ of 5

Infield back—score him _____ of 5

Reads at second base _____ of 5

Reads at third base _____ of 5

Your score _____ of 25

Moving Runners and Scoring Drill 2
Simulated Team Intrasquad

Intrasquad is a great live setting to practice moving runners and scoring. This drill is run like a live game. The base runners should work on proper timing and technique. They should be looking for signs from the base coaches to see what they should do. They should also be reading the pitches and watching the hitter.

TO DECREASE DIFFICULTY

- Have the pitchers throw only fastballs

Success Check

- The runner should make the right decision based on his read of the situation, and he should also be keeping an eye on the base coaches for guidance.
- The hitter should hit the ball properly and place it correctly to advance the runner.

Score Your Success

Runner on second base and no outs—move him _____ of 2

Infield in—score him _____ of 2

Infield back—score him _____ of 2

Reads at second base _____ of 2

Reads at third base _____ of 2

Your score _____ of 10

SUCCESS CHECK

Situational offense is important in defining a team and their capabilities. The team that can use these skills based on their personnel, putting each player in the best scenario to be successful, will be a team that defenses do not like to face. By rating your success, you can determine where you will be most successful within your team's offense and what you can work on to help your team become more complete.

Bunting Drills

1. Breakdown _____ out of 10
2. Batting practice rounds with bunts _____ out of 10
3. Bunt only intrasquad _____ out of 20

Hit and Run and Run and Hit Drills

1. Batting practice rounds _____ out of 20
2. Intrasquad _____ out of 10

First-and-Third Offense Drills

1. Team offense—baserunning without a hitter _____ out of 10
2. Simulated team intrasquad _____ out of 10

Moving Runners and Scoring Drill

1. Batting practice with base runners _____ out of 25
2. Simulated team intrasquad _____ out of 10

Total _____ **out of 125**

A score of 75 or higher is an outstanding score that should give you confidence as a team player. This score proves your ability to focus and execute during pressure situations and shows that you have the baseball IQ to adjust to each play. If your score is low in certain areas, you can work on that part of your game to help you and your team become more complete.

Glossary

at-bat—Appearance by a hitter.

ball—Pitch called outside the strike zone that the hitter doesn't swing at.

base—Bag or plate located at each corner of the infield.

base coach—When a team is batting, the coach allowed to occupy a box close to first and third bases.

base hit—Hit that allows the batter to reach base.

baseman—Fielders positioned near first, second, and third bases.

base paths—Areas between the base pads marked with dirt. A runner cannot run outside the base paths to avoid a tag.

batter—Member of the hitting team currently at the plate.

batter's box—Either side of home plate, in which the batter has to stand when he tries to hit the baseball.

blocking—Whenever there is a close play at home plate, meaning the ball and runner arrive at the plate at about the same time, the catcher squats in front of the plate to block the runner's path.

breaking ball—Pitch that moves into or away from or suddenly drops as it reaches the hitter.

bunt—Attempt to hit the ball by simply dropping it close to the hitter, usually as a surprise tactic.

changeup—Slower pitch thrown with the same action as a fastball.

center field—Middle part of the outfield.

cheat—Slightly move but not to an extreme for it to be noticed.

chopper—Ground ball that initially hits the ground close to home plate, which causes the initial hop to be much higher than it is on any other ground ball.

corner infielder—First baseman and third baseman.

crow hop—Technique used to incorporate the maximum amount of energy and direction into a throw.

curveball—Off-speed breaking ball that drops sharply at the plate.

cutoff man—Infielder who gets into position to line up a throw from the outfield. If the throw from the outfielder is off line to the base it's intended to go to, the cutoff man catches it.

cutter—Pitch thrown with the same arm speed as the fastball; therefore, the velocity should not be very much lower than that of the fastball. The spin should be tight, and the cut action, a slight flat movement of the ball, should be small and late.

delivery—Pitcher throwing the ball to the hitter.

dirt ball—Ball thrown in the dirt in front of defender. A ground ball is not the same as a dirt ball because a ground ball is a hit ball on the ground.

double—Base hit that allows the hitter to reach second base.

double play (DP)—Fielding play in which two offensive players are called out.

double-play depth—Fielding alignment where the infielders field closer than usual, hoping to field a ground ball and throw out runners going to both second and first bases.

double steal—Play when two runners try to steal bases at the same time.

drag bunt—Bunt for a hit that is placed close to or on the third-base line and have it stop about halfway to third base or little farther.

dugout—Area in which the players, manager, and coaches sit when they aren't on the field of play or in the bullpen.

error—Fielding mistake that is officially charged against the fielder.

fair—Ball hit by the batter that stays within the foul lines between first and third base.

fast ball—Pitch thrown as hard and fast as possible.

fielder—Defensive player. The fielding team has nine fielders, one of whom is the pitcher.

fly ball—Ball hit into the air. If a fielder catches the ball, it's known as a fly-out.

force-out—Out in which the runner is put out having been forced to run to a base.

foul—Ball hit by the batter that falls outside of the foul lines between first and third bases.

foul lines—Lines that extend from home base through first and third bases to the outfield walls.

four-seam grip—Most common way to throw a baseball, and it is the suggested grip for all position players to use because it allows the thrower the most control of where the ball will go.

fungo—Thin bat used for a person to hit ground balls or fly balls for practice; it's not to be used to hit a thrown ball.

ground ball (or grounder)—Ball hit along the ground.

hit and run—Play in which the runner sets off early, gambling on the batter making a base hit.

holding the runner—Baseman who stands close to a base to prevent a runner from taking too big a lead away from the base.

home plate—Base located at home, over which a strike must be thrown and a runner must touch to score a run.

hop—Bounce of the ball.

infield—Area of the field inside the bases and base paths.

infielder—Defensive player who fields in and around the infield.

inning—Period of the game. Each team has nine innings in which to score runs. The visiting team hits in the top of the inning and the home team hits in the bottom of the inning.

leading off—Base runner takes a few steps off the base while waiting for the pitcher to pitch.

left field—Side of the outfield behind third base.

long hop—Thrown ball that hits ground and bounces one smooth time to the fielder.

no doubles—Playing the outfielders deeper (farther away from infield) than normal to allow better angles on batted balls and to keep batted balls in front of outfielders. This would be used in late innings in close games to reduce the chance of a batter's hitting a double.

out—When a hitter or runner is removed from the field of play by the fielding side.

outfield wall or fence—Wall or fence that marks the outer boundary of the field.

outfield—Area of the field beyond the infield.

outfielder—Fielder who occupies the outfield.

passed ball—Pitched ball that should have been caught by the catcher but was not; because of the missed ball by the catcher, a runner or runners advance a base.

PFP—Pitcher's fielding practice.

pick—Catching a short hopped thrown ball.

pickoff—Pitcher or catcher throws to an infielder at an occupied base (runner on base) to try to get the base runner out.

pitch—Throw made by a pitcher to the hitter.

pitcher's mound—Mound in the center of the field from which the pitcher throws to the hitters.

plate—Base at home over which pitchers have to throw the ball to get a strike.

pop-up—Fly ball in the infield.

pump fake—With ball in hand, moving arm in a throwing motion without releasing the ball.

push bunt—Bunt for a hit where the batter places the bunt in the triangle area between the first baseman, second baseman, and past pitcher.

ready position—Athletic position with the hands off the knees and in front of the body.

right field—Side of the outfield behind first base.

routine ground ball—Ground ball that stays on the same angle through the hops and glove stays on continued angle (soft).

rundown—Runner caught between bases and chased down by two fielders to make a tag on him.

sacrifice—Hitter deliberately sacrificing his out to advance at least one runner a base.

safe—Runner reaching base without being tagged.

safety squeeze—Type of squeeze bunt where the runner waits to see where the bunt goes before committing himself to trying to score.

scoring position—Base runner on second or third base who can normally be expected to score on a single.

shading—Positioning the outfielder a little to the left or right of his normal position, which would be used to match the tendencies of a hitter.

short-hop dig—Thrown ball that bounces near the fielder's feet and fielder must catch it out of the dirt.

single—Base hit that allows the hitter to reach first base.

slide—Attempt to get on base where the runner goes in feetfirst (hook slide) or headfirst.

slider—Pitch that drops away from the hitter while also moving away from him.

squaring up the baseball—Hitting the ball on the same trajectory as it was delivered.

split-fingered fastball—Pitch that looks like a fastball, but it is slower and dips at the hitter.

squeeze bunt—Bunt on which a runner from third base tries to reach home base.

steal—Runner moving from one base to the next without the batter's hitting the ball.

stretch—Pitcher's set position for delivering the ball to home plate.

strike—Pitch that the umpire rules is within the strike zone or swung at and missed by the hitter.

strike zone—Area above the hitter's knees, below the midpoint between the hitter's waist and shoulders, and over the plate.

strikeout—Out in which the pitcher retires the hitter with three strikes.

suicide squeeze—Type of squeeze bunt in which the runner on third takes off as the ball is pitched, which if the bunt goes wrong means an out for the runner.

tag—Out in which the fielder catches a runner trying to reach base.

tandem—A way that the defense can control a ball thrown from the outfield and relay it quickly to the infield.

two-seam grip—Common fastball grip for pitchers because, with only two seams rotating, the ball is likely to drift from side to side.

walk—Base on balls.

wild pitch—Pitched ball that was thrown in a manner that the catcher had no chance of catching; because of the ball getting by the catcher, a runner or runners advance a base.

windup—Pitcher's motion in throwing to home base.

working through the catch—Outfielder catching a fly ball while moving toward infield and direction he will throw the ball.

About the Authors

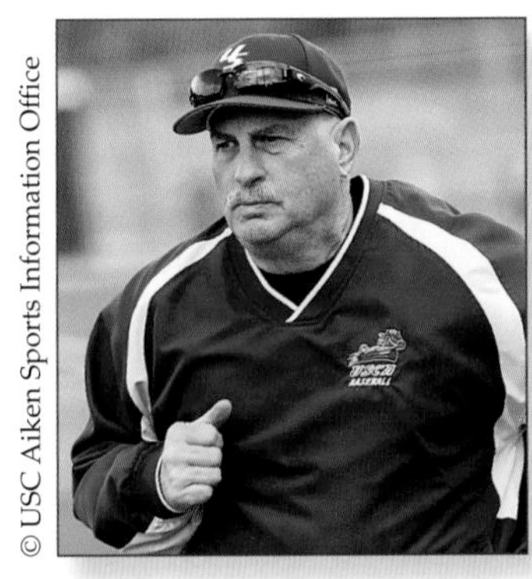
© USC Aiken Sports Information Office

Since becoming the head coach of the University of South Carolina Aiken baseball program in 2000, **Kenny Thomas** has re-established the Pacers as a force in the Peach Belt Conference and a perennial top 25 team in NCAA Division II.

As of the start of the 2017 season, Thomas has 1,139 career wins, including 619 at the USC Aiken helm. His record is currently 1,139-562 in 29 seasons as a college head coach. He ranks in the top 40 among active NCAA Division II coaches for wins. His .643 winning percentage as the Pacer skipper places him in the top 30 among active NCAA Division II head coaches. Thomas has led the Pacers to eight NCAA Tournament appearances (2005, 2006, 2007, 2008, 2009, 2013, 2014, and 2016) in the past 11 seasons.

Thomas has coached 67 players who have been drafted and signed in the Major League Baseball free agent draft. He's coached 102 All-Conference players, 17 All-Americans, six conference Players of the Year, one Southeast Region Player of the Year, and one National Player of the Year. Under Thomas's direction, USC Aiken has had five straight years (2012-2016) with a player selected within the first 15 rounds of the MLB draft.

As a player at Trevecca University in Nashville, Tennessee, Thomas was named All-Conference three times, All-District two times, team captain three times, and an NAIA All-American catcher his senior year.

DJ King spent three seasons as associate head coach and recruiting coordinator at Andrew College in Georgia. He also spent three seasons at Kennesaw State University as the volunteer assistant coach. He spent three seasons at the University of South Carolina Aiken, where he was the pitching coach for two years as well as a recruiter, strength and conditioning coach, alumni coordinator, and stadium supervisor.

King was the head coach of the Dubuque Waves in the River Valley League in Iowa for one summer, where he was selected to manage the league's all-star team. For two summers he was also the head coach of the Waynesboro Generals in the Valley Baseball League in Virginia; the team won the Valley League Championship in 2014 and fell just short in 2015, losing in the semifinal round.

Before his coaching career, King won back-to-back state championships at Parkview High School, where he played for legendary coach Hugh Buchanan. He played collegiate ball at Chattahoochee Valley, where he was an All-Conference pitcher. He concluded his playing career at Shorter College.